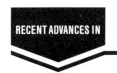

RECENT ADVANCES IN

Gastroenterology

RECENT ADVANCES IN GASTROENTEROLOGY

Contents of Number 8

Inflammatory bowel disease
R. N. Allan, H. J. F. Hodgson
Enteric infections
M. J. G. Farthing
Molecular genetics in gastroenterology
I. Forgacs
Peptide regulatory factors in the gut
Y. R. Mahida, P. D. E. Jones, T. K. Daneshmend, C. J. Hawkey
The oesophagus
J. R. Bennett
Upper gastrointestinal bleeding
R. P. Walt
Duodenal ulceration
R. E. Pounder, C. U. Nwokolo
AIDS and the gut
I. McGowan, I. Weller
Enteral and parenteral nutrition
S. P. Allison, R. C. Spiller
Liver transplantation
A. K. Burroughs, K. Rolles
The hepatotrophic viruses causing acute and chronic viral
hepatitis: a compendium from A to E
G. Dusheiko
Autoimmune liver disease
H. C. Mitchison, M. F. Bassendine
Reviews and leaders
M. C. Allison

ISBN 0 443 04324 8

You can place your order by contacting your local medical bookseller or
The Sales Promotion Department, Robert Stevenson House,
1–3 Baxter's Place, Leith Walk, Edinburgh EH1 3AF, UK

Tel: (031) 556 2424; Telex: 727511 LONGMN G; Fax: (031) 558 1278

Look out for *Recent Advances in Gastroenterology 10* in September 1994

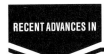
RECENT ADVANCES IN

Gastroenterology

Edited by

Roy Pounder MA MD FRCP
Professor of Medicine,
Chairman, Academic Division of Clinical Science,
Consultant Physician and Gastroenterologist,
The Royal Free Hospital and School of Medicine, London, UK

NUMBER NINE

CHURCHILL LIVINGSTONE
EDINBURGH LONDON MADRID MELBOURNE NEW YORK AND TOKYO
1992

CHURCHILL LIVINGSTONE
Medical Division of Longman Group UK Limited

Distributed in the United States of America by Churchill
Livingstone Inc., 650 Avenue of the Americas, New York,
N.Y. 10011, and by associated companies, branches and
representatives throughout the world.

First published 1992

ISBN 0 443 046743
ISSN 0 141-5581

British Library Cataloguing in Publication Data
A catalogue record for this book is available from the British
Library

Library of Congress Cataloging in Publication
is available

Printed in Great Britain by The Bath Press, Avon

Contents

1. Inflammatory bowel disease   1
   R. N. Allan, H. J. F. Hodgson

2. Helicobacter pylori   27
   A. T. R. Axon

3. Irritable bowel syndrome   49
   K. W. Heaton

4. Functional gastrointestinal disorders: psychological factors in aetiology and management   63
   G. G. Lloyd

5. Molecular gastroenterology   73
   J. A. Summerfield

6. Pancreatic disease   85
   J. P. Neoptolemos

7. Duodenal ulceration   105
   R. E. Pounder, A. G. Fraser

8. Paediatric gastroenterology   119
   R. Nelson

9. Upper-gastrointestinal haemorrhage   135
   C. P. Swain

10. Colorectal oncology   151
    H. J. W. Thomas

11. The pharmacotherapy of portal hypertension   171
    A. K. Burroughs, P. A. McCormick

12. Hepatitis C virus   195
    G. M. Dusheiko

13. Variants of hepatitis B virus   217
    W. F. Carman

14. Reviews and leaders 231
M. C. Allison

Index 251

Preface

Once again, it has been a pleasure to prepare a further issue of Recent Advances in Gastroenterology. Each of the authors provided an excellent manuscript on time which allowed the whole book to go to press immediately. The book will be published 24 weeks after receipt of the last manuscript. Nothing is more frustrating than the delayed publication of an up-to-date manuscript, hence our thanks must go to Catherine Hawes and her colleagues at Churchill Livingstone.

In *Recent Advances in Gastroenterology 9* there is a split between two major themes: clinical gastroenterology and the scientific basis of gastrointestinal disease.

The clinical topics are: inflammatory bowel disease, *Helicobacter pylori*, functional bowel disease and psychiatric aspects of gastrointestinal disease, pancreatic disease, duodenal ulceration, paediatric gastroenterology, gastrointestinal haemorrhage, and the management of portal hypertension. Chapters with a more scientific approach relate to a description of molecular biology and its role in gastroenterology, gastrointestinal oncology, hepatitis C, and the variants of hepatitis B. Unfortunately, not every topic can be brought up-to-date in only 13 chapters, but Dr Miles Allison has again prepared 'Reviews and Leaders'—an indexed collection of most of the important review articles concerning gastrointestinal topics published in the last two years.

Once again, my great thanks go to my secretary Miss Doris Elliott, who administered the preparation of this book.

London 1992   R.P.

Contributors

Robert N. Allan MD PhD FRCP
Consultant Physician, Gastroenterology Unit, General Hospital,
Birmingham, UK

Miles C. Allison MD MRCP
Consultant Physician, Royal Gwent Hospital, Newport, Gwent, UK

Anthony T. R. Axon MD FRCP
Consultant Physician and Gastroenterologist, The General Infirmary,
Leeds, UK

Andrew K. Burroughs MBChB MD FRCP
Senior Lecturer in Medicine and Honorary Consultant Physician,
Hepato-Biliary and Liver Transplantation Unit, The Royal Free Hospital
School of Medicine, London, UK

W. F. Carman MBBCh MMed MRCPath
Senior Lecturer and Honorary Consultant, Department of Virology,
University of Glasgow, Glasgow, UK

Geoffrey M. Dusheiko FCP(SA) FRCP
Reader in Medicine, Royal Free Hospital School of Medicine,
London, UK

Alan G. Fraser MBChB FRACP
Research Fellow in Gastroenterology, Royal Free Hospital School of
Medicine, London, UK

K. W. Heaton MA MD FRCP
Reader in Medicine, University of Bristol; Honorary Consultant
Physician, Bristol United Health Care Trust, Bristol, UK

H. J. F. Hodgson DM FRCP
Professor of Gastroenterology, Department of Medicine, Royal
Postgraduate Medical School, Hammersmith Hospital, London, UK

Geoffrey G. Lloyd MD FRCP FRCPsych
Consultant Psychiatrist, Royal Free Hospital, London, UK

P. Aiden McCormick MB BCR BAO MRCP(UK)
Lecturer in Medicine, Royal Free Hospital School of Medicine,
London, UK

Robert Nelson MBChB FRCP DCH
Consultant Paediatrician, Royal Victoria Infirmary, Newcastle upon
Tyne, UK

J. P. Neoptolemos MA MD FRCS
Reader in Surgery, University of Birmingham; Honorary Consultant
Surgeon, Dudley Road Hospital, Birmingham, UK

Roy Pounder MA MD FRCP
Professor of Medicine, Chairman, Academic Division of Clinical Science,
Consultant Physician and Gastroenterologist, Royal Free Hospital
and School of Medicine, London, UK

John A. Summerfield MD FRCP
Reader in Medicine, St Mary's Hospital Medical School, and Imperial
College, London, UK

C. Paul Swain MD FRCP
Senior Lecturer and Consultant Gastroenterologist, Royal London
Hospital, London, UK

Huw J. W. Thomas MA PhD MRCP
Senior Registrar in Gastroenterology, St Mary's Hospital, London, UK

Inflammatory bowel disease

R. N. Allan   H. J. F. Hodgson

In this chapter we have selected and summarized important advances in our understanding and management of inflammatory bowel disease, principally in the last two years. The review is intended to have broad appeal for physicians and those in training with an interest in gastroenterology, in addition to the specialist gastroenterologist.

PATHOGENESIS

There has been no dramatic breakthrough in our understanding of the aetiology of these diseases, and those who traditionally begin their review articles with the statement that 'the aetiology of inflammatory bowel disease remains unknown' may for the time being continue to do so. Immunological observations relevant to the expression of damaging immune responses in the gastrointestinal mucosa in these diseases continue to be reported, and a number of reviews have appeared.[1-3]

Epidemiology

The strong association between non-smoking and ulcerative colitis,[4] and between smoking and Crohn's disease,[5] are still being explored. Two studies refine the association of smoking with Crohn's disease by finding a higher relapse rate ($1.6 \times$ approximately) over 6 months in a group of diagnosed Crohn's disease sufferers who smoked compared with those who did not.[6] In trying to understand these associations, researchers investigated the effect of smoking on the production of prostaglandins and leucotrienes by colonic mucosal biopsies in normal individuals; the results suggested that eicosanoid production was diminished in smokers.[7] While this association between inflammatory bowel disease and smoking is persistently being confirmed, community-based, controlled studies did not confirm previous weak associations between oral contraceptives and either ulcerative colitis[8] or Crohn's disease.[9] A number of studies, for example Stow et al 1990,[10] suggest that the rising incidence of Crohn's disease in the 1960s and 1970s may have peaked or even declined in the 1980s, although this is an area where 'time will tell'.

Genetics

Familial clustering of inflammatory bowel disease is of course well recognized, and if both parents have such a condition, the risk in children is very high (12 out of 33 children born to 19 couples[11]). Such a strong association cannot, of course, fully exonerate environmental causes.

The intriguing possibility that altered intestinal permeability might be the genetic factor predisposing to Crohn's disease – as indicated by previous studies in unaffected relatives – has been obscured by the fact that the permeability increase reported with one marker (PEG 400) was not shown with three other permeability markers.[12] While pedigree analysis in ulcerative colitis suggests that a rare single gene with incomplete penetrance (of about 20%) may cause the disease,[13] we are no nearer knowing what that gene is or what it codes for. The demonstration of a fivefold increase above expectation of ulcerative colitis among the relatives of patients with coeliac disease[14] suggests an enhanced immune responsiveness to gut-associated antigens as one possibility.

Infectious agents

Atypical mycobacteria of more than one type have again[15] been cultured from tissues of a minority of patients with Crohn's disease. In regard to *Mycobacterium paratuberculosis*, however, there was no evidence of an IgM[16] or T cell[17] response to this bacterium which would have suggested active infection, nor could bacteria be detected in the tissues.[16] Further work is currently appearing in abstract form identifying *M. paratuberculosis* in bowel tissues, and the jury is currently out on whether the association of this bacterium with Crohn's disease is a primary event or merely a secondary phenomenon. Among other clues relevant to a possible infectious aetiology is the demonstration of enhanced antibody responses to a particular form of baker's yeast in Crohn's disease but not in ulcerative colitis or normals.[18, 19]

The nude mouse finding – the identification within the lymph nodes of nude mice who had been injected with tissue from Crohn's disease patients of antigens which cross-reacted with the Crohn's disease patients' sera – was initially taken as evidence of the growth in that immunodeficient animal of an infectious agent. This finding has not been confirmed as specific for injected Crohn's tissue,[20] although cross-reactivity is more common with sera from Crohn's disease patients than those of ulcerative colitis patients or controls.[21] While further work is still in progress,[22] it seems unlikely that this approach will lead to identification of a single agent specific for Crohn's disease.

Immune mechanisms of inflammation

Why there is an inflammatory process mounted against the gut, or at least within the gut mucosa causing adjacent damage, remains unclear. The possibility that it is against an infectious agent has already been discussed. The possibility that in ulcerative colitis the immune response is mounted against a specific 40 000 mol. wt, colon-associated protein continues to receive attention, particularly as this antigen can block antibody-dependent cytolysis of colon-derived cells by ulcerative colitic sera.[23] Evidence of autoantibodies against small intestinal and colonic epithelial cell-associated antigens is also found in relatives of patients with inflammatory bowel disease, both ulcerative colitis and Crohn's disease, suggesting that the phenomenon may be primary rather than a consequence of inflammation.[24]

Much evidence has been produced concerning the nature of the inflammatory process in these diseases, in investigating mechanisms that can mediate the inflammatory process, although why they arise remains a mystery. In the latter respect, an interesting study[25] investigated local humoral immunity in the histologically uninvolved jejunum in Crohn's disease by a perfusion technique, and showed a significant reduction in jejunal IgA secretion and the density of IgA-containing cells. This primary deficit in local immunity might permit increased penetration of antigen to the gut mucosa and initiate the disease. This phenomenon was not found in patients with ulcerative colitis.

The definition by basic immunologists at the molecular level of a series of pro-inflammatory cytokines – notably the interleukin (IL) series – has prompted description of their involvement in the inflammatory processes of ulcerative colitis and Crohn's disease. Mononuclear cells from the gut of patients with Crohn's disease produce increased quantities of IL-1β[26] and interferon,[27] and the enhanced amounts produced by cultured mucosa of patients with ulcerative colitis and Crohn's disease are depressed by prednisolone.[28] Within the circulation of patients with Crohn's disease, IL-2, and a soluble form of the T-cell IL-2 receptor, increase in amount.[29] Cytokines not only promote local inflammation but also amplify specific immune responses, and they probably mediate systemic features such as fever, and the generation of acute phase reactants (for example, orosomucoid and C-reactive protein) from the liver. In addition, interferon can lead to changes in the surface membranes characteristic of colonic epithelial cells, which in inflamed tissue can express HLA antigens.

Once expressing HLA, such cells have the potential to become antigen-producing cells,[30–32] a function which could give a further twist to the process of developing damaging immune responses to the gut and gut-associated antigens. Other alterations in the epithelium favouring inflammation are the increased expression of adhesion molecules[33] and local synthesis of complement.[34]

The role of polymorphonuclear leucocytes as modulators of inflammation continues to attract attention, particularly as the production of toxic oxygen metabolites, such as superoxide, by these cells and by monocytes is a potential mechanism of tissue damage.[35, 36] Circulating products of polymorphonuclear leucocytes such as lactoferrin, may be useful markers of inflammation.[37] The availability of blockers of various activators of inflammation, varying from superoxide dismutase, which inactivates such active oxygen metabolites, or the IL-1β-receptor antagonist, may offer therapeutic hope for the future, and some blockers have already been explored in experimental inflammatory situations.[38]

A new insight into the pathogenesis of Crohn's disease was provided by a study of the microvasculature of resected specimens of gut fixed after resin casting, an investigation which suggested that vascular injury and focal arteritis were early pathological events in Crohn's disease, leading to microinfarction[39] and which indicated that the majority of granulomas in Crohn's disease form within the walls of blood vessels.[40] While this does not define the initiating factors for the condition, it directs attention away from the mucosa, and indicates an important area for further studies.

The possibility that abnormal metabolic pathways in the mucosa may underlie the development of inflammatory bowel disease continues to receive attention.[41, 42]

Experimental and naturally occurring models

The cotton-top tamarin, which in colonies develops a colitis reminiscent of ulcerative colitis, also shows evidence of autoimmune reactions against the colon, although it remains open to speculation whether this is merely a secondary change.[43]

Granulomatous inflammation can be caused in the small and large bowels of guinea-pigs by injection of myobacterial antigens, whether the organisms are alive or dead.[44] Further exploration of the similarities of inflammatory bowel disease to a number of other experimental models – carrageen in injection, with[45] or without[46] alteration of bacterial flora, and graft-versus-host disease[47] – has been pursued.

CLINICAL ASSESSMENTS OF INFLAMMATORY BOWEL DISEASE

Endoscopy. For those who wish, reproducibly, to describe and quantify endoscopic appearances in the colon, the GETAID French multicentre assessment of nine definite lesions (ranging from frank erythema to ulcerated stenosis) in five segments between the rectum and the terminal ileum provides a reproducible formula, and offers the opportunity of calculating an endoscopic incidence of severity. This may be helpful if endoscopic changes are the chosen end-point in clinical trials, although there was, in fact, surprisingly little change between, before, and after a clinically effective course of corticosteroids.[48]

Leucocyte scanning. In the search for alternative isotopic techniques, which give one as much information about disease extent distribution and activity as ^{111}In leucocyte scanning or TcHMPAO scanning, the effect of scanning after ^{99}Tc-labelled nanocolloid injection has been studied by two groups. Both found the technique to be substantially less sensitive than ^{111}In-autologous leucocyte scanning.[49, 50] Tc-labelled immunoglobulin[51] and ^{111}In-labelled monoclonal antibodies[52] are also being explored, presumably because current cell-labelling isotope techniques are acknowledged to be useful but technically demanding, as they require cell separation. While little more has emerged on the use of CT scanning or ultrasound, it has been suggested that magnetic resonance imaging may offer a new approach to the diagnosis and mapping of fistulas and sinus tracts in Crohn's disease, reflecting the extraordinary capacity of this technique for soft-tissue mapping.[53] Quantitation of disease activity by leucocyte scans has been compared with a number of clinical and laboratory indices in 58 patients, and the objective presence of inflammation, as shown by leucocytes and faecal excretion, correlated poorly with clinical activity indices.[54]

The message that the clinical activity indices beloved of clinical trials reflect severity of symptoms, rather than, necessarily, the activity of the inflammatory process, is being more generally accepted.[55] If one is seeking another objective parameter of inflammatory activity, faecal α-1-antitrypsin clearance has proved effective in a group of patients with Crohn's disease followed prospectively after gut resection.[56]

THE NEW SALICYLATES

Pharmacokinetics

Sulphasalazine has been the mainstay of medical treatment in ulcerative colitis for many years. It consists of a carrier (sulphapyridine) linked by a diazo bond to the active component (5-aminosalicylic acid). When taken orally, most of the drug is delivered to the colon intact. A small amount is absorbed in the small intestine, undergoes entero-hepatic circulation, and is excreted in the bile, so that plasma concentrations are very low. The diazo bond is split in the colon by anaerobic bacterial action, liberating sulphapyridine and 5-aminosalicylic acid. Sulphapyridine is responsible for many of the side-effects of sulphasalazine, including headache, nausea, vomiting, skin rashes, and impaired fertility in men.[57]

The new formulations eliminate the carrier sulphapyridine and have been developed to deliver 5-aminosalicylate (5-ASA) to either the small or large intestine or to both, depending on the formulation.[58]

Olsalazine (Dipentum) most closely resembles the parent molecule since two 5-aminosalicylate molecules are linked by the diazo bond, thus eliminating the carrier sulphapyridine and its associated side-effects. In the colon 5-aminosalicylic acid is released by anaerobic bacterial action as for sulphasalazine.[59]

In other preparations the delivery of 5-aminosalicylate is achieved by mechanical or pH-dependent release, which has two important implications. It increases the small-intestinal delivery and reduces the colonic delivery of 5-ASA, and secondly it alters 5-ASA pharmacokinetics. For example, Asacol is 5-ASA coated with eudragit-S that dissolves at a pH above 7, and 5-ASA is thus released in the distal small bowel and colon. The ethylcellulose coating of Pentasa granules dissolves gradually during passage through the small bowel. Thus, with these preparations, free 5-ASA is released in both the small bowel and colon. In both sites 5-ASA is acetylated by the epithelium.

In the small bowel this process can be overloaded by rapid release of 5-ASA, which allows an appreciable amount of non-acetylated 5-ASA to be absorbed. This, unlike acetylated 5-ASA, is nephrotoxic in experimental animals. Rapid release of 5-ASA is more likely in the small bowel with Asacol than with the slow-release Pentasa.

Other 5-ASA preparations include a slow-release system achieved by compressing 5-ASA with sodium carbonate and glycerine, and protecting this core with an enteric coating of eudragit-L. 5-ASA is released from this preparation at a pH greater than 5.5 (Claversal and Salofalk). Other preparations include a core surrounded by an envelope of resin which dissolves at different pH levels predominantly in the terminal ileum and caecum (Rowasa).[60]

Mechanism of action

The mechanism by which 5-ASA exerts its anti-inflammatory action is uncertain. The most likely mechanisms are an inter-relationship between local production of eicosanoids and reactive oxygen metabolites in conjunction with activated neutrophils, though the nature of the initial triggering factors remains to be determined. Bacterial derived chemotactic peptides, such as ethylene-P, may act as a trigger factor, as they are potent inhibitors of IL-1 production.[61] There may also be an underlying defect in mucosal permeability.

Clinical studies

Sulphasalazine is an established, proven, cost-effective treatment for mild to moderate exacerbations of ulcerative colitis and Crohn's disease and for the maintenance of remission in patients with ulcerative colitis. Its use is limited by the side-effects caused by the carrier sulphapyridine, including headache, nausea, vomiting, skin rash, and impaired fertility in men. There are now good data comparing the new salicylates with sulphasalazine, particularly in ulcerative colitis. There is, as yet, little available evidence in Crohn's disease. Several excellent summaries of published clinical trials of the new aminosalicylates have been published recently.[60, 62]

Active ulcerative colitis

Controlled trials have clearly shown that the new aminosalicylates are superior to placebos and equivalent to sulphasalazine, but with fewer side-effects. The newer preparations studied include Asacol, Dipentum, Mesasal, Rowasa, and Pentasa.

For example, a double-blind, triple-centre controlled trial studied 37 patients presenting with a first attack of distal colitis. The patients were randomly allocated to either olsalazine 2 g daily or sulphasalazine 3 g daily for 4 weeks. The assessment included symptoms, sigmoidoscopic appearances, and histological evaluation of rectal biopsies. Both groups showed a similar decrease in stool frequency and bloating, although stools remained looser in the olsalazine group. Sigmoidoscopic, histological appearances and clinical activity improved significantly and to a similar extent in both groups. Intolerance was higher using sulphasalazine ($n = 4$), as compared with olsalazine ($n = 2$). Olsalazine was at least as effective as sulphasalazine and rather better tolerated.[63]

Inactive ulcerative colitis

There is good evidence that sulphasalazine 2 g daily is effective in maintaining patients with ulcerative colitis in remission. The newer therapies have all been evaluated in controlled trials, and Asacol, Dipentum, Mesasal, and Pentasa are all equivalent to sulphasalazine for maintenance therapy of patients with ulcerative colitis.[60, 62]

Local treatment

A number of controlled studies albeit with small numbers of patients have shown that 5-ASA enemas are effective and well tolerated in the treatment of active left-sided ulcerative colitis and proctitis.[64]

In an uncontrolled study of a large series of patients with active left-sided colitis, unresponsive to or intolerant of conventional therapy (sulphasalazine, steroid enemas, or oral steroids), 87% of patients, of whom 54% were asymptomatic and in remission, had improved with treatment using 5-ASA enemas after a 12-week course.[65]

Active Crohn's disease

Sulphasalazine is significantly better than placebo for the treatment of active Crohn's disease but it is not effective as maintenance therapy. Since most of the newer 5-ASA compounds are released in both the small and large bowels, depending on the formulation, rather than in the colon alone, we might reasonably expect the new salicylates to be useful in both the treatment of active Crohn's disease and the maintenance of remission.

However, in a study of slow-release 5-ASA (Pentasa) in the treatment of 40 patients with active Crohn's disease allocated to receive either 5-aminosalicylate 1.5 g daily or placebo for 6 weeks, there was no significant difference in clinical activity or laboratory indices. There were no serious side-effects.[66]

There was, however, a significant benefit, as compared with placebo in the treatment of active Crohn's disease, when the dose of 5-ASA (Pentasa) was increased to 4 g daily,[67] although the benefit was not dramatic.

Maintenance treatment for Crohn's disease

The role of 5-ASA in maintenance treatment is not yet established, but it may benefit certain subgroups of patients. In the management of Crohn's disease in remission, 5-ASA 0.5 g t.d.s. was compared with placebos over 12 months. There was no major differences except for a reduction in the ileal disease relapse rates in patients taking 5-ASA as compared with those taking placebos.[68]

In a series of 161 patients with inactive Crohn's disease, 5-ASA (Pentasa) 2 g daily was compared with placebo over 2 years. There was no overall benefit, but there was a significant reduction in relapse rates in patients, particularly those with ileal disease, treated early after induction of remission.[69]

Side-effects of 5-ASA

Serious nephrotoxicity following ingestion of 5-aminosalicylate compounds has been reported in nine patients in the UK.[70] The mechanism of the nephrotoxicity is unknown, but is probably related to absorption of 5-ASA from the small intestine. There have been no reports so far of nephrotoxicity associated with ingestion of olsalazine (Dipentum), which, like its parent compound, sulphasalazine, is largely released in the large intestine, or with Pentasa, probably because of the slow release of 5-ASA, which can be acetylated in the small intestine and inactivated.

Olsalazine (Dipentum) may induce watery diarrhoea in some patients. This effect can be minimized by using a low starting dose, which can then be increased gradually over 1–2 weeks. The proportion of patients with intolerance of this preparation from all causes is similar to that with other aminosalicylates.[59]

Summary

Sulphasalazine has been used for many years. Its safety profile and side-effects are well understood, and it is cost-effective. Some physicians now use the new salicylates as first-line therapy for active ulcerative colitis and as maintenance therapy in preference to sulphasalazine. However, others, because of the occasional nephrotoxic effects of 5-aminosalicylates, use sulphasalazine as the drug of first choice, reserving the newer 5-aminosali-cylates for those patients intolerant of sulphasalazine or for men planning a family where sulphasalazine infertility might be a problem. On present evidence, olsalazine (Dipentum) or slow-release 5-ASA (e.g. Pentasa) should minimize the nephrotoxic risks.

The role of 5-ASA in the treatment of active and inactive Crohn's disease is as yet unknown. Further studies in the next few years should define the indications for its use and the incidence of severe side-effects.

NEW CORTICOSTEROIDS AND IMMUNOSUPPRESSIVE THERAPY

The ideal corticosteroid drug for inflammatory bowel disease – either rapidly effective non-absorbed or so rapidly metabolized that it does not cause systemic effects – has not yet reached the market! Studies have been performed with enema preparations – particularly in ulcerative colitis – and oral preparations. Beclomethasone – which is rapidly metabolized first-pass by the liver – was clinically as effective in a 1-mg enema formation as the systemically absorbed agent betamethasone – 5 mg – in distal ulcerative colitis, without depressing the hypothalamic pituitary adrenal axis. Histo-logical improvement after 28 days was, however, slightly less than that seen with the systemic drug.[71] In a similar trial versus prednisolone, beclo-methasone enemas at a higher dose (2–3 mg) were, clinically and histologi-cally, as effective as 30 mg of prednisolone enema. Again, the systemic steroid markedly suppressed endogenous cortisol, but beclomethasone did not.[72] It is conjectural whether similar results will be obtained with oral formulations. An open trial of the poorly absorbed and rapidly metabolized oral agent fluticasone, in a small group of patients with large- and small-intestinal Crohn's disease, has suggested a favourable outcome, but con-trolled data are needed.[73]

The role of immunosuppressive agents in inflammatory bowel disease has been reviewed.[74] Attention continues to be focused – naturally – on side-effects, and the full survey of the New York experience of the toxicity of 6-mercaptopurine has been published.[75] The most common side-effects were pancreatitis (3.3%), bone marrow depression (2.2%), allergy (2.0%), and infections (7.4%) of which a quarter were severe. One neoplasm, from an experience of 396 patients, was tentatively attributed to the drug's toxicity, and its overall toxicity was asserted to be low enough for its use in the treatment of intractable inflammatory bowel disease. This drug has never been as widely used in the UK as azathioprine. It is reassuring that 16 pregnancies, in patients with inflammatory bowel disease, occurring during treatment with azathioprine had a successful outcome with delivery of normal children,[76] although most physicians and patients would rather avoid such drugs during pregnancy. Methotrexate has been advocated for severe inflammatory bowel disease, but as yet without information from controlled studies.[77]

Most interest in the field of immunosuppression has centred on the use of cyclosporin (CyA), and this has been reviewed.[78] The main event was the publication of the placebo-controlled randomized trial of 3 months' oral CyA (5.0–7.5 mg/kg) in steroid-resistant or -dependent patients with Crohn's disease. Of 37 patients on CyA, 59% improved over 3 months, as compared with 32% of 34 placebo-treated patients, a significantly greater proportion.[79] If improvement occurred in response to CyA, it was fairly rapid – within 2 weeks – and no serious side-effects of the drug were noted. Although this drug has risks of acute and chronic toxicity, it seems to have a beneficial effect in active Crohn's disease in patients resistant to or intolerant of steroids, even though it is clear that it is not always effective[80] in these circumstances. It has been suggested that its use should be limited to clinical trials, or at least to centres with access to experience with the use of the drug and in particular with the capacity to monitor blood levels. Absorption may be unpredictable.[79] It does not seem likely that low doses will prevent relapse after withdrawal,[81] and in fact the tendency for relapse to occur on reducing or stopping this drug, as persistently reported anecdotally, makes decisions on the role of the drug difficult.

Additional circumstances in which the drug has been recommended include treatment of severe ulcerative colitis resistant to high-dose corticosteroids, where intravenous CyA has been thought to induce a remission after about a week of inadequate response to a severe regimen for colitis.[82] There are no controlled data available to support this as yet. In addition, in distal ulcerative colitis resistant to other forms of treatment, there have been some hopeful reports of an effect of CyA given in enema form.[83, 84]

NICOTINE

The association between non-smoking and ulcerative colitis is well recognized, and several case reports suggest that symptoms may improve with smoking and deteriorate when the nicotine source is removed.

A small double-blind, randomized cross-over trial of nicotine gum was evaluated in seven non-smoking patients with ulcerative colitis who chewed up to 10 squares daily (20 mg) nicotine gum or placebo gum for 2 weeks. The treatment was crossed over every 2 weeks for the 8 weeks of the trial. Three of the seven patients studied responded to a degree which justified adding this therapy to their current regimen[85].

ELEMENTAL AND ENTERAL DIET

The immediate and long-term outcome of treating patients with acute

Crohn's disease at Northwick Park Hospital, Middlesex, has been evaluated in a large retrospective study. Remission was induced in 96 of the 113 patients (85%) who followed the diet successfully. A good response was found regardless of age, sex, and site or severity of disease. Most other studies have suggested that patients with small-bowel disease respond better than those with large-intestinal disease. The relapse rate was 22% at 6 months, and thereafter the annual relapse rate was 8–10%. The relapse rate was particularly high following treatment for perianal disease and fistula formation. There was no apparent difference in outcome between remission induced by elemental diet or oral prednisolone.[86]

The efficacy of a liquid defined-formula diet has been compared with 6-methyl prednisolone (48 mg daily initially, reducing the dose weekly over 6 weeks to 12 mg daily) and sulphasalazine 3 g daily in a 6-week randomized prospective multicentre trial of 95 patients with active Crohn's disease. Of the 44 randomized to receive drug treatment, 32 showed improvement in CDAI, as compared with 21 of 51 receiving an oral defined-formula diet ($P < 0.05$). The proportion of withdrawals was much higher in the formula diet group, mostly because the liquid diet was unpalatable. In those who completed the study, the formula diet and drug treatment were equally effective. The effectiveness is well established in those who can tolerate the regime.[87]

In a similar study carried out by the European Co-operative Crohn's disease study group, the results suggested that enteral nutrition was less effective than a combination of 6-methyl prednisolone and sulphasalazine in the treatment of active Crohn's disease.[88] Polymeric and elemental diets have been evaluated in a small randomized prospective study. The outcome was significantly better using the elemental diet, suggesting that polymeric diets are not an effective alternative to elemental diets.[89] The long-term outcome after completion of a course of elemental diet in the treatment of active Crohn's disease is of particular interest. Most patients (80%) with colonic disease relapsed by 6 months, while the relapse rate was much lower with small-bowel disease alone (27%). One-third of the total patients had a prolonged remission (12–36 months).[90] A critical review of the dietary and nutritional management of Crohn's disease has been published recently.[91]

TOTAL PARENTERAL NUTRITION

The pendulum has swung back against the short-term use of total parenteral nutrition (TPN) since the benefits are limited and may even cause harm by inducing considerable intestinal mucosal atrophy with a breakdown of the normal gut mucosal barrier, thus allowing ingress of bacteria and endotoxins. Enteral or oral feeding provides energy sources for the intestinal epithelium and minimizes the risk of infection from ingress of bacteria and endotoxins.[92]

In a study from Chicago, Hanauer et al examined the effects of preoperative total parenteral nutrition on patients with Crohn's disease undergoing bowel resection, as compared with a historical cohort assembled from among 103 patients undergoing resection during 1982–84 by a single surgical team. The length of small-intestinal resection was rather less in those patients receiving TPN, but there was little difference among those undergoing ileocaecal or colonic resections, while the average duration of stay was prolonged by 13.5 d[93] in the TPN group.

THERAPY WITH DIETARY FISH OILS

The efficacy of fish oil containing 3-omega fatty acids which are inhibitors of leucotriene synthesis has been evaluated in a rat model of granulomatous colitis. The rats exposed to 3-omega fatty acids in the form of cod-liver oil supplements were protected from the effects of inflammatory colitis induced by intracolonic administration of trinitro-benzene-sulphonic acid.[94]

A 7-month, double-blind, placebo-controlled crossover trial of dietary supplementation with fish oils has been carried out in 39 patients with chronic inflammatory bowel disease. In the treatment group the arachidonic acid-derived prostanoid generation was reduced by fish oil supplementation, and there was a moderate reduction in inflammatory lipid mediators by dietary n-3-omega fatty acids. There was limited morphological improvement, and the clinical benefits were small and confined to patients with ulcerative colitis.[95]

In an open study of patients with ulcerative colitis, some modest improvement was demonstrated using fish oil n-3-omega fatty acids supplementation in 10 patients with mild to moderate ulcerative colitis who had failed on or refused conventional therapy. Surprisingly, all patients tolerated the fish oil supplement in the diet. Seven patients had moderate to marked improvement, and the steroid dose was reduced in four or five patients taking prednisolone. Three patients had little or no improvement, but in none of the patients was the situation worse. It was felt that these results in this open study justified a double-blind controlled trial.[96]

SURGERY FOR ULCERATIVE COLITIS

The surgical alternatives for the surgical treatment of ulcerative colitis have been reviewed recently.[97] Colectomy and ileorectal anastomosis may sometimes be appropriate and were an option taken in 12% of a large Scandinavian series. The cumulative probability of having an intact ileorectal anastomosis in these selected patients at 10 years was 51%. The commonest cause of proctectomy was persistent symptoms from recurrent inflammation in the rectum and occasionally from dyplasia or postoperative complications. Patients with relative rectal sparing at the time of surgery compared favourably with those who had moderate rectal diseases at the time of surgery.[98]

The outcome among 758 patients with ulcerative colitis treated by ileal pouch–anal anastomosis, including a comparison with 94 patients undergoing the same operation for familial adenomatous polyposis, provides an excellent account of the present situation. There was an operative mortality among the colitis patients of only 0.3%. The overall outcome was remarkably good. A few patients in the colitis group developed sepsis and required reoperation (6%).

Patients undergoing surgery for ulcerative colitis had rather more daytime stools (mean 5.8 daily) and more night-time faecal spotting (40%); pouchitis was more common (22%) than in the patients undergoing treatment for polyposis. This paper draws attention to the small but significant price that has to be paid to avoid a permanent stoma in the surgical management of patients with ulcerative colitis.[99]

Twenty-five patients among the series of 362 consecutive ulcerative colitis patients undergoing ileal pouch–anal anastomosis were subsequently found to have Crohn's disease. After a mean follow-up of 38 months, 16 patients have a functioning pouch, seven have required pouch excision, one is diverted and one has died. Only one of nine patients in whom there were any clinical features suggestive of Crohn's disease has a functioning pouch, whereas 15 or 16 patients with no preoperative features suggesting Crohn's disease still have an intact pouch with good results.[100]

A similar experience is emerging in the surgical management of children with ulcerative colitis where ileo-anal anastomosis is the surgical treatment of choice for chronic symptomatic ulcerative colitis.[101]

The question of whether a covering loop ileostomy is needed after restorative proctocolectomy is currently being evaluated since there is a small but definite morbidity associated with closure. In a series of 40 patients undergoing closure, 36 had an uncomplicated recovery. One patient developed a superficial wound infection, and small-bowel obstruction occurred in three patients, of whom two required further laparotomy. In this series there were no enterocutaneous fistulas of incisional hernia, which have occurred previously.[102]

There is good evidence that the metabolism of body water and electrolytes after surgery for ulcerative colitis, whether by conventional ileostomy or J-pouch, is satisfactory,[103] and in patients with ulcerative colitis treated by ileo-anal J-pouch, total body fat, total body protein, and total body water had returned to preoperative levels within 3 months of operation.[104]

SURGERY IN CROHN'S DISEASE

The present situation has been well summarized by Alexander-Williams.[105] The principal indication for surgery in the small intestine for Crohn's disease is to overcome the effects of fibrous stenosis and its sequelae, fistula and abscess formation. Unresponsive acute colitis may necessitate colectomy, but early effective medical therapy has reduced the need for emergency surgery. For socially inconvenient Crohn's disease colitis (diarrhoea with frequency and urgency, or chronic ill health), colectomy and ileorectal anastomosis are appropriate, providing that the rectum is not grossly diseased and there is sufficient anal sphincter function. Otherwise, panproctocolectomy is advised.

The outcome using this strategy for the management of distal ileal Crohn's disease has produced a good long-term outcome. Among 139 patients with a mean follow-up of 10 years, 11 patients died (10 of unrelated causes), and among 128 living patients, 114 are fit and well, of whom only two are taking specific medication. Fourteen are unwell, of whom six need or have refused further surgery.[106]

Rutgeerts et al have continued their important studies of recurrent Crohn's disease after ileal resection by regular colonoscopy of the neoterminal ileum.[107] Endoscopic lesions of the neoterminal ileum can be seen in 75% of these patients within 1 year of surgery, although only a small proportion of the patients are symptomatic. After 3 years the endoscopic recurrence rate increases to 85% with symptomatic recurrence in 34%. Severe early postoperative lesions, endoscopically detected, have proved to be the best predictors of recurrent disease. In 22 patients included in this study, the neoterminal ileum was carefully examined during surgery, and multiple biopsies were taken. The resection margin was normal both macroscopically and microscopically. However, recurrent disease still occurred in this group, suggesting that early lesions of the neoterminal ileum after Crohn's disease resection do not originate from microscopic inflammation present in the bowel segment at the time of surgery, but arise de novo.[107] The segments of neoterminal ileum did, however, contain an increased number of HLA-DR$^+$, ATPase, and dendritic cells in the lamina propria, suggesting that immunological processes may play a role in the development of recurrent lesions.[108]

A European multicentre study comparing radical and conservative resections for Crohn's disease has shown that conservative resections are associated with a lower recurrence rate. The recurrence rate was even lower following treatment with sulphasalazine 3 g daily for 2 years. This is the first study to suggest that sulphasalazine may have some effect in reducing recurrent disease following resection for Crohn's disease, contrary to earlier findings.[109]

Fazio[110, 111] has both summarized his own experience of strictureplasty and provided an excellent overview. Strictureplasty is particularly appropriate where there are multiple strictures in the small bowel. Short strictures have been treated by Heinecke-Mikulicz strictureplasty and longer strictures by Finney side-to-side strictureplasty. There was no mortality, but there were occasional complications, including enterocutaneous fistulas, intra-abdominal sepsis, and haemorrhage. Strictureplasty may be appropriate for short strictures in association with a resection of more extensive disease elsewhere in the small intestine. Other centres have reviewed strictureplasty as a surgical option in patients with Crohn's disease with symptomatic small-bowel stricture.[112]

The surgical treatment of enterovesical fistulas, which are usually associated with ileal or ileocolonic Crohn's disease, has been analysed. Resection of the diseased bowel, drainage of any associated abscess, and oversewing of the defect with drainage produce an effective outcome in nearly all patients.[113]

Recto-vaginal fistulas pose a problem in the management of Crohn's disease. Some patients require panproctocolectomy, while others with minimal symptoms may never require surgical treatment. In a few patients local surgical repair of fistulas may be attempted with a covering loop ileostomy or colostomy. Of five patients treated in this way, closure of the colostomy was eventually possible in three. Results of this analysis suggest that in the setting of quiescent rectal disease an attempt to repair the fistula can be expected to have a reasonable chance of success, particularly in the presence of a diverting loop ileostomy.[114]

Good results have been obtained in the trans vaginal repair of recto-vaginal fistulas in patients with Crohn's disease. After diverting ileostomy, repair was effected by using a transvaginal approach with closure of the diverting ileostomy within 6 months. After a mean follow-up of 55 months in 14 patients only one fistula has recurred.[115]

In those few patients with symptomatic segmental colonic skip lesions, segmental colonic resection is an appropriate operation without resorting to colectomy. The 10-year reoperation rates of 66% are higher than those following colectomy and ileorectal anastomosis (23%). However, the findings suggest that when a patient with Crohn's disease has a short segment of diseased large bowel, a segmental resection is both feasible and safe.[116]

Hughes in Cardiff has reported his experience of proctectomy for perianal disease, which comprises fewer than half the patients with Crohn's disease coming to abdominal perineal excision. The principal indications for proctectomy in this group were high fistulas, stricture, and recto-vaginal fistulas. There was a tendency, both in this series and perhaps in others, for prolonged delay before inevitable surgical treatment for severe perianal disease was accepted by the patient.[117]

A study of the surgical treatment of Crohn's disease in childhood has emphasized the good outcome in patients undergoing ileocaecal resection and in those having a subtotal colectomy with ileostomy. In addition to symptomatic relief, the principal early benefit of surgery was improved growth.[118]

Balloon dilatation

Endoscopic balloon dilatation has been attempted in a few patients with

Crohn's disease. Among seven patients treated in one study, five had strictures from recurrent disease at the site of ileal transverse anastomosis, one had duodenal stenosis, and one had a colonic stricture. The procedure was performed under sedation on from one to four occasions (median two). Sustained improvement over a period of 18–24 months was achieved in five patients, but dilatation was unsuccessful in two cases. There was no related morbidity. The thickened, fibrous stricture associated with obstructive lesions in Crohn's disease, seen at laparotomy, does not look readily amenable to endoscopic dilatation. Further studies are needed, particularly in respect of morbidity and duration of the resolution of symptoms.[119]

MALIGNANCY IN ULCERATIVE COLITIS

There are now adequate data to establish the risk of developing colorectal cancer in ulcerative colitis, a risk which is a function of time in patients with extensive or total colitis, particularly in those with early onset disease. Apart from the biliary tree, there is no evidence of excess cancer risk at any other site.

Recent studies have challenged a number of these assumptions. A Scandinavian study has suggested that the colorectal cancer risk was similar in patients with pancolitis and left-sided colitis and that in females there was an excess of extraintestinal cancer in patients with colitis.[120] This is at variance with all previously published work which has scrutinized both these aspects carefully.

A Danish study reported a very low colorectal cancer risk in a cohort of 783 regional patients with ulcerative colitis.[46] This low estimate of risk may in part be related to the small number of patients with extensive or total colitis and the short duration of follow-up. With increasing length of follow-up, this patient group should provide one of the best estimates of colorectal cancer risk in a population-based series of patients with colitis.[121]

Screening for colorectal cancer

In patients with extensive or total colitis of more than 10 years' duration following an initial negative screen by colonoscopy and multiple biopsies, the incidence of developing severe dysplasia or colorectal cancer is small, being of the order of 0.5% per year. While this figure is significantly in excess of the risk in the general population matched for age and sex, the absolute numbers are still small. The returns from any screening programme in terms of detection of dysplasia or carcinoma are therefore likely to be small. This challenging viewpoint has been considered in a leader which finds screening for colorectal cancer in ulcerative colitis to be of dubious benefit at high cost.[122] Much has been achieved recently to quantify the potential benefit of surveillance programmes.

The overall results of a remarkable surveillance programme show that the cumulative probability of developing carcinoma was 3% at 15 years, 5% at 20 years, and 9% at 25 years among patients with extensive colitis. The equivalent figures for developing precancer or carcinoma or both were 4%, 7%, and 13% respectively. It is of interest that of the five patients who died of colorectal carcinoma, two were under regular observation, and three developed cancer 4–6 years after their last attendance.[123]

In a Scandinavian study, 12 of 72 patients with total ulcerative colitis developed definite dysplasia after a mean review period of 15 years. Low-grade dysplasia was detected in seven patients, high-grade in four, and Duke's A carcinoma in one patient at operation. The cumulative risk of developing at least a low-grade dysplasia was estimated at 14% after 25 years from the onset of disease.[124]

A US study has confirmed these findings in patients with total colitis. The risk of developing high-grade dysplasia or cancer in patients with total colitis from the onset of symptoms was 2.5% at 20 years, 4.0% at 25 years, 7.0% at 30 years, 13.0% at 35 years, and 20.0% at 40 years.[125]

An interesting study from North America has compared two groups of patients with total colitis, one of which had undergone screening while the other group had not. There were actually more cancer deaths in the surveillance group, but fewer overall deaths, presumably because those who were not screened did not attend for regular follow-up either, and died of other causes related to their colitis. Benefit was therefore derived from screening, perhaps by regular hospital review and treatment, but the improvement was not related to the anticipated benefits of improved survival of cancer.[126]

Nugent et al[127] has published the results of their own cancer surveillance programme among 213 patients with a mean follow-up of 13 years, revealing the following important features. The initial screen identified 18 patients who had dysplasia, of whom 15 underwent colectomy and seven had unsuspected carcinoma, supporting earlier observations that the initial screen of a previously unscreened population with total colitis produces important benefits. However, after this only 11 more patients developed dysplasia, of whom seven had colectomy, but in only one was there evidence of carcinoma.

The authors conclude that the returns beyond the initial screening are small. There were few examples of false negative reports in this series, suggesting that multiple biopsies with no evidence of dysplasia imply that the short-term risk for developing carcinoma in patients with negative biopsy results is low. The other surprising feature in this study was the observation that the risk of developing colorectal carcinoma was similar in patients with extensive colitis and left-sided disease.[127]

The development of alternative markers to detect premalignant disease has not yet been a resounding success. Abnormal biopsy specimens showing dysplasia from patients with ulcerative colitis and samples from other parts of the large bowel have been subject to flow cytometric DNA analysis.

All three patients with high-grade dysplasia showed aneuploidy (abnormal DNA stem lines). However, this work still relies on morphological detection of dysplasia, and it is uncertain whether this has general application. A great deal more work is required before it can be used in clinical practice.[128]

In other studies aneuploidy has been detected without concomitant dysplasia and might therefore be an appropriate early marker. Such studies have only been carried out in small numbers of patients, and prospective studies are needed before the clinical significance of these findings can be determined.[129]

Other markers that have been explored include tumour-associated glycoproteins.[130] Attempts have been made to identify c-Ki-*ras* genes in dysplasia associated with ulcerative colitis by direct sequencing of polymerase chain-reaction products, but so far without success.[131]

CANCER IN CROHN'S DISEASE

In a large Scandinavian study of 1655 patients with Crohn's disease under long-term review, 12 colorectal cancers were detected, with an overall excess risk of 2.5. The excess risk was similar for males and females, and, perhaps surprisingly, the duration of follow-up did not seem to affect the risk.

The relative risk of developing malignancy when Crohn's disease involved the terminal ileum was 1.0; for terminal ileum and proximal colon involvement, 3.2; and for the colon alone, 5.6. Patients in whom Crohn's colitis developed before the age of 30 had a much higher relative risk (20.9), than those diagnosed at an older age (2.2).[132]

SCLEROSING CHOLANGITIS

The association of inflammatory bowel disease with sclerosing cholangitis has been described in editorials[133] and by observation. In an unusual paper, liver biopsy appearances in 50 patients with ulcerative colitis without clinical or biochemical evidence of liver disease were reviewed, and three showed classical onion-skin fibrosis around the ducts, suggestive of sclerosing cholangitis. Eighteen years later, over 85% of the patients were reviewed. Only two patients had developed frank liver disease, and neither of these two had had abnormal histology at the first liver biopsy. The authors concluded that morphological change is of little help in predicting future risk of an associated hepatic complaint in inflammatory bowel disease.[134]

When sclerosis cholangitis does occur with inflammatory bowel disease, it tends to have a presentation different from that when it occurs without,[135] but, surprisingly, these differences seem merely to reflect greater awareness of the potential of liver disease in inflammatory bowel disease, when the diagnosis can be made without the need for frank hepatic presentation such as jaundice. It is of interest that in this group of patients who had both sclerosing cholangitis and inflammatory bowel disease, 39 had ulcerative colitis and eight had Crohn's disease. It remains uncertain whether sclerosing cholangitis should be regarded as an autoimmune condition, but the association of a relatively newly described autoantibody with ulcerative colitis and with sclerosing cholangitis 'gives food for thought', as does a strong HLA association with sclerosing cholangitis.[136]

Antineutrophil nuclear antibodies were found in 84% of patients with sclerosing cholangitis, and in 86% of patients with inflammatory bowel disease, but at lower titres in the absence of liver disease.[136] Strong associations with an antineutrophil cytoplasmic antibody and sclerosing cholangitis, with and without inflammatory bowel disease, and ulceration on its own were reported.[137]

The precise significance of such autoantibodies needs to be defined, and it is difficult to say more at the moment than that they may be useful diagnostic pointers[138] pertaining to pathogenesis.

In terms of treatment of sclerosing cholangitis, the variable rates of progression and the absence of any clearly effective medical treatment that alters the prognosis remain apparent, and the arguments against short-term surgical intervention or therapeutic endoscopy that may induce infective complications are strengthened by the reports of excellent results from liver transplantation in that group of patients with progressive severe liver disease.[139]

REFERENCES

1 Lowes JR, Jewell DP. The immunology of inflammatory bowel disease. Springer Semin Immunopathol 1990; 121: 251–268
2 Fiocchi C. Immune events associated with inflammatory bowel disease. Scand J Gastroenterol (suppl)1990; 172: 4–12
3 Jewell DP. Aetiology and pathogenesis of ulcerative colitis and Crohn's disease. Postgrad Med J 1989; 65: 718–719
4 Calkins BM. A meta-analysis of the role of smoking in inflammatory bowel disease. Dig Dis Sci 1989; 34: 1841–1854
5 Duffy LC, Zielezny MA, Marshall JR et al. Cigarette smoking and risk of clinical relapse in patients with Crohn's disease. Am J Prev Med 1990; 6: 161–166
6 Sutherland LR, Ramcharan S, Bryant H, Fick G. Effect of cigarette smoking on recurrence of Crohn's disease. Gastroenterology 1990; 98: 1123–1128
7 Motley RJ, Rhodes J, Williams G, Tavares IA, Bennett A. Smoking, eicosanoids and ulcerative colitis. J Pharm Pharmacol 1990; 42: 288–289
8 Lashner BA, Kane SV, Hanauer SB. Lack of association between oral contraceptive use and Crohn's disease: a community-based matched case-control study. Gastroenterology 1989; 97: 1442–1447
9 Lashner BA, Kane SV, Hanauer SB. Lack of association between oral contraceptive use and ulcerative colitis. Gastroenterology 1990; 99: 1032–1036
10 Stow SP, Redmond SR, Stormont JM et al. An epidemiologic study of inflammatory bowel disease in Rochester, New York. Hospital incidence. Gastroenterology 1990; 98: 104–110
11 Bennett RA, Rubin PH, Present DH. Frequency of inflammatory bowel disease in offspring of couples both presenting with inflammatory bowel disease. Gastroenterology 1991; 100: 1638–1643

12 Katz KD, Hollander D, Vadheim CM et al. Intestinal permeability in patients with Crohn's disease and their healthy relatives. Gastroenterology 1989; 97: 921–931

13 Monsen U, Iselius L, Johansson C, Hellers G. Evidence for a major additive gene in ulcerative colitis. Clin Genet 1989; 36: 411–414

14 Shah A, Mayberry JF, Williams G, Holt P, Loft DE, Rhodes J. Epidemiological survey of coeliac disease and inflammatory bowel disease in first-degree relatives of coeliac patients. Q J Med 1990; 74: 283–288

15 Gitnick G, Collins J, Beaman B et al. Preliminary report on isolation of mycobacteria from patients with Crohn's disease. Dig Dis Sci 1989; 34: 925–932

16 Tanaka K, Wilks M, Coates PJ, Farthing MJ, Walker-Smith JA, Tabaqchali S. *Mycobacterium paratuberculosis* and Crohn's disease. Gut 1991; 32: 43–45

17 Seldenrijk CA, Drexhage HA, Meuwissen SG, Meijer CJ. T-cellular immune reactions (in macrophage inhibition factor assay) against *Mycobacterium paratuberculosis*, *Mycobacterium Kansasil*, *Mycobacterium tuberculosis*, *Mycobacterium avium* in patients with chronic inflammatory bowel disease. Gut 1990; 31: 529–535

18 McKenzie H, Main J, Pennington CR, Parratt D. Antibody to selected strains of *Saccharomyces cerevisiae* (baker's and brewer's yeast) and *Candida albicans* in Crohn's disease. Gut 1990; 31: 536–538

19 Barnes RM, Allan S, Taylor-Robinson CH, Finn R, Johnson PM. Serum antibodies reactive with *Saccharomyces cerevisiae* in inflammatory bowel disease: is IgA antibody a marker for Crohn's disease? Int Arch Allergy Appl Immunol 1990; 92: 9–15

20 Walvoort HC, Fazzi GE, Pena AS. Seroreactivity of patients with Crohn's disease with lymph nodes of primed nude mice is independent of the tissue used for priming. Gastroenterology 1989; 97:1097–1100

21 Zuckerman MJ, Williams SE, Bura R, Das KM, Sachar DB. Sera-reactivity in inflammatory bowel disease: frequency of recognition of Crohn's disease tissue primed nude mouse lymphoid tissue in an interinstitutional blinded study. J Clin Gastroenterol 1989 11: 639–644

22 Das KM, Vecchi M, Novikoff A, Mazumdar S, Novikoff PM. Hybridomas using athymic nude mouse injected with Crohn's disease (CD) tissue filtrate. Immunoreactivity of the hybridomas with CD sera. Am J Pathol 1990; 136: 1375–1382

23 Das KM, Sakamaki S, Vecchi M. Ulcerative colitis: specific antibodies against a colonic epithelial Mr 40,000 protein. Immunol Invest 1989; 18: 459–472

24 Fiocchi C, Roche JK, Michener WM. High prevalence of antibodies to intestinal epithelial antigens in patients with inflammatory bowel disease and their relatives. Ann Intern Med 1989; 15; 110: 786–794

25 Marteau P, Colombel JF, Nemeth J, Vaerman JP, Dive JC, Rambaud JC. Immunological study of histologically non-involved jejunum during Crohn's disease: evidence for reduced in vivo secretion of secretory IgA. Clin Exp Immunol 1990; 80: 196–201

26 Mahida YR, Wu K, Jewell DP. Enhanced production of interleukin 1-beta by mononuclear cells isolated from mucosa with active ulcerative colitis of Crohn's disease. Gut 1989; 30: 835–838

27 Fais S, Capobianchi MR, Pallone F et al. Spontaneous release of interferon gamma by intestinal lamina propria lymphocytes in Crohn's disease. Kinetics of in vitro response to interferon gamma inducers. Gut 1991; 32: 403–407

28 Ligumsky M, Simon PL, Karmeli F, Rachmilewitz D. Role of interleukin-1 in inflammatory bowel disease-enhanced production during active disease. Gut 1990; 31: 686–689

29 Brynskov J, Tvede N. Plasma interleukin-2 and a soluble/shed interleukin-2 receptor in serum of patients with Crohn's disease. Effect of cyclosporin. Gut 1990; 31: 795–799

30 Chiba M, Iizuka M, Horie Y, Igarashi K, Masamune O. HLA-DR antigen expression in macroscopically uninvolved areas of intestinal epithelia in Crohn's disease. Gastroenterol Jpn 1989; 24: 365–372

31 Mayer L, Eisenhardt D, Salomon P, Bauer W, Plous R, Piccinini L. Expression of class II molecules on intestinal epithelial cells in humans. Differences between normal and inflammatory bowel disease. Gastroenterology 1991; 100: 3–12

32 Fais S, Pallone F. Ability of human colonic epithelium to express the 4F2 antigen, the common acute lymphoblastic leukemia antigen, and the transferrin receptor. Studies in

inflammatory bowel disease and after in vitro exposure to different stimuli. Gastroenterology 1989; 97:1435–1441

33 Malizia G, Calabrese A, Cottone M et al. Expression of leukocyte adhesion molecules by mucosal mononuclear phagocytes in inflammatory bowel disease. Gastroenterology 1991; 100: 150–159

34 Ahrenstedt O, Knutson L, Nilsson B, Nilsson-Ekdahl K, Odlind B, Hallgren R. Enhanced local production of complement components in the small intestines of patients with Crohn's disease. N Engl J Med 1990; 322: 1345–1349

35 Williams JG, Hughes LE, Hallett MB. Toxic oxygen metabolite production by circulating phagocytic cells in inflammatory bowel disease. Gut 1990; 31: 187–193

36 Curran FT, Allan RN, Keighley MR. Superoxide production by Crohn's disease neutrophils. Gut 1991; 32: 399–402

37 Adeyemi EO, Hodgson HJF. Lactoferrin: a correlate of disease activity in inflammatory bowel disease. Eur J Gastro & Hepatol 1991; 3: 51–56

38 Cominelli F, Nast CC, Clarke BD et al. Interleukin-1 gene expression, synthesis, and effect of specific IL-1 receptor blockade in rabbit immune complex colitis. J Clin Invest 1990; 86: 972–980

39 Wakefield AJ, Sawyerr AM, Dhillon AP et al. Pathogenesis of Crohn's disease: multifocal gastrointestinal infarction. Lancet 1989; 2: 1057–1062

40 Wakefield AJ, Sankey EA, Dhillon AP et al. Granulomatous vasculitis in Crohn's disease. Gastroenterology 1991; 100[Pt 1]: 1279–1287

41 Ramakrishna BS, Roberts-Thomson IC, Pannall PR, Roediger WE. Impaired sulphation of phenol by the colonic mucosa in quiescent and active ulcerative colitis. Gut 1991: 32: 46–49

42 Roediger WE, Nance S. Selective reduction of fatty acid oxidation in colonocytes: correlation with ulcerative colitis. Lipids 1990; 25: 646–652

43 Winter HS, Crum PM Jr, King NW, Sehgal PK, Roche JK. Expression of immune sensitisation to epithelial cell-associated components in the cotton-top tamarin: a model of chronic ulcerative colitis. Gastroenterology 1989; 97: 1075–1082

44 Mitchell IC, Turk JL. An experimental animal model of granulomatous bowel disease. Gut 1989; 30: 1371–1378

45 Oestreicher P, Nielsen ST, Rainsford KD. Inflammatory bowel disease induced by combined bacterial immunisation and oral carrageenan in guinea-pigs. Model development, histopathology, and effects of sulfasalazine. Dig Dis Sci 1991; 36: 461–470

46 Moyana TN, Lalonde JM. Carrageenan-induced intestinal injury in the rat – a model for inflammatory bowel disease. Ann Clin Lab Sci 1990; 20: 420–426

47 Eigenbrodt ML, Elgenbrodt EH, Thiele DL. Histologic similarity of murine colonic graft-versus-host disease (GVHD) to human colonic GVHD and inflammatory bowel disease. Am J Pathol 1990; 137: 1065–1076

48 Mary JY, Modigliani R. Development and validation of an endoscopic index of the severity for Crohn's disease: a prospective multicentre study. Groupe d'Etudes Thérapeutiques des Affections Inflammatoires du Tube Digestif (GETAID). Gut 1989; 30: 983–989

49 Wheeler JG, Slack NF, Duncan A, Palmer M, Harvey RF. ^{99}Tcm-nanocolloid imaging in inflammatory bowel disease. Nucl Med Commun 1990; 11: 127–133

50 Arndt JW, van der Sluys Veer A, Blok D et al. Technetium-99m nanocolloid for the scintigraphic assessment of inflammatory bowel disease in the colon: its value in comparison with indium-111-labelled granulocytes. Eur J Radiol 1991; 12: 30–34

51 Buscombe JR, Lui D, Ensing D, de-Jong R, Ell PJ. ^{99m}Tc-human immunoglobulin (HIG) – first results of a new agent for the localisation of infection and inflammation. Eur J Nucl Med 1990; 16: 649–655

52 Bares R, Fass J, Truong S, Buell U, Schumpelick V. Radioimmunoscintigraphy with 111-In-labelled monoclonal antibody fragments against CEA. Nucl Med Commun 1989; 10: 627–641

53 Koelbel G, Schmiedl U, Majer MC et al. Diagnosis of fistulae and sinus tracts in patients with Crohn's disease: value of MR imaging. AJR 1989; 152: 999–1003

54 Crama-Bohbouth G, Pena AS, Biemond I et al. Are activity indices helpful in assessing active intestinal inflammation in Crohn's disease? Gut 1989; 30: 1236–1240

55 Goebell H, Wienbeck M, Schomerus H, Malchow H. Evaluation of the Crohn's Disease

Activity Index (CDAI) and the Dutch Index for severity and activity of Crohn's disease. An analysis of the data from the European Co-operative Crohn's Disease Study. Dig Dis Sci 1991; 36: 573–576

56 Boirivant M, Pallone F, Ciaco A, Leoni M, Fais S, Torsoli A. Usefulness of fecal alpha 1-antitrypsin clearance and fecal concentration as early indicator of postoperative asymptomatic recurrence in Crohn's disease. Dig Dis Sci 1991; 36: 347–352

57 Hayllar J, Bjarnason I. Sulphasalazine in ulcerative colitis: in memoriam? Gut 1991; 32: 462–463

58 Ireland A, Jewell DP. Mechanism of action of 5-aminosalicyclic acid and its derivatives. Clin Sci 1990; 78: 119–125

59 Staerk Laursen L, Stokholm M, Bukhave K, Rask-Madsen J, Lauritsen K. Disposition of 5-aminosalicyclic acid by olsalazine and three mesalazine preparations in patients with ulcerative colitis: comparison of intraluminal colonic concentrations, serum values, and urinary excretion. Gut 1990; 31: 1271–1276

60 Jarnerot G. Newer 5-aminosalicyclic acid based drugs in chronic inflammatory bowel disease. Drugs 1989; 37: 73–86

61 Mahida YR, Lamming CE, Gallagher A, Hawthorne AB, Hawkey CJ. 5-aminosalicyclic acid is a potent inhibitor of interleukin-1 beta production in organ culture of colonic biopsy specimens from patients with inflammatory bowel disease. Gut 1991; 32: 50–54

62 Thomson ABR. New developments in the use of 5-aminosalicyclic acid in patients with inflammatory bowel disease. Aliment Pharmacol Therap 1991; 5: 449–470

63 Rao SS, Dundas SA, Holdsworth CD, Cann PA, Palmer KR, Corbett CL. Olsalazine or sulphasalazine in first attacks of ulcerative colitis? A double blind study. Gut 1989; 30: 675–679

64 Jacobsen BA, Abildgaard K, Rasmussen HH et al. Availability of mesalazine (5-aminosalicyclic acid) from enemas and suppositories during steady-state condition. Scand J Gastroenterol 1991; 26: 374–378

65 Biddle WL, Miner PB Jr. Long-term use of mesalamine enemas to induce remission in ulcerative colitis. Gastroenterology 1990; 99: 113–118

66 Mahida YR, Jewell DP. Slow-release 5-aminosalicyclic acid (Pentasa) for the treatment of active Crohn's disease. Digestion 1990; 45: 88–92

67 Law R, Hanauer S, Rick G. Multicentre open label long-term cohort study of oral Pentasa in Crohn's disease. Gastroenterology 1990; 98: A185

68 Thomson ABR, on behalf of the International Mesalazine Study Group. Coated oral 5-aminosalicyclic acid versus placebo in maintaining remission of inactive Crohn's disease. Aliment Pharmacol Therap 1990; 4: 55–64

69 Gendie JP, Mary JY, Florent C. Does Pentasa prevent relapses in quiescent Crohn's disease? Gastroenterology 1990; 98: A171

70 Committee on Safety of Medicines. Current problems. 30 December 1990

71 Halpern Z, Sold O, Baratz M, Konikoff F, Halak A, Gilat T. A controlled trial of beclomethasone versus betamethasone enemas in distal ulcerative colitis. J Clin Gastroenterol 1991; 13: 38–41

72 Mulder CJ, Endert E, van der Heide H et al. Comparison of beclomethasone dipropionate (2 and 3 mg) and prednisolone sodium phosphate enemas (30 mg) in the treatment of ulcerative proctitis. An adrenocortical approach. Neth J Med 1989; 35: 18–24

73 Carpani de Kaski M, Peters AM, Lavender JP, Hodgson HJF. Fluticasone propionate in Crohn's disease. Gut 1991; 32: 657–662

74 Hawthorne AB, Hawkey CJ. Immunosuppressive drugs in inflammatory bowel disease. A review of their mechanisms of efficacy and place in therapy. Drugs 1989; 38: 267–288

75 Present DH, Meltzer SJ, Krumholz MP, Wolke A, Korelitz BI. 6-Mercaptopurine in the management of inflammatory bowel disease: short- and long-term toxicity. Ann Intern Med 1989; 111: 641–649

76 Alstead EM, Ritchie JK, Lennard-Jones JE, Farthing MJ, Clark ML. Safety of azathioprine in pregnancy in inflammatory bowel disease. Gastroenterology 1990; 99: 443–446

77 Kozarek RA, Paterson DJ, Gelfand MD et al. Methotrexate induces clinical and histological remission in patients with refractory inflammatory bowel disease. Ann Intern Med 1989; 110: 353–356

78 Hodgson HJF. Cyclosporin in inflammatory bowel disease. Aliment Pharmacol Therap 1991; 5: 343–350
79 Brynskov J, Freund L, Rasmussen SN et al. A placebo-controlled, double blind, randomized trial of cyclosporine therapy in active chronic Crohn's disease. N Eng J Med 1989; 321: 845–850
80 Lofberg R, Angelin B, Einarsson K, Gabrielsson N, Ost L. Unsatisfactory effect of cyclosporin A treatment in Crohn's disease: a report of five cases. J Intern Med 1989; 226: 157–161
81 Lobo AJ, Juby LD, Rothwell J, Poole TW, Axon AT. Long-term treatment of Crohn's disease with cyclosporine: the effect of a very low dose of maintenance of remission. J Clin Gastroenterol 1991; 13: 42–45
82 Lichtinger S, Present DH. Cyclosporin in treatment of severe active ulcerative colitis. Lancet 1990; 336: 16–19
83 Brynskove J, Freund L, Ostergaard Thomsen O, Andersen CB, Norby Rasmussen S, Binder V. Treatment of refractory ulcerative colitis with cyclosporine enemas. Lancet 1989; 1: 721–722
84 Ranzi T, Campanini MC, Velio P et al. Treatment of chronic proctosigmoiditis with cyclosporine enemas. Lancet 1989; 2: 97
85 Lashner BA, Hanauer SB, Silverstein MD. Testing nicotine gum for ulcerative colitis patients. Experience with single-patient trials. Dig Dis Sci 1990; 35: 827–832
86 Teahon K, Bjarnason I, Pearson M, Levi AJ. Ten years' experience with an elemental diet in the management of Crohn's disease. Gut 1990; 31: 1133–1137
87 Malchow H, Steinhardt HJ, Lorenz-Meyer H et al. Feasibility and effectiveness of a defined-formula diet regimen in treating active Crohn's disease. European Co-operative Crohn's Disease Study III. Scand J Gastroenterol 1990; 25: 235–244
88 Lochs H, Steinhardt HJ, Klaus-Wentz B et al. Comparison of enteral nutrition and drug treatment in active Crohn's disease. Results of the European Co-operative Crohn's Disease Study IV. Gastroenterology 1991; 101: 881–888
89 Giaffer MH, North G, Holdsworth CD. Controlled trial of polymeric versus elemental diet in treatment of active Crohn's disease. Lancet 1990; 335: 816–819
90 Giaffer MH, Cann P, Holdsworth CD. Long-term effects of elemental and exclusive diets for Crohn's disease. Aliment Pharmacol Therap 1991; 5: 115–126
91 Russell RI. Dietary and nutritional management of Crohn's disease. Aliment Pharmacol Therap 1991; 5: 211–226
92 Maynard ND, Bihari DJ. Postoperative feeding. BMJ 1991; 303: 1007–1008
93 Lashner BA, Evans AA, Hanauer SB. Preoperative total parenteral nutrition for bowel resection in Crohn's disease. Dig Dis Sci 1989; 34: 741–746
94 Vilaseca J, Salas A, Guarner F, Rodriguez R, Martinez M, Malagelada JR. Dietary fish oil reduces progression of chronic inflammatory lesions in a rat model of granulomatous colitis. Gut 1990; 31: 539–544
95 Lorenz R. Supplementation with n-3 fatty acids from fish oil in chronic inflammatory bowel disease. J Intern Med Suppl 1989; 225: 225–232
96 Salomon P, Kornbluth AA, Janowitz HD. Treatment of ulcerative colitis with fish oil n-3-omega-fatty acid: an open trial. J Clin Gastroenterol 1990; 12: 157–161
97 Jagelman DG. Surgical alternatives for ulcerative colitis. Med Clin N Am 1990; 74: 155–167
98 Leijonmarck CE, Lofberg R, Ost A, Hellers G. Long-term results of ileorectal anastomosis in ulcerative colitis in Stockholm County. Dis Colon Rectum 1990; 33: 195–200
99 Dozois RR, Kelly KA, Welling DR et al. Ileal pouch–anal anastomosis: comparison of results in familial adenomatous polyposis and chronic ulcerative colitis. Ann Surg 1989; 210: 268–271; Discussion 272–273
100 Hyman NH, Fazio VW, Tuckson WB, Lavery IC. Consequences of ileal pouch–anal anastomosis for Crohn's colitis. Dis Colon Rectum 1991; 34: 653–657
101 Orkin BA, Telander RL, Wolff BG, Perrault J, Ilstrup DM. The surgical management of children with ulcerative colitis. The old vs. the new. Dis Colon Rectum 1990; 33: 947–955
102 Lewis P, Bartolo DC. Closure of loop ileostomy after restorative proctocolectomy. Ann R Coll Surg Engl 1990; 72: 263–265

103 Christie PM, Knight GS, Hill GL. Metabolism of body water and electrolytes after surgery for ulcerative colitis: conventional ileostomy versus J pouch. Br J Surg 1990; 77: 149–151

104 Christie PM, Hill GL. Return to normal body composition after ileoanal J-pouch anastomosis for ulcerative colitis. Dis Colon Rectum 1990; 33: 584–586

105 Alexander-Williams J. Surgical aspects of inflammatory bowel disease. Scand J Gastroenterol Suppl 1990; 172: 39–42

106 Andrews HA, Keighley MR, Alexander-Williams J, Allan RN. Strategy for management of distal ileal Crohn's disease. Br J Surg 1991; 78: 679–682

107 Rutgeerts P, Geboes K, Vantrappen G, Beyls J, Kerremans R, Hiele M. Predictability of the postoperative course of Crohn's disease. Gastroenterology 1990; 99: 956–963

108 Vantrappen G, Rutgeerts P. Recurrence of Crohn's lesions in the neoterminal ileum after ileal resection and ileocolonic anastomosis. Verh K Acad Geneeskd Belg 1990; 52: 373–382

109 Ewe K, Herfarth C, Malchow H, Jesdinsky HJ. Postoperative recurrence of Crohn's disease in relation to radicality of operation and sulfazalazine prophylaxis: a multicentre trial. Digestion 1989; 42: 224–232

110 Fazio VW. Conservative surgery for Crohn's disease of the small bowel: the role of strictureplasty. Med Clin N Am 1990; 74: 169–181

111 Fazio VW, Galandiuk S, Jagelman DG, Lavery IC. Strictureplasty in Crohn's disease. Ann Surg 1989; 210: 621–625

112 Pritchard TJ, Schoetz DJ Jr, Caushaj FP et al. Strictureplasty of the small bowel in patients with Crohn's disease. An effective surgical option. Arch Surg 1990; 125: 715–717

113 McNamara MJ, Fazio VW, Lavery IC, Weakley FL, Farmer RG. Surgical treatment of enterovesical fistulas in Crohn's disease. Dis Colon Rectum 1990; 33: 271–276

114 Cohen JL, Stricker JW, Schoetz DJ Jr, Coller JA, Veidenheimer MC. Rectovaginal fistula in Crohn's disease. Dis Colon Rectum 1989; 32: 825–828

115 Sher ME, Bauer JJ, Gelernt I. Surgical repair of rectovaginal fistulas in patients with Crohn's disease: transvaginal approach. Dis Colon Rectum 1991; 34: 641–648

116 Allan A, Andrews H, Hilton CJ, Keighley MR, Allan RN, Alexander-Williams J. Segmental colonic resection is an appropriate operation for short skip lesions due to Crohn's disease in the colon. World J Surg 1989; 13: 611–614

117 Williams JG, Hughes LE. Abdominoperineal resection for severe perianal Crohn's disease. Dis Colon Rectum 1990; 33: 402–407

118 Davies G, Evans CM, Shand WS, Walker-Smith JA. Surgery for Crohn's disease in childhood: influence of site of disease and operative procedure on outcome. Br J Surg 1990; 77: 891–894

119 Williams AJ, Palmer KR. Endoscopic balloon dilatation as a therapeutic option in the management of intestinal strictures resulting from Crohn's disease. Br J Surg 1991; 78: 453–454

120 Kvist N, Jacobsen O, Kvist HK et al. Malignancy in ulcerative colitis. Scand J Gastroenterol 1989; 24: 497–506

121 Binder V. Incidence of colonic cancer in inflammatory bowel disease. Scand J Gastroenterol (suppl)1989; 170: 78; Discussion 81–82

122 Gyde S. Screening for colorectal cancer in ulcerative colitis: dubious benefits and high costs. Gut 1990; 31: 1089–1092

123 Lennard-Jones JE, Melville DM, Morson BC, Ritchie JK, Williams CB. Precancer and cancer in extensive ulcerative colitis: findings among 401 patients over 22 years. Gut 1990; 31: 800–806

124 Lofberg R, Brostrom O, Karlen P, Tribukait B, Ost A. Colonoscopic surveillance in long-standing total ulcerative colitis – a 15-year follow-up study. Gastroenterology 1990; 99: 1021–1031

125 Lashner BA, Silverstein MD, Hanauer SB. Hazard rates for dysplasia and cancer in ulcerative colitis. Results from a surveillance programme. Dig Dis Sci 1989; 34: 1536–1541

126 Lashner BA, Kane SV, Hanauer SB. Colon cancer surveillance in chronic ulcerative colitis: historical cohort study. Am J Gastroenterol 1990; 85: 1083–1087

127 Nugent FW, Haggitt RC, Gilpin PA. Cancer surveillance in ulcerative colitis Gastroenterology 1991; 100[Pt 1]: 1241–1248

128 Rutegard J, Ahsgren L, Stenling R, Roos G. DNA content and mucosal dysplasia in ulcerative colitis. Flow cytometric analysis in patients with dysplastic or indefinite morphologic changes in the colorectal mucosa. Dis Colon Rectum 1989; 32: 1055–1059

129 Lofberg R, Caspersson T, Tribukait B, Ost A. Comparative DNA analyses in long-standing ulcerative colitis with aneuploidy. Gut 1989; 30: 1731–1736

130 Thor A, Itzkowtiz SH, Schlom J, Kim YS, Hanauer S. Tumor-associated glycoprotein (TAG-72) expression in ulcerative colitis. Int J Cancer 1989; 43: 810–815

131 Meltzer SJ, Mane SM, Wood PK et al. Activation of c-Ki-ras in human gastrointestinal dysplasias determined by direct sequencing of polymerase chain reaction products. Cancer Res 1990; 50: 3627–3630

132 Ekbom A, Helmick C, Zack M, Adami HO. Increased risk of large bowel cancer in Crohn's disease with colonic involvement. Lancet 1990; 336: 357–359

133 Sachar DB. Ulcerative colitis and sclerosing cholangitis: does 'IBD' mean 'inflamed bile ducts'? [Editorial]. Gastroenterology 1991; 100[Pt 1]: 1469–1470

134 Broome U, Glaumann H, Hultcrantz R. Liver histology and follow-up of 68 patients with ulcerative colitis and normal liver function tests. Gut 1990; 31: 468–472

135 Rabinovitz M, Gavaler JS, Schade RR, Dindzans VJ, Chien MC, Van Thiel DH. Does primary sclerosing cholangitis occurring in association with inflammatory bowel disease differ from that occurring in the absence of inflammatory bowel disease? A study of sixty-six subjects. Hepatology 1990; 11: 7–11

136 Snook JA, Chapman RW, Fleming K, Jewell DP. Anti-neutrophil nuclear antibody in ulcerative colitis, Crohn's disease and primary sclerosing cholangitis. Clin Exp Immunol 1989; 76: 30–33

137 Duerr RH, Targan SR, Landers CJ et al. Neutrophil cytoplasmic antibodies: a link between primary sclerosing cholangitis and ulcerative colitis. Gastroenterology 1991; 100[Pt 1]: 1385–1391

138 Saxon A, Shanahan F, Landers C, Gaz T, Targan S. A distinct subset of antineutrophil cytoplasmic antibodies is associated with inflammatory bowel disease. J Allergy Clin Immunol 1990; 86: 202–210

139 Marsh JW, Iwatsuki S, Makowka L et al. Orthotopic liver transplantation for primary sclerosing cholangitis. Ann Surg 1988; 207: 21–25

2

Helicobacter pylori

A. T. R. Axon

Helicobacter pylori (H. pylori) inhabits the mucus layer which overlies gastric epithelial cells. It occurs naturally only in man and other primates and is responsible for the common form of chronic gastritis which affects over 50% of the world's population. The organism is infective and causes an initial acute hypochlorhydric gastritis which, in most individuals, progresses to chronic gastritis. It is considered to be the major factor in the multifactorial disease, duodenal ulcer,[1] it may also be responsible for many gastric ulcers, and recent work suggests that it could be implicated in the pathogenesis of gastric cancer.

THE ORGANISM

When originally isolated,[2] *H. pylori* was thought to be a member of the genus *Campylobacter*, but subsequent work has shown it to be the first member of the new genus *Helicobacter*.[3] A number of different species have been identified and are classified under the name of the relevant host, e.g. *H. felis* (cat), *H. mustelae* (ferret), and *H. acinonyx* (cheetah). One of the characteristics of *H. pylori* is the possession of a powerful urease, which may be responsible for its ability to survive in the acidic environment of the gastric lumen. The ammonia produced raises the pH in its immediate vicinity and may protect it[4] during the critical period after it has been ingested and before it reaches the sanctuary zone beneath the gastric mucus where the pH approaches neutral.

Having reached its ecological niche,[5] it attaches itself to the gastric epithelial cell where it is anchored by strands of electron-dense material,[6] and an adhesion pedestal may form,[7] reminiscent of that seen with pathogenic *E. coli*. It probably adheres to specific carbohydrate-associated receptors on the gastric epithelial cell.[8,9] Cells of other lineage, such as goblet cells and enterocytes, probably do not possess the appropriate receptor because the organism cannot colonize them, and within the stomach it is unable to infect areas of intestinal metaplasia.

The organism is strongly antigenic and stimulates a severe inflammatory response, but, in spite of this, the infection often persists throughout the life of the host. It is possible that the local inflammatory reaction host may actually work to the organism's advantage, stimulating the exudation of essential nutrients.

Detection of *H. pylori*

ELISA methods reliably detect serum antibodies to *H. pylori* with acceptable sensitivity and specificity. After eradication, antibody levels fall over a period of months; thus, they are not helpful in assessing short-term eradication. They may also be misleading in anergic elderly patients.

Histological examination of two antral biopsies by an expert pathologist is as effective as any other test. Negative and equivocal biopsies should be stained by the Giemsa method.

The urease secreted by *H. pylori* has been exploited into two ways. Endoscopic biopsies are placed in a solution of urea with a pH indicator. If *H. pylori* is present, ammonia is released, the pH rises, and the indicator changes colour. Commercially prepared tests are readily available. The $^{13}C^{10-12}$ and ^{14}C breath tests[13] are alternative non-invasive techniques. Carbon-labelled urea is taken by mouth and expired air is collected. Gastric *H. pylori* degrades the urea and labelled carbon dioxide is detected in the breath. ^{13}C is not radioactive and is therefore totally non-invasive; its disadvantage is that it is relatively expensive to measure.

The culture of endoscopic biopsies gives excellent results and is probably the most sensitive and specific technique for detecting *H. pylori*. It has the advantage that antibiotic sensitivities can be obtained; however, results are very dependent on the expertise of the laboratory.

The most sensitive and specific technique becoming available is PCR;[14,15] this will be the 'gold standard' in due course.

Epidemiology

H. pylori has a worldwide[16] distribution, but it is more common in the developing world, where infection occurs early in childhood[17] and may rise to over 80% in young adults. In developed countries childhood infection is uncommon, but the prevalence rises after the age of 40 (Fig. 2.1).

There are two possible explanations for the consistent relationship between increasing age and infection. It could be that the organism is acquired gradually throughout life; alternatively, it may be a cohort effect. The pattern of infection in the UK 40–50 years ago may have been closer to that found today in developing countries, the change being due to improvements in living standards. If this is the case, when the present generation of children reach 60, this cohort will continue to have a low prevalence.

In developed countries there is an association between infection and lower socio-economic[18] and educational attainment, and certain ethnic minorities and immigrants.[19] A study from Houston, Texas,[20] shows (Fig. 2.2) Afro-Americans to be infected earlier in life than whites, although by

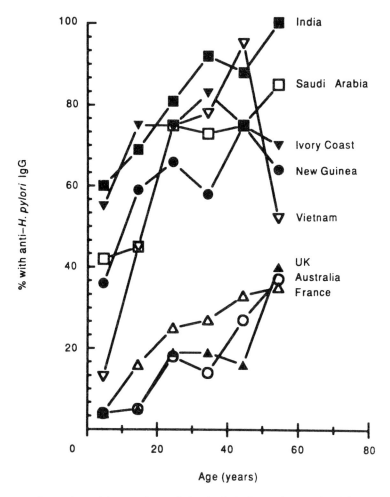

Fig. 2.1 Comparison of the prevalence of *H. pylori* infection in developed and developing countries. (Reproduced with permission from Graham et al 1991.)

the age of 60–70 the prevalence is similar. The curves can be superimposed by moving the white data 25 years to the left. Unlike the whites, socio-economic differences in Afro-Americans did not affect prevalence (Fig. 2.3). These discrepancies might be explained by infection arising during childhood and the socio-economic status of the parent determining the risk of infection.

Transmission

Iatrogenic transmission of *H. pylori* is well recognized. Two epidemics of acute hypochlorhydric gastritis have been attributed to this organism,

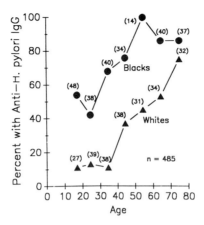

Fig. 2.2   The prevalence of *H. pylori* infection in blacks and whites in relation to age. (Reproduced with permission from Graham et al 1991.)

infection occurring during research on normal individuals using pH electrodes which had been inadequately disinfected. Since then there have been documented cases of endoscopic transmission,[21] this route of transfer being probably commoner than is at present recognized. A postendoscopy syndrome reported in Japan[22] was probably caused by *H. pylori*. Two volunteers became infected after taking the organism by mouth. These data and the increased prevalence of infection in endoscopists[23] suggest that infection may follow contact with gastric secretions.

Most epidemiological data support a faeco-oral route of transmission, inadequate hygiene being commoner in developing countries and among the socially disadvantaged. Parents of infected children have a higher

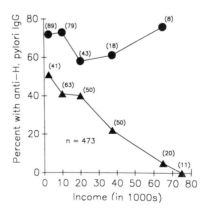

Fig. 2.3   The relationship between income and the prevalence of *H. pylori* infection. *H. pylori* infection was inversely related to income in whites (▲——▲) but not in blacks (●——●). (Reproduced with permission from Graham et al 1991.)

prevalence of infection than those of negative controls,[24-26] and DNA and RNA[27] typing of *H. pylori* confirms an identity of strain within some families. An alternative or additional route of transfer may be oral–oral, because the organism has been recovered from saliva and dental plaque.[28-30] A study from Peru[31] has linked infection to water supply. *H. pylori* is able to survive in water for long periods.[32] Infection may be transmitted in different ways depending upon environment, hygienic practices, and social interrelationships. The organism may disappear spontaneously following infection. This was so in one of the two volunteers who took the organism by mouth.

Mechanisms of pathogenicity

H. pylori secretes a number of enzymes and chemicals[33] and is intensely antigenic. It is unclear which of its properties are mainly responsible for damaging the host.[34] Research has focused on urease[35,36] because ammonia is toxic to gastric and other epithelia.[37-39] However, the organism also secretes a vacuolating cytotoxin[40-42] which damages cells in culture. A 120-KDa component has been identified in certain organisms, and mucosal IgA recognition of this appears to be associated with more significant pathology.[43] A second possibility is that the organism may exert a direct pathogenic effect by attachment to the epithelial cell. Electron micrographs show degenerative changes[7,44,45] in infected cells which may be invaded.[46] Alternatively, the organism may not itself be directly responsible for cellular disruption, which may result from the host's response. Neutrophils and macrophages generate cytokines and potentially pathogenic products such as hyperoxygen radicals. This is an attractive hypothesis when considering the long-term damage which affects not only the superficial epithelial cells but also the gastric pits and glands. The latter are infiltrated by acute and chronic inflammatory cells and over many years may lead to atrophic changes and eventually to metaplasia and dysplasia.

Acute hypochlorhydric gastritis

Sir William Osler described acute hypochlorhydric gastritis in the early part of this century. This disease occurred in chidren or adults and was characterized by a furred tongue, fetor, flatulence, salivation, nausea, and vomiting; when tested, the vomit did not contain acid. The disease was usually self-limiting. The symptoms of acute *H. pylori* infection are similar, and it is probable that this infection was commoner in Britain at the end of the last century when living standards were lower.

Figure 2.4 shows the histological appearance of gastric mucosa 7 d after the onset of symptoms in a young gastroenterologist who diagnosed *H. pylori* infection in himself.[47] It shows severe degeneration of the superficial gastric epithelial cells and a generalized inflammatory reaction throughout

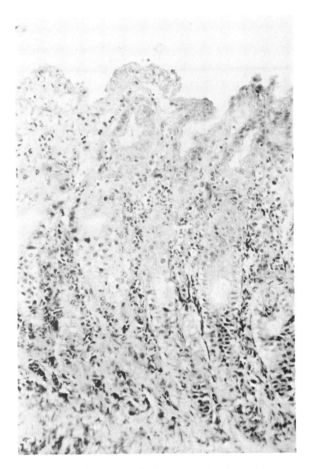

Fig. 2.4   H & E section showing acute *Helicobacter*-associated gastritis.

the lamina propria with infiltration of acute inflammatory cells. A second biopsy two weeks later showed similar changes, but Figure 2.5 shows the appearances 10 weeks later; there has been considerable resolution of the degenerative changes in the superficial epithelium, but a heavy infiltration with inflammatory cells remains. Polymorphs are still present, but the majority are now chronic inflammatory cells. This is the typical appearance of chronic gastritis with activity, the hallmark of *Helicobacter*-associated gastritis. During the acute phase the patient developed complete achlorhydria, but by the time the second biopsy was taken, gastric secretion had resumed.

Chronic gastritis

The discovery of *H. pylori* has led to a reappraisal of gastric pathology.[48]

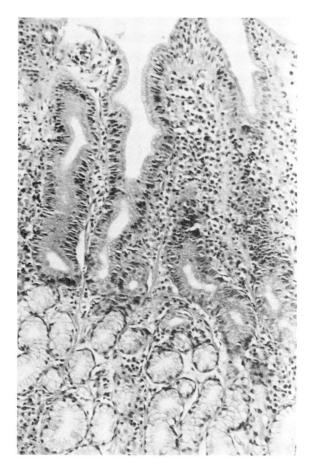

Fig. 2.5   H & E section showing *Helicobacter*-associated gastritis 10 weeks following infection.

Helicobacter-associated gastritis is so common that the histological changes now known to be the result of infection were formerly thought to be part of the normal process of ageing. The realization that the formerly 'idiopathic' type B gastritis is in fact the result of *H. pylori* infection has enabled pathologists to reclassify mucosal inflammation of the stomach aetiologically. A small number of individuals have autoimmune gastritis, a lesion which primarily affects the body of the stomach, usually with antral sparing, which causes pernicious anaemia, and which is associated with positive parietal cell antibodies. Reactive (reflux-type) gastritis is commoner,[49] has a typical histological appearance, and is associated with chemical injury such as occurs with ingestion of NSAIDs and bile reflux.

There are rarer forms of gastritis, such as eosinophilic gastritis and lymphocytic gastritis, Menetrier's disease, etc., the aetiologies of which remain speculative, but by far the commonest cause of chronic gastritis is that associated with *H. pylori*.[48] The distribution of the inflammation may be predominantly antral or represent a pangastritis which is often patchy. The severity and activity of the inflammation varies and is assessed on the number and type of inflammatory cells present. The typical appearance is an infiltration with chronic inflammatory cells, but with ongoing activity recognized by the presence of polymorphonuclear leucocytes. The infiltration may be limited to the superficial mucosa or extend to the deeper areas of the lamina propria, where there may be associated atrophy of the glandular elements. This atrophic gastritis may progress until the appearance is similar to that seen in pernicious anaemia, and it may occasionally be impossible to distinguish between the two. This atrophic appearance is frequently associated with intestinal metaplasia and hypochlorhydria.

The association of intestinal metaplasia and hypochlorhydria leads to diminution, or even disappearance, of *H. pylori*. The reason for this is not clear, but the organism is unable to colonize intestinal type cells, and hypochlorhydria leads to colonization of the stomach with other organisms which compete with *H. pylori*. The occurrence of hypochlorhydria means that locally produced ammonia is no longer neutralized, and the organism may undergo 'autodestruction' by toxic ammonia. With the disappearance of the organism, plasma antibodies may occasionally disappear too. Circumstantial evidence suggests that the atrophic appearance is the result of long-standing infection, but few longitudinal studies have been published.

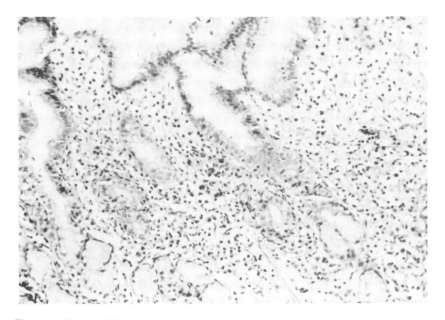

Fig. 2.6   Chronic *Helicobacter*-associated gastritis with activity. Note epithelial cell degeneration.

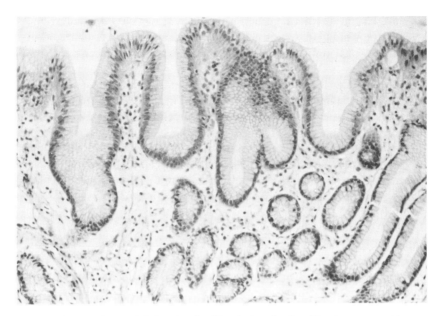

Fig. 2.7   Same patient as 2.6, 6 weeks after *H. pylori* eradication. Note improvement in chronic inflammatory infiltration and improvement in the gastric epithelial cells.

With the exception of autoimmune gastritis, which can usually be differentiated from *H. pylori*-associated gastritis, no other preatrophic lesion has been identified. The distribution of the gastritis may be of critical importance[50] to other pathologies in the upper gastrointestinal tract.

The most telling proof that *H. pylori* causes gastritis is that its eradication leads to complete resolution.[51] Figure 2.6 shows a gastric biopsy from a patient with *Helicobacter*-associated gastritis; Figure 2.7 shows a biopsy from the same patient 6 weeks after *H. pylori* eradication. There is a diminution in the chronic inflammatory cells in the lamina propria, and the epithelial cells have changed from a degenerate, flattened appearance to a more columnar morphology with well-orientated nuclei and good mucus retention. It may take many months for the chronic inflammatory cells to disappear entirely. The effects of eradication on atrophy and intestinal metaplasia have not yet been assessed, but on basic principles, these alterations are probably permanent.

Duodenitis and duodenal ulcer

The role of *H. pylori* in duodenal ulcer is still controversial although the evidence favouring *H. pylori* as the most important aetiological factor in duodenal ulcer disease is regarded by many as overwhelming.[1] The main criticisms advanced against this hypothesis are that duodenal ulcer can be healed by acid suppression alone and therefore the organism is not relevant;

that 50% of the world's population is infected, but only a small minority develop duodenal ulcer; and that *H. pylori* can infect only gastric epithelial cells, so how can it cause duodenal disease? Recent research can now answer these criticisms.

Duodenal ulcer is almost invariably associated with antral gastritis. The reason for this is that over 95% of duodenal ulcer patients are infected by *H. pylori*. This association is not as impressive in countries where most of the 'normal' population is infected, but in developed countries where the prevalence is below 40% (as in the UK), a 95% prevalence in duodenal ulcer means that less than half the population accounts for nearly all cases. This association is so powerful that it can be put to practical use; if young dyspeptic patients are screened by serology, those negative for *H. pylori* antibodies are very unlikely to have a peptic ulcer.[52]

The association of gastric acid and duodenal ulcer is also powerful ('no acid, no ulcer'). Treatment by acid decreasing operations or drugs heals ulcers, and when acid secretion is permanently reduced, recurrence is uncommon. However, nearly everyone secretes gastric acid, but only a few develop ulcers, and cytoprotective drugs heal ulcers without affecting acid secretion. Thus, acid, although essential in the pathogenesis of peptic ulceration, is not the only factor involved. Virtually all vertebrates secrete gastric acid, and it would be surprising if evolutionary mechanisms had not developed to protect vulnerable epithelia from acid/pepsin damage. These mechanisms include 'non-wetability', the mucus layer, secretion of an alkali, rapid cellular regeneration, and an effective mucosal blood supply.[53, 54] If one or more of these protective mechanisms are impaired, the balance between acid attack and mucosal defence is upset. Slight derangement may not be important in an individual with medium or low acid secretion, but could be critical if acid secretion is above average. Severe impairment of mucosal defence, however, might lead to damage at average or low acid levels.

Duodenal ulcer arises in a field of mucosal inflammation, and after healing, the underlying mucosal abnormality remains. Duodenal inflammation appears to be the precursor of ulceration, not the effect, and it is likely to be the lesion which undermines the mucosal defence mechanism. The association between gastric metaplasia in the duodenum and duodenal ulcer is also well recognized. Small areas of gastric metaplasia are found in 20–30% of normal individuals in developed countries,[55, 56] but are absent in hypochlorhydria. This change of native duodenal mucosa to an epithelium with the characteristics of gastric cells can be induced in animals by increasing acid output, is found in individuals with higher than normal acid secretion,[57] and is common in the Zollinger-Ellison syndrome.

The relationship between duodenitis and intestinal metaplasia was unclear until the discovery of *H. pylori*. Two factors appear to be necessary for the development of duodenitis; firstly, a gastric-type epithelium must be present within the duodenum; secondly, the individual must be infected by *H. pylori*.[58] Given that up to 30% of people in the UK have gastric metaplasia and about 30–40% are infected with *H. pylori*, it follows that duodenitis will be present in about 10%. It is this minority who are at risk of duodenal ulcer. Figure 2.8 shows the duodenal histology in a patient with duodenal ulcer 1 month following *H. pylori* eradication and 13 months later. There is a marked improvement with normalization of the epithelial cells and diminution in the number of inflammatory cells.

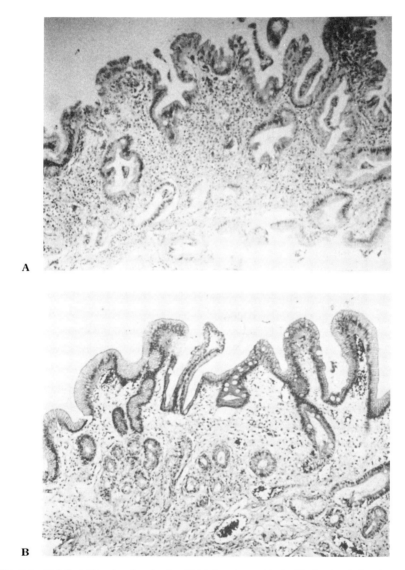

Fig. 2.8 H & E section showing duodenal histology in a patient with duodenal ulcer 1 month following *H. pylori* eradication (**A**) and 13 months later (**B**).

The most convincing evidence that *H. pylori* is the primary pathological cause of duodenal ulcer is that eradication of the organism leads to a change in the natural history of the disease. When ulcers are healed by H_2 receptor antagonists or sucralfate, the 12-month recurrence rate is around 80%. However, a number of recent trials have confirmed that when *H. pylori* is eradicated, 12-month recurrence rates are below 10% and that a significant proportion of these failures are due to incomplete eradication with recrudescence of the original infection. These impressive results have not arisen because of the use of cytoprotective drugs. The study in which both arms included colloidal bismuth subcitrate[59] demonstrated that the better results were obtained only in those in whom the organisms were eradicated.

The hypothesis that *H. pylori* is responsible for duodenal ulcer accounts for many previously unexplained observations, which include the association between duodenal ulcer and antral gastritis, duodenitis, and gastric metaplasia in the duodenum, and, more recently, the close association with *H. pylori* infection in the stomach and in the duodenum. This hypothesis takes account of the role of gastric acid. As gastric metaplasia in the duodenum is uncommon in children and very rare in patients with hypochlorhydria,[55] it accounts for the low incidence of ulcer in these groups. There is, of course, a small minority of duodenal ulcers where *H. pylori* is not involved. If mucosal defence is impaired by treatment with NSAIDs or by other inflammatory lesions such as Crohn's disease, *H. pylori* negative ulcers may arise; similarly, excessive acid secretion in the Zollinger-Ellison syndrome may induce ulceration. It seems likely that the enigma of duodenal ulcer is finally explained.

Gastric ulcer (GU)

The evidence favouring *H. pylori* as the main aetiological factor in gastric ulcer is less persuasive than with duodenal ulcer (DU). Although the organism is present in over 70% of GU patients, its prevalence in normal individuals of the GU age group is higher than in the DU age group, and differences between GU patients and age-matched controls are not as dramatic. Furthermore, a higher percentage of elderly patients receive treatment with NSAIDs, and mucosal ischaemia may be more important. Only one controlled trial has compared eradication with standard treatment,[60] but the results are in line with those reported in DU; that is, if *H. pylori* is eradicated, ulcer relapse is unlikely, whereas, if *H. pylori* remains, recurrence is the rule. It is too early to attribute gastric ulceration to *H. pylori*, but it seems likely that a proportion is caused by the infection.

Non-ulcer dyspepsia (NUD)

Studies designed to demonstrate a higher incidence of *H. pylori* in NUD are unconvincing because of a lack of controls matched for age and socio-economic status. However, around 40% of patients are not infected, so if *H. pylori* is responsible for NUD it is in a small minority of patients. Attempts to identify specific symptoms or syndrome complexes have been generally unsuccessful[61] and have not usually been controlled for such factors as age, drinking, or smoking.[62]

Controlled trials[63, 64] have been badly designed,[65, 66] with small numbers and poor control.[67] There have been problems in the selection of treatment arms.

No authoritative statement can be made as to whether or not *H. pylori* is responsible for a proportion of individuals with NUD.

Gastric cancer

The close association between chronic atrophic gastritis, and gastric cancer has caused speculation that *H. pylori* may be an aetiological factor. Only one longitudinal study of *H. pylori* and atrophic gastritis has been reported.[68] However, the changes in *H. pylori*-associated gastritis occurring with age suggest that in some patients the natural course of events is for chronic, active inflammation to develop gradually into an atrophic state in which the organism may spontaneously disappear.

Pernicious anaemia is associated with gastric cancer,[69] but here gastric atrophy results from immune damage, not from infection with *H. pylori*, supporting the concept that gastric atrophy may predispose to cancer, but at the same time striking a cautionary note as to the necessary involvement of *H. pylori*.

There is a close relationship between *H. pylori* infection and communities with a high prevalence of gastric cancer.[70−73] Three recent studies[74−76] investigated patients in whom serum samples had been stored some years previously. The results, given in Table 2.1, show that the odds ratio for cancer for infected individuals ranged from 3 to 6. This is the most persuasive evidence supporting an aetiological role for *H. pylori*, but it does not prove cause and effect.

If *H. pylori* is an aetiological factor, it is unlikely to be the only one. Other causes of gastritis, duodenogastric reflux,[77] and dietary and genetic factors may also play a role. It is possible that some of these may potentiate the effect of *H. pylori* infection, either by inducing atrophy or metaplasia in a stomach rendered susceptible by *H. pylori* infection, or by acting as a mutagenic agent on an already damaged or hyperplastic tissue.

If, as seems likely, *H. pylori* is responsible for mucosal atrophy, a number of mechanisms might lead to malignant transformation. The gastric process induces a hyperproliferative state, implying that the chance of mutation is thereby increased. The hypergastrinaemia known to be associated with *H. pylori* infection[78, 79] may further increase cell turnover. The inflammatory cells provoked by the infection produce potentially damaging chemicals, such as cytokines[80] and hyperoxygen radicals,[80, 81] which may

Table 2.1   Studies relating *H. pylori* status to carcinoma of the stomach

Reference	No. of patients	No. with gastric cancer	Date of venesection	Age (years) Entry	Age (years) Diagnosis	% +ve for H. pylori Test controls	Odds ratio (95% confidence limits)
Forman et al[76]	22 000	29	1975–82	54	60	69	47	2.77 (0.04–7.97)
Nomura et al[75]	5 908	109	1967–70	59	72	94	76	6.00 (2.1–17.3)
Parsonnet et al[74]	128 922	186	1964–69	54	67	84	61	3.60 (1.8–7.3)

cause DNA damage. Intestinal metaplasia may be less responsive to the local influences normally exercised over native gastric cells. With the development of atrophic gastritis, gastric pH rises, leading to bacterial colonization with organisms capable of converting dietary nitrate to nitrite and possibly to potentially carcinogenic N-nitroso compounds. Intraluminal bacteria may produce other, as yet unrecognized, mutagens. A recent hypothesis[14] suggests that in the normal stomach, gastric acid may destroy premalignant cells which lack the normal mucosal defence mechanisms. This natural protection will be lost in hypochlorhydria.

Epidemiological studies show gastric cancer to be associated with a low intake of ascorbic acid. Pretreatment with ascorbic acid reduces the mutagenic activity of gastric juice[82] and prevents DNA damage[83] in vitro. Ascorbic acid is a powerful reducing agent capable of scavenging nitrite and free oxygen radicals. In these reactions ascorbic acid is oxidized to inactive dehydroascorbic acid. The normal stomach secretes ascorbic acid against a concentration gradient[84, 85] such that the luminal concentration is about three times that of plasma. When the stomach is inflamed, its ability to secrete ascorbic acid is inactivated[86] and with hypochlorhydria ($> pH 4$) the small amount of intragastric vitamin C still present is in the form of inactive dehydroascorbic acid.[85, 87] The dramatic effect of *H. pylori* infection on gastric ascorbic acid is shown in Figure 2.9. A research worker[47] had studied his own gastric ascorbic acid both resting and after intravenous loading. Immediately after chance infection with *H. pylori*, repeat studies showed that fasting ascorbic acid virtually disappeared and did not rise on loading. Seven months later, resting levels remained negligible and there was only a marginal response to intravenous loading even though gastric acid secretion had by then recommenced (see Fig. 2.9).

The link between *H. pylori* infection and gastric cancer is circumstantial

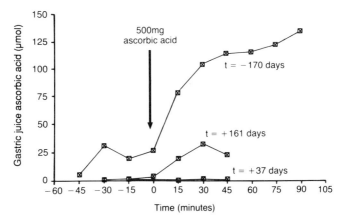

Fig. 2.9 Gastric juice ascorbic acid concentrations before and after intravenous injection of 500 mg ascorbic acid, 170 days before and 37 and 161 days after acute *H. pylori* infection.

and theoretical. It is too early for eradication studies to demonstrate a fall in cancer incidence, but a tentative hypothesis favouring *Helicobacter* as an aetiological factor in gastric cancer is now supported by substantial experimental work.

A recent paper[88] has reported a 92% incidence of *H. pylori* in patients with primary B-cell gastric lymphoma, suggesting that this uncommon malignancy may also be attributed to infection with this organism.

PATTERN OF *H. PYLORI* INFECTION ON GASTRIC PHYSIOLOGY AND ITS RELATIONSHIP TO GASTRODUODENAL PATHOLOGY[89, 90]

Duodenal ulcer, gastric ulcer, and gastric cancer are very uncommon in individuals with otherwise normal gastric mucosa. Duodenal ulcer is almost invariably associated with antral gastritis and gastric ulcer with pangastritis, while gastric cancer arises predominantly in stomachs which have undergone atrophy and intestinal metaplasia. *H. pylori* was identified less than a decade ago, and there has been insufficient time to elucidate the factors which influence its severity, distribution, extent, and change with time. These factors include the virulence of the infecting strain, the age at which infection occurs, and the host response. Individuals whose acid secretion is in the higher range of normal may be better able to protect the corpus of the stomach from local involvement,[90] and these relative hypersecretors will also be likely to develop gastric metaplasia in the duodenum and therefore be at greater risk of duodenitis and duodenal ulcer. Gastric metaplasia is very uncommon in children; therefore, if *H. pylori* is acquired at an early age, as appears to be the case in the developing world, gastric atrophy and hypochlorhydria may supervene before adulthood, thus protecting them from duodenal ulcer.

Subjects whose acid secretion is in the lower range or those infected with a more virulent strain of *H. pylori* may develop pangastritis, and in a proportion, for reasons not as yet understood, gastric ulcer may occur. It seems likely that with the passage of time the inflamed mucosa progresses to atrophy with a diminution in acid secretion. In some individuals an initial antral gastritis may gradually extend proximally and also lead to pangastritis.

These concepts might account for the different prevalence of duodenal ulcer, gastric ulcer, and gastric cancer found in the developed as opposed to the undeveloped parts of the world. Extraneous factors such as bile reflux, dietary habits, and other environmental factors may also influence the physiological status of a stomach which has been colonized by *H. pylori*.

Treatment of *H. pylori*

H. pylori is sensitive to a wide range of antibiotics in vitro, but few are effective in vivo. The most useful drugs are the bismuth compounds, metronidazole, amoxycillin, tetracycline, and omeprazole. None of them used singly are very effective, but combinations may give eradication rates of over 90%. Eradication is defined as the absence of the organism as assessed by *a validated method* at least *1 month* after the end of the course of treatment.

At present the recommended regimen is triple therapy with a bismuth compound, e.g. colloidal bismuth subcitrate 120 mg four times daily, tetracycline hydrochloride 500 mg 4 times daily, and metronidazole 400 mg three times daily[91] for 2 weeks. With this combination eradication rates in developed countries are usually over 85%. Failure is due to metronidazole resistance or poor compliance. Some physicians have used shorter treatment periods with success.[92] The problem with metronidazole resistance is greater in developing countries where this antibiotic is commonly used. There are significant side-effects comprising nausea, malaise, sore mouth, sore tongue, and diarrhoea. Monotherapy is usually ineffective and dual therapy, for example, bismuth and metronidazole, may lead to the emergence of resistant strains.[93, 94] Omeprazole 40 mg daily with amoxycillin for 2 weeks has produced eradication rates of around 50%,[95] though figures vary from 0[96] to 90%.[97]

Treatment of peptic ulcer and non-ulcer dyspepsia

If *H. pylori* is responsible for duodenal ulcer disease, it is logical to heal the ulcer first, and then give triple therapy to eradicate the organism. Those who remain sceptical about the aetiological role of *H. pylori* may have misgivings about this approach. However, the figures in Table 2.2 show that 12-month recurrence is reduced by a factor of 8 following eradication. Therefore, while not being convinced, they may feel eradication therapy to be a reasonably practical solution to a recurrent, painful, expensive, and sometimes devastating condition.

There are as yet insufficient data to advocate the general use of eradication therapy in gastric ulcer, and eradication therapy is not recommended in non-ulcer dyspepsia.

Table 2.2   One-year duodenal ulcer relapse rates, depending on *H. pylori* status

	Hp +ve	%	*Hp* −ve	%
Coghlan et al[98]	24	79	15	27
Marshall et al[99]	44	84	26	23
Smith et al[100]	25	92	19	26
Rauws & Tytgat[59]	21	81	17	0
George et al[101]	0	?	40	13
Patchett et al[102]	0	?	62	0
Hentschel et al[103]	52	79	51	2
Oderda et al[104]	0	?	48	2

ACKNOWLEDGEMENTS

I am grateful to Dr M. F. Dixon for his helpful advice, and to both Dr Dixon and Dr J. I. Wyatt for providing histological figures. I would like to thank Mrs O. Bell and Miss J. Mackintosh for typing the manuscript.

REFERENCES

1 *Helicobacter pylori*: causal agent in peptic ulcer disease? Working Party Report to the World Congresses of Gastroenterology, Sydney 1990. J Gastroenterol Hepatol 1991; 6: 103–140
2 Marshall BJ. History of the discovery of *C. pylori*. In: Blaser M, ed. *Campylobacter pylori* in gastritis and peptic ulcer disease. New York: Igaku-Shoin, 1989: pp 7–23
3 Goodwin CS, Armstrong JA, Chilvers TL et al. Transfer of *Campylobacter pylori* and *Campylobacter mustelae* to *Helicobacter* gen. nov. as *Helicobacter pylori* comb. nov. and *Helicobacter mustelae* comb. nov., respectively. Int J Syst Bacteriol 1989; 39: 397–405
4 Marshall BJ, Barrett L, Prakash C, McCallum RW, Guerrant RL. Urea protects *C. pylori* from the bactericidal effect of acid. Gastroenterology 1990; 99: 697–702
5 Lee A. II. *Helicobacter pylori*; causal agent in peptic ulcer. Microbiological aspects. J Gastroenterol Hepatol 1991; 6: 115–120
6 Thomsen LL, Gavin JB, Tasman-Jones C. Relation of *Helicobacter pylori* to the human gastric mucosa in chronic gastritis of the antrum. Gut 1990; 31: 1230–1236
7 Goodwin CS, Armstrong JA, Marshall BJ. *Campylobacter pyloridis*, gastritis, and peptic ulceration. J Clin Pathol 1986; 39: 353–365
8 Lingwood CA, Pellizzari A, Law H, Sherman P, Drumm B. Gastric glycerolipid as a receptor for *Campylobacter pylori*. Lancet 1989; 2: 238–241
9 Emody L, Carlsson A, Ljungh A, Wadstrom T. Mannose-resistant haemagglutination by *Campylobacter pylori*. Scand J Infect Dis 1988; 20: 353–354
10 Graham DY, Klein PD, Evans DJ. *Campylobacter pylori* detected non-invasively by the ^{13}C-urea breath test. Lancet 1987; 2: 1174–1177
11 Dill S, Payne-James JJ, Misiewicz JJ et al. Evaluation of ^{13}C-urea breath test in the detection of *Helicobacter pylori* and in monitoring the effect of tripotassium dicitratobismuthate in non-ulcer dyspepsia. Gut 1990; 31: 1237–1241
12 Logan RPH, Dill S, Bauer FE et al. The European ^{13}C-urea breath test for the detection of *Helicobacter pylori*. Eur J Gastroenterol Hepatol 1991; 3: 915–921
13 Weil J, Bell GD. The ^{14}C breath test. In: Rathbone BJ, Heatley RV, eds. *Campylobacter pylori* and gastroduodenal disease. Oxford; Blackwell Scientific Publications, 1989: pp 83–93
14 Seery JP. Achlorhydria and gastric carcinogenesis. Lancet 1991; 2: 1508–1509
15 Mapstone NP, Lynch D, Lewis FA, Axon ATR, Dixon MF, Quirke P. The polymerase chain reaction in the diagnosis of *Helicobacter* infection (IV Workshop Gastroduodenal Pathology and *Helicobacter pylori*, Bologna, November 1991). Ital J Gastroenterol 1991; 23 (suppl 2): 4 (Rome: International University Press)
16 Graham DY. *Helicobacter pylori*: its epidemiology and its role in duodenal ulcer disease. J Gastroenterol Hepatol 1991; 6: 105–113
17 Sullivan PB, Thomas JE, Wight DGD et al. *Helicobacter pylori* in Gambian children with chronic diarrhoea and malnutrition. Arch Dis Child 1990; 65: 189–191
18 Sitas F, Forman D, Yarnell JWG et al. *Helicobacter pylori* infection rates in relation to age and social class in a population of Welsh men. Gut 1991; 32: 25–28
19 Dwyer B, Kaldor J, Tee W, Raios K. The prevalence of *Campylobacter pylori* in human populations. In: Rathbone BJ, Heatley RV, eds. *Campylobacter pylori* and gastroduodenal disease. Oxford: Blackwell Scientific Publications, 1989: pp 190–196
20 Graham DY, Malaty HM, Evans DG, Evans DJ, Klein PD, Adam E. Epidemiology of *Helicobacter pylori* in an asymptomatic population in the United States. Effect of age, race, and socioeconomic status. Gastroenterology 1991; 100: 1495–1501
21 Langenberg W, Rauws EAJ, Oudbier JH, Tytgat GNJ. Patient-to-patient transmission of *Campylobacter pylori* infection by fiberoptic gastroduodenoscopy and biopsy. J Infect Dis 1990; 161: 507–511

22 Sugiyama T, Takayama Y, Awakawa T et al. Is *Helicobacter pylori* responsible for the post-endoscopic acute gastric mucosal lesions? (The 4th International Symposium on *Helicobacter pylori* and its Diseases). Tokyo: Taisho Pharmaceutical, Uehara Memorial Foundation, 1991: Abstract III-28, p 30

23 Mitchell HM, Lee A, Carrick J. Increased incidence of *Campylobacter pylori* infection in gastroenterologists. Scand J Gastroenterol 1989; 24: 396–400

24 Mitchell HM, Bohane TD, Berkowicz J, Hazell SL, Lee A. Antibody to *Campylobacter pylori* in families of index children with gastrointestinal illness due to *C. pylori*. Lancet 1987 2: 681–682

25 Katelaris PH, Zoli G, Norbu P, Tippett G, Lowe D, Farthing MJG. An evaluation of factors affecting *Helicobacter pylori* prevalence in a defined population from a developing country (IV Workshop Gastroduodenal Pathology and *Helicobacter pylori*, Bologna, November 1991). Ital J Gastroenterol 1991; 23 (suppl 2): 12 (Rome: International University Press)

26 Oderda G, Vaira D, Holton J et al. *Helicobacter pylori* in children with peptic ulcer and their families. Dig Dis Sci 1991; 36: 572–576

27 Tee W, Dwyer B, Smallwood R, Ross B, Schembri M, Lambert J. Ribo-typing of *Helicobacter pylori* from clinical specimens (IV Workshop Gastroduodenal Pathology and *Helicobacter pylori*, Bologna, November 1991). Ital J Gastroenterol 1991; 23 (suppl 2): 4 (Rome: International University Press)

28 Majmudar P, Shah SM, Dhungbhoy KR, Desai HG. Isolation of *Helicobacter pylori* from dental plaque in healthy volunteers. Indian J Gastroenterol 1990; 9: 271–272

29 Khandaker MAK, Scott A, Eastwood MA, Palmer KR. Do teeth predispose to duodenal ulcer relapse? Gut 1991; 32: A1207

30 Shames B, Krajden S, Fuksa M, Babida C, Penner JL. Evidence for the occurrence of the same strain of *Campylobacter pylori* in the stomach and dental plaque. J Clin Microbiol 1989; 27: 2849–2850

31 Klein PD, Gastrointestinal Physiology Working Group, Graham DY, Gaillour A, Opekun AR, Smith EO. Water source as risk factor for *Helicobacter pylori* infection in Peruvian children. Lancet 1991; 1: 1503–1506

32 Shahamat M, Paszko-Kolva C, Yamamoto H, Mia U, Pearson AD, Colwell RR. Ecological studies of *Campylobacter pylori*. Klin Wochenschr 1989; 67 (suppl 18): 62–63

33 Marshall BJ. Virulence and pathogenicity of *Helicobacter pylori*. J Gastroenterol Hepatol 1991; 6: 121–124

34 Vaira D, Holton J, Miglioli M, Barbara L. Pathogenic mechanisms of acid-related diseases: *Helicobacter* and other spiral organisms. Curr Opin Gastroenterol 1991; 7: 881–887

35 Kim H, Park C, Jang WI et al. The gastric juice urea and ammonia levels in patients with *H. pylori*. Am J Clin Pathol 1990; 94: 187–191

36 Sidebotham RL, Batten JJ, Karim QN, Spencer J, Baron JH. Breakdown of gastric mucus in the presence of *H. pylori*. J Clin Pathol 1991; 14: 52–57

37 Murakami M, Yoo JK, Teramura S et al. Generation of ammonia and mucosal lesion formation following hydrolysis of urea by urease in the rat stomach. J Clin Gastroenterol 1990; 12 (suppl 1): S104–S109

38 Kawano S, Tsujii M, Fusamoto H, Sato N, Kamada T. Chronic effects of intragastric ammonia on gastric mucosal structures in rats. Dig Dis Sci 1990; 36: 3–38

39 Xu JK, Goodwin CS, Cooper M, Robinson J. Intracellular vacuolization caused by the urease of *Helicobacter pylori*. J Infect Dis 1990; 161: 1302–1304

40 Leunk RD, Johnson PT, David BC, Kraft WG, Morgan DR. Cytotoxic activity in broth-culture filtrates of *Campylobacter pylori*. J Med Microbiol 1988; 26: 93–99

41 Figura N, Guglielmeti P, Rossolini A et al. Cytotoxin production by *Campylobacter pylori* strains isolated from patients with peptic ulcers and from patients with chronic gastritis only. J Clin Microbiol 1989; 27: 225–226

42 Cover TL, Dooley CP, Blaser MJ. Characterization of and human serologic response to proteins in *Helicobacter pylori* broth culture supernatants with vacuolizing cytotoxin activity. Infect Immun 1990; 58: 603–610

43 Crabtree JE, Taylor JD, Wyatt JI et al Mucosal IgA recognition of *Helicobacter pylori* 120 kDa protein, peptic ulceration, and gastric pathology. Lancet 1991; 2: 332–335

44 Hessey SJ, Spencer J, Wyatt JI et al. Bacterial adhesion and disease activity in *Helicobacter*-associated chronic gastritis. Gut 1990; 31: 134–138

45 Caselli M, Figura N, Trevisani L et al. Patterns of physical modes of contact between *Campylobacter pylori* and the gastric epithelium: implications about bacterial pathogenicity. Am J Gastroenterol 1989; 84: 511–513

46 Anderson LP, Holick S. Possible evidence of invasiveness of *Helicobacter (Campylobacter) pylori*. Eur J Clin Microbiol Infect Dis 1990; 9: 135–138

47 Sobala GM, Crabtree JE, Dixon MF et al. Acute *Helicobacter pylori* infection: clinical features, local and systemic immune response, gastric mucosal histology, and gastric juice ascorbic acid concentrations. Gut 1991; 32: 1415–1418

48 The Sydney System: a new classification of gastritis. Working Party Report to the World Congresses of Gastroenterology, Sydney 1990. J Gastroenterol Hepatol 1991; 67: 207–252 (Melbourne: Blackwell Scientific Publications)

49 Sobala GM, King, RFG, Axon ATR, Dixon MF. Reflux gastritis in the intact stomach. J Clin Pathol 1990; 43: 303–306

50 Sipponen P, Seppälä K, Aärynen M, Helske T, Kettunen P. Chronic gastritis and gastroduodenal ulcer: a case control study on risk of coexisting duodenal or gastric ulcer in patients with gastritis. Gut 1989; 30: 922–929

51 Valle J, Seppälä K, Sipponen P, Kosunen T. Disappearance of gastritis after eradication of *Helicobacter pylori*. A morphometric study. Scand J Gastroenterol 1991; 26: 1057–1065

52 Sobala GM, Crabtree JE, Pentith JA et al. Screening dyspepsia by serology to *Helicobacter pylori*. Lancet 1991; 2: 94–96

53 Wallace JL. Gastroduodenal mucosal defense. Curr Opin Gastroenterol 1991; 7: 870–875

54 Brown CM, Rees WDW. Gastroduodenal mucosal defence. Curr Opin Gastroenterol 1990; 6: 867–872

55 Wyatt JI, Rathbone BJ, Sobala GM et al. Gastric epithelium in the duodenum: its association with *Helicobacter pylori* and inflammation. J. Clin Pathol 1990; 43: 981–986

56 Fitzgibbons PL, Dooley CP, Cohen H, Appleman MD. Prevalence of gastric metaplasia, inflammation and *Campylobacter pylori* in the duodenum of members of a normal population. Am J Clin Pathol 1988; 90: 711–714

57 Axon ATR. *Campylobacter pylori*. In: Pounder RE, Recent advances in gastroenterology. Vol 7. Edinburgh: Churchill Livingstone, 1988; pp 225–244

58 Wyatt JI, Rathbone BJ, Dixon MF, Heatley RV. *Campylobacter pyloridis* and acid-induced gastric metaplasia in the pathogenesis of duodenitis. J Clin Pathol 1987; 40: 841–848

59 Rauws EAJ, Tytgat, GNJ. Eradication of *Helicobacter pylori* cures duodenal ulcer. Lancet 1990; 1: 1233–1235

60 Seppälä K, Pikkarainen P, Karvonen A-L, Lehtola J, Gormsen MH, the FGUSG. A double-blind study to compare the efficacy of De-Nol in combination with metronidazole versus De-Nol or ranitidine in combination with metronidazole placebo in the treatment of gastric ulcers (Hepatogastroenterology, Abstracts of the European Digestive Disease Week, Amsterdam, 20–26 October). Stuttgart: Georg Thieme Verlag, 1991: abstract 175, p 43

61 Veldhuyzen van Zanten SJO, Tytgat KMAJ, Jalali S, Goodacre RL, Hunt RH. Can gastritis symptoms be evaluated in clinical trials? An overview of treatment of gastritis, non-ulcer dyspepsia and *Campylobacter*-associated gastritis. J Clin Gastroenterol 1989; 11: 496–501

62 Sobala GM, Dixon MF, Axon ATR. Symptomatology of *Helicobacter pylori*-associated dyspepsia. Eur J Gastroenterol Hepatol 1990; 2: 445–449

63 Patchett S, Beattie S, Leen E, Keane C, O'Morain C. Eradicating *Helicobacter pylori* and symptoms of non-ulcer dyspepsia. Br Med J 1991; 303: 1238–1240

64 Lambert JR, Dunn K, Borromeo M, Korman MG, Hansky J. *Campylobacter pylori* – a role in non-ulcer dyspepsia? Scand J Gastroenterol 1989; 24 (suppl 160): 7–13

65 Axon ATR. Is non-ulcer dyspepsia improved by treating *Helicobacter pylori* infection? In: Malfertheiner P, Ditschuneit H, eds. *Helicobacter pylori*, gastritis and peptic ulcer. Berlin: Springer-Verlag, 1990: pp 434–437

66 Colin-Jones DG. *Campylobacter pylori*. An advance in understanding of dyspepsia and gastritis. J Clin Gastroenterol 1989; 11 (suppl 1): S39–S42

67 Gad A, Hradsky M, Furugård K, Malmodin B, Nyberg O. *Campylobacter pylori* and non-ulcer dyspepsia. 2. A prospective study in a Swedish population. Scand J

Gastroenterol 1989; 24 (suppl 167): 44–48

68 Villako K, Maards H, Tammur R et al. *Helicobacter (Campylobacter) pylori* infestation and the development and progression of chronic gastritis: results of long-term follow-up examinations of a random sample. Endoscopy 1990; 22: 114–117

69 Brinton LA, Gridley G, Hrubec Z, Hoover R, Fraumeni JF. Cancer risk following pernicious anaemia. Br J Cancer 1989; 59: 810–813

70 Forman D, Sitas F, Newell DG et al. Geographic association of *H. pylori* antibody prevalence and gastric cancer mortality in rural China. Int J Cancer 1990; 46: 608–611

71 Correa P, Fox J, Fonthan E et al. *H. pylori* and gastric carcinoma: serum antibody prevalence in populations with contrasting cancer risks. Cancer 1990; 66: 2569–2574

72 Fox JG, Correa P, Taylor NS et al. *Campylobacter pylori*-associated gastritis and immune response in a population at increased risk of gastric carcinoma. Am J Gastroenterol 1989; 84: 775–781

73 Talley NJ, DiMagno E, Zinsmeister AR, Perez-Perez GI, Blaser M. *Helicobacter pylori and gastric cancer: a case-control study*. Rev Esp Enferm Apar Dig 1990; 78: suppl S7–S8

74 Parsonnet J, Friedman GD, Vandersteen DP et al. *Helicobacter pylori* infection and the risk of gastric carcinoma. N Engl J Med 1991; 325: 1127–1131

75 Nomura A, Stemmermann GN, Chyou P-H, Kato I, Perez-Perez GI, Blaser MJ. *Helicobacter pylori* infection and gastric carcinoma among Japanese-Americans in Hawaii. N Engl J Med 1991; 325: 1132–1136

76 Forman D, Newell DG, Fullerton F et al. Association between infections with *H. pylori* and risk of gastric cancer: evidence from a prospective investigation. Br Med J 1991; 302: 1302–1305

77 Taylor PR, Mason RC, Filipe MI et al. Gastric carcinogenesis in the rat induced by duodenogastric reflux without carcinogens: morphology, mucin histochemistry, polyamine metabolism, and labelling index. Gut 1991; 32: 1447–1454

78 Levi S, Haddad G, Ghosh P, Beardshall K, Playford R, Calam J. *Campylobacter pylori* and duodenal ulcers; the gastrin link. Lancet 1989; 1: 1167–1168

79 Chittajallu RS, Neithercut WD, Macdonald AMI, McColl KEL. Effect of increasing *Helicobacter pylori* ammonia production by urea infusion on plasma gastrin concentrations. Gut 1991; 32: 21–24

80 Mai UE, Perez-Perez GI, Wahl LM, Blaser MJ, Smith PD. Soluble surface protein from *H. pylori* activates monocyte/macrophage by lipopolysaccharide independent mechanism. J Clin Invest 1991; 87: 894–900

81 Davies GR, Simmonds NJ, Stevens TRS, Grandison A, Rampton DS. Enhanced production of reactive oxygen species by gastric antral mucosa infected with *H. pylori*. Gut 1991; 32: A564

82 O'Connor HJ, Habibzedah N, Schorah CJ, Axon ATR, Riley SE, Garner RC. Effect of increased intake of vitamin C on the mutagenic activity of gastric juice and intragastric concentrations of ascorbic acid. Carcinogenesis 1985; 6: 1675–1676

83 Brambilla G, Cavanna M, Faggin P et al. Genotoxic effects in rodents given high oral doses of ranitidine and sodium nitrite. Carcinogenesis 1983; 4: 1281–1285

84 Rathbone BJ, Johnson AW, Wyatt JI, Kelleher J, Heatley RV, Losowsky MS. Ascorbic acid: a factor concentrated in human gastric juice. Clin Sci 1989; 76: 237–241

85 Sobala GM, Schorah CJ, Sanderson M et al. Ascorbic acid in the human stomach. Gastroenterology 1989; 97: 357–363

86 O'Connor HJ, Schorah CJ, Habibzedah N, Axon ATR, Cockel R. Vitamin C in the human stomach: relation to gastric pH, gastroduodenal disease, and possible sources. Gut 1989; 30: 436–442

87 Schorah CJ, Sobala GM, Sanderson M, Collis N, Primrose JN. Gastric juice ascorbic acid: effects of disease and implications for gastric carcinogenesis[1-3]. Am J Clin Nutr 1991; 53: 287S–293S

88 Wotherspoon AC, Ortiz-Hidalgo C, Falzon MR, Isaacson PG. *Helicobacter pylori*-associated gastritis and primary B-cell gastric lymphoma. Lancet 1991; 2: 1175–1176

89 Sipponen P, Kekki M, Siurala M. The Sydney System: epidemiology and natural history of chronic gastritis. J Gastroenterol Hepatol 1991; 6: 244–251

90 Dixon MF. *Helicobacter pylori* and peptic ulceration: histopathological aspects. J Gastroenterol Hepatol 1991; 6: 125–130

91 Axon ATR. *Helicobacter pylori* therapy: effect on peptic ulcer disease. J Gastroenterol Hepatol 1991; 6: 131–137

92 Logan RPH, Gummett PA, Misiewicz JJ, Karim QN, Walker MM, Baron JH. One-week eradication regimen for *Helicobacter pylori*. Lancet 1991; 2: 1249–1252
93 Bell GD, Weil J, Powell K et al. *Helicobacter pylori* treated with combinations of tripotassium dicitrato and metronidazole: efficacy of different treatment regimens and some observations on the emergence of metronidazole resistance. Eur J Gastroenterol Hepatol 1991; 3: 819–822
94 Glupczynski Y, Burette A. Drug therapy for *Helicobacter pylori* infection: problems and pitfalls. Am J Gastroenterol 1990; 85: 1545–1551
95 Unge P, Gad A, Gnarpe H, Olsson J. Does Omeprazole improve antimicrobial therapy directed towards gastric *Campylobacter pylori* in patients with antral gastritis? A pilot study. Scand J Gastroenterol 1989; 24 (suppl 167); 49–54
96 De Koster E, Nyst JF, Deprez C et al. HP treatment: disappointing results with amoxicillin plus omeprazole (IV Workshop Gastroduodenal Pathology and *Helicobacter Pylori*, Bologna, November 1991). Ital J Gastroenterol 1991; 23 (suppl 2): 105 (Rome: International University Press)
97 Labenz J, Gyenes E, Rühl GH, Börsch G. Amoxicillin-omeprazole treatment for eradication of *Helicobacter pylori*. Eur J Gastroenterol Hepatol 1991; 3 (suppl 1): S10
98 Coghlan JG, Gilligan D, Humphries H et al. *Campylobacter pylori* and recurrence of duodenal ulcers: a 12 months follow-up study. Lancet 1987; 2: 1109–1111
99 Marshall BJ, Goodwin CS, Warren JR et al. Prospective double-blind trial of duodenal ulcer relapse after eradication of *Campylobacter pylori*. Lancet 1988; 2: 1437–1442
100 Smith AC, Price AB, Borriello P, Levi AJ. A comparison of ranitidine and tripotassium dicitratobismuthate (TDB) in relapse rates of duodenal ulcer. The role of *Campylobacter pylori (C. p.)*. Gastroenterology 1988; 94: A431
101 George L, Hyland L, Morgan A et al. Smoking does not contribute to duodenal ulcer relapse after eradication. Gastroenterology 1990; 98: A48
102 Patchett S, O'Riordan TO, Leen E, Keane C, O'Moraine CO. A prospective study of *Helicobacter pylori* eradication in duodenal ulcer. Gastroenterology 1990; 98: A104
103 Hentschel E, Nemec K, Schutze K et al. Duodenal ulcer recurrence and *Helicobacter pylori*. Lancet 1991; 2: 569
104 Oderda G, Forni M, Dell'Olio D, Ansaldi N. Cure of peptic ulcer associated with eradication of *Helicobacter pylori*. Lancet 1990; 1: 1599

3

Irritable bowel syndrome

K. W. Heaton

DEFINITIONS OF FUNCTIONAL BOWEL DISEASE

International working teams meeting in Rome have produced a new set of definitions[1-4] to help doctors define their patients' problems more precisely and to aid research. A functional gastrointestinal (GI) disorder is defined as a variable combination of persistent or recurrent GI symptoms not explained by structural or biochemical abnormalities. *Functional bowel disorders* are such disorders in which the symptoms are attributable to the mid- or lower intestine. They are divided into irritable bowel syndrome (IBS), functional abdominal bloating, functional constipation, and functional diarrhoea. There is, of course, overlap in symptoms and pathophysiology. Functional abdominal pain is a separate entity – it is often blamed on the gut, but with little justification, and its main characteristic is pain behaviour.[4]

The Rome meeting defined IBS as a functional bowel disorder in which abdominal pain is associated with defecation or a change in bowel habit; there are also features of disordered defecation, very often with abdominal bloating or distension. Note that pain is necessary to the diagnosis though some doctors dispute this. Functional abdominal bloating consists of symptoms traditionally ascribed to excess gas or abnormal movement of gas in the intestine, chiefly bloating or distension and full feelings, but borborygmi (audible bowel sounds) and excessive farting (voiding of gas per anum) may also be complained of. The term 'flatulence' is ambiguous and should be dropped. Functional constipation is defined as persistent symptoms of difficult, infrequent, or seemingly incomplete evacuation; abdominal pain or episodes of diarrhoea are absent (otherwise, IBS is diagnosed). Functional diarrhoea is defined as persistence of frequent and/or urgent passage of *unformed* stool; abdominal pain is absent and hard or lumpy stools are never passed.

The Rome documents[2-4] contain detailed criteria for diagnosing each of the functional bowel disorders and much else besides. They are essential reading for serious students of the subject.

The present chapter concentrates on IBS, which is the commonest and most troublesome of the functional bowel disorders, as well as the most studied.

VALIDATION OF IBS AS A SYNDROME

In 1978 Manning et al in Bristol[5] reported that four out of 15 GI symptoms were significantly commoner in patients with IBS than in patients with organic GI disease attending the same clinic, and two more were of borderline significance. These six symptoms were found to cluster together in a survey of GI symptoms in apparently healthy people.[6] Recently, the six symptoms, now known as the Manning criteria, have been rigorously tested for their diagnostic value. In a large study at the Mayo clinic all six criteria were found to be reliable.[7] When 82 patients found to have IBS were compared with 101 patients with organic GI disease, the sensitivity of the Manning criteria was only 58%, but the specificity was 74%. The criteria seem to be particularly good at distinguishing IBS from upper GI problems such as peptic ulcer[8] and non-ulcer dyspepsia.[7] Probably the only organic disease which mimics IBS at all closely is colitis,[8] and this is easily distinguished by the history and examination including sigmoidoscopy.

Whitehead et al[9] did cluster analysis on the occurrence of 23 GI symptoms in 500 healthy women. The main cluster consisted of the four original Manning criteria (relief of abdominal pain with defecation, looser stools with pain onset, more frequent stools with pain onset, and visible bloating) plus GI reactions to food.

The Manning criteria seem to be less diagnostically useful in men than in women.[7] One group has reported they do not help at all in men,[10] but more data are needed, with care being taken to classify patients correctly, before this conclusion can be accepted.

Positive diagnosis

It is now widely accepted that the diagnosis of IBS should, if possible, be made on the characteristic symptom pattern (assuming of course that symptoms and signs of organic bowel disease are absent) rather than by negative investigations.[1, 4] Migraine makes a useful analogy. Confidence comes from experience but also from knowing that it is rarely necessary to revise the diagnosis. In the Netherlands 224 patients diagnosed as having functional GI complaints were followed up for 2 years; only one needed a new diagnosis.[11] Another confidence-boosting fact is that GI symptoms are useless in screening for cancer.[12]

The defecatory symptoms of IBS

The terms 'constipation' and 'diarrhoea' mean different things to different people and when used by a patient should not be taken at face value. A patient can have frequent, urgent defecations but a normal transit time and solid, even lumpy stools.[13] Presumably such a patient's pseudodiarrhoea is due to an irritable rectum which overreacts to the arrival of faeces. There

Table 3.1   The Bristol stool-form scale

Type 1	Separate, hard lumps, like nuts
Type 2	Like a sausage but lumpy
Type 3	Like a sausage or snake, with a cracked surface
Type 4	Like a sausage or snake, with a smooth surface
Type 5	Soft blobs with clear-cut edges
Type 6	Fluffy pieces with ragged edges; a mushy stool
Type 7	Watery; no solid pieces

are also patients who strain for a long time to defecate though there is no apparent need to strain, their stools being normal or even loose.[14] Such patients say they are constipated, but what is really bothering most of them are feelings of incomplete evacuation[15] with, perhaps, unproductive calls to stool (a common but poorly researched symptom). Again the root of the problem is probably a supersensitive or irritable rectum.

Thus, the clinician must be able to distinguish pseudoconstipation from true constipation and pseudodiarrhoea from true diarrhoea. One way to do this is to measure the intestinal transit time. However, this is cumbersome and involves irradiating the abdomen or collecting stools. A simpler way is to get patients to record the form of their stools on a chart, since stool form correlates well with transit time, provided a validated scale is used, such as the 7-point Bristol scale (Table 3.1).[13] This scale corresponds not only with transit time but also with symptoms of urgency and straining,[15] and it is well understood by ordinary people.

Prevalence of IBS in the community

It has been known since 1980[6] that symptoms of IBS are common in the community, but only recently have figures become available from random samples of the general population. In Bristol one or more of nine IBS symptoms were admitted to by 47% of women and 27% of men; two or more by 24% and 11%; and three or more, which was considered diagnosable IBS, by 13% and 5%, respectively.[16] Abdominal pain with another feature of IBS was admitted to by 20% of women and 10% of men. The prevalence of individual symptoms is shown in Table 3.2. Similar results have been published from Southampton[17] and from Rochester, Minnesota,[18] except that, in those locations, IBS was nearly as common in men as in women. There is no consistent relation of IBS symptoms to age.

The above figures probably understate the true incidence of IBS symptoms in the community. When 27 healthy women who had recently denied getting abdominal pain were followed closely for a month, no fewer than 81% experienced one or more non-menstrual abdominal pains and 93% experienced bloating.[15] Most of them had at least one episode of urgent defecation or runny stools, and all had at least one occasion when they felt evacuation was incomplete. Thus, it seems that symptoms of IBS are

Table 3.2   Prevalence of nine IBS symptoms in a random sample of the Bristol population[16]

	Percentage who admitted symptom	
Symptom	Women aged 25–69 years (n = 1038)	Men aged 40–69 years (n = 858)
Recurrent* abdominal pain (RAP), often relieved by defecation	10.3	5.6
RAP associated with looser stools	6	3
RAP associated with more frequent stools	5	2.3
Frequent† bloated feelings	15	6
Frequent feelings of incomplete evacuation	13	4.5
Frequent urgency of defecation	14	8
Frequent runny/watery stools	2.5	3
Frequent straining to finish defecating	5	2
Passage of mucus (ever)	15	5
Any one or more of the above	47	27
Two or more of the above	24	11
Three or more of the above	13	5

* 'Recurrent' was defined as more than six times in the previous 12 months. There is, of course, overlap between the three categories of recurrent abdominal pain.
† For each symptom, 'frequent' was defined as ⩾1/4 days or occasions

experienced by all women from time to time and, doubtless, by most men. Since most people deny having the symptoms, they must usually be ignored or forgotten. When they *are* noticed and remembered, they are usually not taken to a doctor. In surveys of healthy people, only 14–66% of those with IBS symptoms have consulted a doctor, usually less than half.[16–19]

It is tempting to conclude that patients with IBS are whingers, or hypochondriacs, that is, people who notice, remember, and complain about bodily sensations more than the rest of us. The reality is more complex and subtle. To appreciate this, two lines of evidence must be considered – pain thresholds, and the differences between consulters or complainers, that is, patients, and non-consulters (non-complainers, non-patients).

Pain thresholds – somatic and visceral

Two research groups have compared the somatic pain thresholds of IBS patients and controls. One found that IBS patients tolerated electric shocks to the hand just as well as patients with Crohn's disease and better than normal subjects.[20] The other found that IBS patients could hold a hand in iced water just as long as normal people or patients with lactose intolerance.[21] The conclusion must be that IBS patients have a normal or even high pain threshold (or that they are unusually brave).

On the other hand, there is much evidence that IBS patients tolerate distension of the gut less well than other people. This is probably true at all levels of the intestine, but most studies have been on the rectum. The rectum not only registers pain at a lower balloon volume than normal but also notices the presence of the balloon earlier.[22] It is altogether more sensitive or alert. It is supersensitive to a normal component of faeces (deoxycholic acid) as well as to mechanical distension.[23]

Thus, patients with IBS have a supersensitive gut and not a general tendency to over-react to discomfort.

Differences between consulters and non-consulters

Two thorough US studies have established beyond reasonable doubt that hospital patients with IBS are more distressed than, and have different personality profiles from, people with IBS symptoms who have not consulted a doctor.[24, 25] According to a standard personality inventory, such patients score far higher for hypochondriasis and higher for depression and hysterical traits, but lower for ego strength.[24] By another psychiatric scoring system the biggest difference between patients and non-patients was in the tendency to translate emotional distress into physical symptoms (somatization).[25]

Although these were impeccable studies in many ways, they do have methodological limitations. The cases (consulters) were not drawn from the same population as the controls (non-consulters) but from the clinics of two physicians well known for their research on IBS. Thus, the patients were selected as needing or demanding referral to a superspecialist (and further selected as wanting to take part in research). They may not be representative of ordinary IBS patients going to their family doctors. Even if they were representative, the studies do not prove that people take their functional bowel symptoms to doctors *just* because they have inadequate personalities or abnormal responses to the stresses of life. Such a conclusion is reasonable only if symptoms are equally severe in consulters and non-consulters and if patients with IBS are psychologically less robust than patients with similar symptoms of organic origin. In fact, neither of these two conditions is met according to recent research. Drossman et al[24] got 64 IBS patients to keep records of all the pains they experienced over a 2-week period, their severity and character being scored in a standard fashion. Compared with non-patients, the patients had nearly three times as many days with pain, and, on average, the pains were rated 50% more severe. Heaton et al[15] recorded the pains experienced by 26 patients over a month. By a weighted pain score the patients suffered over three times as much as non-patients. Among GI symptoms, pain is the most potent at driving patients to a doctor, but diarrhoea is the reason in some.[16, 26] We found that patients experienced more urgency, more loose stools, and more days with frequency of defecation than non-consulters.[15] A total score for intestinal symptoms was nearly three times higher. Clearly, patients have reason to complain. All the same, there was some overlap in the symptom scores of patients and non-patients, a result which leaves room for psychological factors as well.

Psychological factors

For a long time it has been accepted that many, if not most, IBS patients are anxious or depressed. However, practically all studies have been done on hospital patients, who, it can be argued, have good cause for distress since their symptoms are particularly bad and long-standing, and other doctors have already failed to help them. There have been four reports on the psychological state of non-consulters. In one they were normal,[25] in two they were abnormal (though, in one case, less so than consulters),[15, 27] and in the fourth they were abnormal until adjustment was made for symptom severity.[24] It is a moot point whether adjusting for symptom severity is appropriate. If not, then the odds are 3 to 1 that non-consulters are psychologically abnormal. If it is, then the balance is even. Readers must make their own judgement, bearing in mind that association does not prove causation.

In trying to work out the role of psychological factors in IBS, it is pertinent to compare the psychology of IBS patients with that of organic disease patients attending the same clinic. Recently there have been three systematic reports of this kind. Smith et al[28] compared 67 IBS patients and 30 patients with various organic diseases and found no difference in the scores from six psychological scales, the two groups being equally abnormal. Talley et al[29] also studied 67 patients with IBS. Compared with 64 patients with various organic diagnoses, the IBS patients scored similarly for hypochondriasis, hysteria, depression, and neurosis. The validity of Talley et al's scoring system is questionable in people with organic disease,[30] but Bleijenberg & Fennis,[11] using different questionnaires, found no difference in anxiety, depression, self-esteem, and coping behaviour in 227 patients with functional GI complaints and 81 with organic GI disease. Similar findings were reported earlier by Welch et al,[31] but they were not believed.

These startling but consistent findings imply that psychological factors are just as important in determining consulting behaviour in organic disease as in functional disorders.

Stress and its denial; somatization

It is common to see patients with functional bowel disease who deny they are under stress even when it seems they must be – like the single parent with a responsible job, adolescent children, and a dependent granny. There is good evidence that functional abdominal pain is often preceded by a threatening life event – usually the break-up of a close relationship – or is associated with extreme interpersonal tensions in the home,[32] but the patient often denies the existence or relevance of these things. The tendency for such denial can be measured, using the Lie scale of a personality inventory, and three separate studies have shown IBS patients to have high Lie scores.[24, 33, 34] A high score means that patients present themselves in an unrealistically favourable light. One way people can do this is by denying that stress disturbs their mental equilibrium, and another is by complaining of bodily symptoms, which are 'respectable', rather than mental ones, which are not. This denial of emotion (which is akin to alexithymia, or inability to express emotions in the normal way) paves the way for somatization, that is to say, a propensity to express emotional distress in altered bodily functions. Somatization is believed to be the mechanism behind many psychosomatic disorders.[35] In somatizers, bodily pain is preferred to mental pain and is unconsciously substituted for it.[36]

One form of stress which is, sadly, topical is the physical and sexual abuse of children. Preliminary data from North Carolina suggest that women who were abused as children are predisposed to functional abdominal complaints, especially pelvic pain.[37]

Non-gastrointestinal symptoms

Whorwell et al have followed up their demonstration of the high prevalence of non-GI symptoms in IBS[38] with two further intriguing findings. To find out which symptoms bother IBS patients most, they asked 100 consecutive patients to rank 14 symptoms in order of severity. They did this by scattering on a table 14 cards, each labelled with a symptom, and asking the patient to pick them up in order of severity of the symptoms.[39] For each symptom a mean rank score was calculated. After abdominal pain and troublesome bowels, the highest ranking symptom was constant lethargy, and this was considered the worst or second worst symptom by a third of the patients (irrespective of their scoring for anxiety and depression). In the second study, the prevalence of non-colonic symptoms was measured in 107 IBS patients and 295 patients with organic GI disease. The IBS patients were 6.7 times more likely to have lethargy and were also twice as likely to have backache, early satiety, nausea, and frequency of micturition.[40] The authors concluded that these symptoms, especially lassitude, can be used to aid the confident diagnosis of IBS. But they kept silent on the mechanisms behind them.

IBS patients are often sent to gynaecological clinics.[41–43] This seems to be due mostly to inappropriate diagnosis of 'pelvic pain', but dyspareunia is common in IBS, and there may be an association with menstrual irregularities.[42]

Mechanism of symptoms

Motility experts agree that there is no motor pattern in the colon unique to patients with IBS.[44, 45] The experts are unlikely to change their minds after reading that pressures were high in the unprepared sigmoid of seven patients,[46] but the report that inducing anger led to more vigorous rectal contractions in IBS than in controls is interesting.[47] The authors claim that anger levels were the same in the two groups.

The pendulum is swinging towards sensory rather than motor mechanisms in IBS. This is true too of other functional GI disorders – e.g. chest pain of oesophageal origin[48] and functional dyspepsia. In the latter a series of studies has shown the most consistent abnormality to be excessive sensitivity of the stomach to balloon distension.[49 – 52] One group has coined the term 'irritable stomach syndrome',[49] and this seems appropriate since there is an overlap in the symptoms of functional dyspepsia and IBS. Furthermore, some patients with functional dyspepsia have an abnormally sensitive jejunum,[50] and some patients with IBS have an abnormally sensitive duodenum.[53] Using prolonged recordings, Kellow et al[14, 53] have shown that IBS patients are abnormally conscious of their duodenums contracting and more often feel pain with the contractions, though these are no stronger than normal.

The idea that the rectum and sigmoid are supersensitive in IBS is not new, but it has been abundantly confirmed.[21, 22] This increased sensitivity is not accompanied by increased tone, so one should think of the irritable bowel as excessively alert rather than inappropriately aroused (although this twitchiness may translate into inappropriate activity when stool arrives). Read[54] has coined the term 'neurotic bowel' but the old term 'irritable' still seems apt. Read suggests that IBS is analogous to bronchial asthma, where the airways become irritable for various reasons, and this is an attractive idea in the light of the recent finding that IBS patients' bronchi react to subnormal doses of methacholine.[55] However, IBS lacks the inflammatory component which is so characteristic of asthma, and there is no statistical link between the two diseases.[17]

Prior et al[22] found evidence of rectal sensitivity in few of their IBS patients with constipation but in most of those who complained of diarrhoea. Anxiety scores were high in the latter, and it is tempting to view rectal sensitivity as an effect of anxiety, especially as experimental stress has been reported to increase rectal sensitivity.[56] This idea could explain why one group found no difference in rectal sensitivity between IBS patients and controls; in their study protocol the measurement was always preceded by a 10-minute stressful interview.[34]

THE SENSORY SYSTEM OF THE INTESTINE

The sensory, or afferent, system of the intestine is simple in the sense that the receptors are just nerve endings in the bowel wall, but it is complicated in every other way.[48, 57, 58] For a start, the receptors are joined to two different kinds of nerve fibre – one that connects only to the enteric nervous system and another that connects via sympathetic nerves to the central nervous system (CNS). It is thought that only the latter kind mediate pain while the former are concerned with local reflex activity. Should the receptors become sensitized, or upregulated (to use the current jargon), a physiological event such as the arrival of digesta or faeces could trigger off increased motor activity as well as pain; in other words, sensitized receptors could explain the main manifestations of IBS. Another way the same thing could happen is through activation of silent pain receptors by persistent damage or inflammation, and this could explain why patients with colitis get IBS-like symptoms.

Knowing the circuitry of the afferent system helps one to understand the curiously wide distribution of intestinal pain and also the role of higher centres, that is, psychological factors. In the spinal cord, afferent messages travelling from the gut to the brain share the same pathway as sensory input from the rest of the body. Heavy traffic up the visceral afferents could be misinterpreted by the CNS as indicating trouble in, say, the back or thighs.[48] The same result could follow if there was upregulation of central synapses on the afferent pathway by messages descending from higher centres. Poor localization of visceral afferent messages might explain the symptoms of bladder irritability which so often co-exist with IBS and even some non-GI manifestations.[57] Stimulation of visceral afferents can evoke a reflex sympathetic discharge to the adrenal medulla and hence the release of adrenaline and enkephalin-like peptides. These could not only cause autonomic symptoms such as faintness, coldness, and sweating, which are a feature of IBS,[17] but also affect gut motility, either directly or indirectly via the release of 5-hydroxytryptamine (5-HT) from gut enterochromaffin cells. 5-HT is one of several neuroactive agents which can enhance the sensitivity of afferents in experimental systems. Hence, a vicious circle could be set up in which sensitized receptors cause symptoms which cause distress which causes sympathetic discharge which causes further sensitization and so further symptoms (Fig. 3.1).

Functional abdominal bloating

Bloating, or distension, is one of the commonest functional abdominal symptoms and sometimes the most troublesome, but it is poorly understood and some doctors even doubt its reality. Recent research has proved that it is genuine. Maxton et al[59] measured the waist circumference of 20 women who had this complaint as part of IBS and found a 4-cm increase between the morning and late afternoon, whereas there was no change in age-matched controls. This finding was confirmed by CT scanning, which also showed no shift in the diaphragm and no increase in the lumbar lordosis. Similar findings have been reported in another group of 12 patients studied by helium dilution and plethysmography.[60] Intestinal gas area was measured in the first study and did not increase, nor did it change

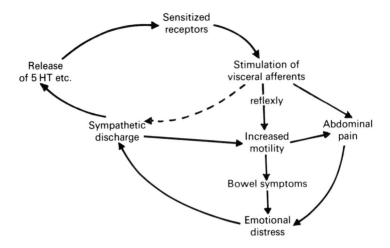

Fig. 3.1   A hypothetical scheme to show how sensitization (upregulation) of sensory receptors in the gut could lead to a vicious circle in IBS. The system becomes self-perpetuating if emotional distress is sustained or afferent stimulation is so intense that, of itself, it causes sympathetic discharge. Increased motility could be mediated in part by local effects of 5-HT. This scheme is based on recent reviews of the afferent visceral system[48, 57, 58] as well as on clinical observations and early results of treatment with 5-HT$_3$ blocking agents. Emotion, attention, and attitude can probably amplify symptoms in other ways (see p 54).

in the X-rays of another 20 IBS patients who were followed prospectively through episodes of bloating.[61] A simple but untested explanation for all these negative findings is that some patients relax their abdominal muscles as an unconscious reaction to their abdominal discomfort.[60]

TREATMENT OF IBS

The debunking of bran, this time corn bran, has continued,[62] and it is time now to think of it as a placebo with a laxative effect. Ispaghula has had a favourable report,[63] but the design of the study can be criticized. In another trial, ispaghula was superior to placebo by global assessment and by feelings of complete evacuation, but no better at relief of pain.[64] A new anti-muscarinic drug, cimetropium, was found to relieve pain in a double-blind trial in Italy.[65] This needs confirmation in view of the dubious results with previous trials of muscle relaxants.[66]

A new class of compounds which is exciting interest is the 5-HT$_3$ antagonists. One of them, granisetron, appears to have the predicted effect of reducing the sensitivity of the rectum (to balloon distension); it also reduces postprandial motor activity.[67] Another one, ondansetron, is said to alleviate the frequency of defecation and looseness of stool of diarrhoea-predominant patients, but it made no difference to the 'difficult' symptoms of IBS, namely, pain and bloating (and lassitude).[68]

The 'difficult' patient who resists simple reassurance, a bulking agent, and perhaps a musculotropic agent, is still every gastroenterologist's bugbear. When diarrhoea is prominent and the patient is intelligent and motivated, an exclusion diet is worth trying,[69] even if it works largely through placebo effect. Otherwise, there is increasing evidence that a psychotherapeutic approach works best. In a useful review, Creed & Guthrie[70] suggest three ways in which psychological treatments may act: by convincing patients their symptoms are stress-related, by helping them to cope with problems and relationships, and by teaching relaxation, which lessens anxiety and tension. The physician may reasonably attempt the first and may have access to a health-care worker who can do the last, but the central element requires a professional psychologist or a committed psychiatrist, and these are rare. Guthrie & Creed,[71] both psychiatrists, have published impressively successful long-term results in 43 patients with resistant IBS who underwent seven sessions of psychotherapy. They agree with others[11] that patients do worse if they have a long history; they disagree in finding that depression (and anxiety) predicts a good outcome, perhaps because their treatment had a psychiatric emphasis. They conclude that, whatever the treatment, the most important ingredient for success is a close doctor–patient relationship.

Doctors who shy away from forming such relationships may be attracted by hypnotherapy. So far, there has been only one small study to support Whorwell's startlingly successful results,[72] and it is the lucky gastroenterologist who has a hypnotherapist at his or her disposal. One attraction of hypnotherapy is that it can be used as a research tool. Already there is evidence that hypnotherapy can be used to desensitize the rectum.[73] Its potential is obvious.

Two practical developments in recent years are the publication of readable and scientifically sound books on IBS for the general public[74, 75] and the setting up of a national self-help organization (IBS Network), which publishes a newsletter *Gut Reaction* (c/o Voluntary Action Sheffield, 69 Division St, Sheffield S1 4GE).

REFERENCES

1 Thompson WG, Dotevall G, Drossman DA, Heaton KW, Kruis W. Irritable bowel syndrome: guidelines for the diagnosis. Gastroenterol Internat 1989; 2: 92–95
2 Drossman DA, Thompson WG, Talley NJ, Funch-Jensen P, Janssens J, Whitehead WE. Identification of sub-groups of functional gastrointestinal disorders. Gastroenterol Internat 1990; 3: 159–172
3 Whitehead WE, Chaussade E, Corazziari E, Kumar D. Report of an international workshop on management of constipation. Gastroenterol Internat 1991; 4: 99–113
4 Thompson WG, Creed F, Drossman DA, Heaton KW, Mazzacca G. Working team report: functional bowel disorders and chronic functional abdominal pain. Gastroenterol Internat 1992; 4: in press
5 Manning AP, Thompson WG, Heaton KW, Morris AF. Towards positive diagnosis of the irritable bowel. Br Med J 1978; 2: 653–654

6 Thompson WG, Heaton KW. Functional bowel disorders in apparently healthy people. Gastroenterology 1980; 79: 283–288

7 Talley NJ, Phillips SF, Melton LJ, Mulvihill C, Wittgen C, Zinsmeister AR. Diagnostic value of the Manning criteria in irritable bowel syndrome. Gut 1990; 31: 77–81

8 Thompson WG. Gastrointestinal symptoms in the irritable bowel compared with peptic ulcer and inflammatory bowel disease. Gut 1984; 25: 1089–1092

9 Whitehead WE, Crowell MD, Bosmajian L et al. Existence of irritable bowel syndrome supported by factor analysis of symptoms in two community samples. Gastroenterology 1990; 98: 336–340

10 Smith RC, Greenbaum DS, Vancouver JB et al. Gender differences in Manning criteria in the irritable bowel syndrome. Gastroenterology 1991; 100: 591–595

11 Bleijenberg G, Fennis JFM. Anamnestic and psychological features in diagnosis and prognosis of functional abdominal complaints: a prospective study. Gut 1989; 30: 1076–1081

12 Farrands PA, Hardcastle JD. Colorectal screening by self-completion questionnaire. Gut 1984; 25: 445–447

13 O'Donnell LJD, Virjee J, Heaton KW. Detection of pseudodiarrhoea by simple clinical assessment of intestinal transit rate. Br Med J 1990; 300: 439–440

14 Kellow JE, Gill RC, Wingate DL. Prolonged ambulant recordings of small bowel motility demonstrate abnormalities in the irritable bowel syndrome. Gastroenterology 1990; 98: 1208–1218

15 Heaton KW, Ghosh S, Braddon FEM. How bad are the symptoms and bowel dysfunction of patients with the irritable bowel syndrome? A prospective, controlled study with emphasis on stool form. Gut 1991; 32: 73–79

16 Heaton KW, O'Donnell LJD, Braddon FEM, Mountford RA, Hughes AO, Cripps PJ. Irritable bowel syndrome in a British urban community: consulters and non-consulters. Gastroenterology 1992: in press

17 Jones R, Lydeard S. Irritable bowel syndrome in the general population. Br Med J 1992; 304: 87–90

18 Talley NJ, Zinsmeister AR, van Dyke C, Melton LJ. Epidemiology of colonic symptoms and the irritable bowel syndrome. Gastroenterology 1991; 101: 927–934

19 Gaburri M, Bassotti G, Bacci G et al. Functional gut disorders and health care seeking behaviour in an Italian non-patient population. Rec Prog Med 1989; 80: 241–244

20 Cook IJ, van Eeden A, Collins SM. Patients with irritable bowel syndrome have greater pain tolerance than normal subjects. Gastroenterology 1987; 93: 727–733

21 Whitehead WE, Holtkotter B, Enck P et al. Tolerance for rectosigmoid distension in irritable bowel syndrome. Gastroenterology 1990; 98: 1187–1192

22 Prior A, Maxton DG, Whorwell PJ. Anorectal manometry in irritable bowel syndrome: differences between diarrhoea and constipation predominant subjects. Gut 1990; 31: 458–462

23 Taylor I, Basu P, Hammond P, Darby C, Flynn M. Effect of bile acid perfusion on colonic motor function in patients with the irritable colon syndrome. Gut 1980; 21: 843–847

24 Drossman DA, McKee DC, Sandler RS et al. Psychosocial factors in the irritable bowel syndrome. A multivariate study of patients and nonpatients with irritable bowel syndrome. Gastroenterology 1988; 95: 701–708

25 Whitehead WE, Bosmajian L, Zonderman AB, Costa PT, Schuster MM. Symptoms of psychologic distress associated with irritable bowel syndrome. Comparison of community and medical clinic samples. Gastroenterology 1988; 95: 709–714

26 Sandler RS, Drossman DA, Nathan HP, McKee DC. Symptom complaints and health care seeking behavior in subjects with bowel dysfunction. Gastroenterology 1984; 87: 314–318

27 Welch CW, Hillman LC, Pomare EW. Psychoneurotic symptomatology in the irritable bowel syndrome: a study of reporters and non-reporters. Br Med J 1985; 291: 1382–1384

28 Smith RC, Greenbaum DS, Vancouver JB et al. Psychosocial factors are associated with health care seeking rather than diagnosis in irritable bowel syndrome. Gastroenterology 1990; 98: 293–301

29 Talley NJ, Phillips SF, Bruce B, Twomey CK, Zinsmeister AR, Melton LJ. Relation among personality and symptoms in non-ulcer dyspepsia and the irritable bowel syndrome. Gastroenterology 1990; 99: 327–333

30 Creed F, Guthrie E. Relation among personality and symptoms in nonulcer dyspepsia and the irritable bowel syndrome. Gastroenterology 1991; 100: 1154–1155
31 Welch CW, Stace NH, Pomare EW. Specificity of psychological profiles of irritable bowel syndrome patients. Aust NZ J Med 1984; 14: 101–104
32 Creed F, Craig T, Farmer R. Functional abdominal pain, psychiatric illness, and life events. Gut 1988; 29: 235–242
33 Toner BB, Garfinkel PE, Jeejeebhoy KN. Psychological factors in irritable bowel syndrome. Can J Psychiatry 1990; 35: 158–161
34 Latimer P, Campbell D, Latimer M, Sarna S, Daniel E, Waterfall W. Irritable bowel syndrome: a test of the colonic hyperalgesia hypothesis. J Behav Med 1979; 2: 285–295
35 Bass CM, ed., Somatization: physical symptoms and psychological illness. Oxford: Blackwell. 1990
36 Brook A. Bowel distress and emotional conflict. J Roy Soc Med 1991; 84: 39–42
37 Drossman DA, Leserman J, Nachman G et al. Sexual and physical abuse in women with functional or organic gastrointestinal disorders. Ann Intern Med 1990; 113: 828–833
38 Whorwell PJ, McCallum M, Creed FH, Roberts CT. Non-colonic features of irritable bowel syndrome. Gut 1986; 27: 37–40
39 Maxton DG, Morris JA, Whorwell PJ. Ranking of symptoms by patients with the irritable bowel syndrome. Br Med J 1989; 299: 1138
40 Maxton DG, Morris J, Whorwell PJ. More accurate diagnosis of irritable bowel syndrome by the use of 'non-colonic' symptomatology. Gut 1991; 32: 784–786
41 Prior A, Whorwell PJ. Gynaecological consultation in patients with the irritable bowel syndrome. Gut 1989; 30: 996–998
42 Prior A, Wilson K, Whorwell PJ, Faragher EB. Irritable bowel syndrome in the gynecological clinic. Survey of 798 new referrals. Dig Dis Sci 1989; 34: 1820–1824
43 Longstreth GF, Preskill DB, Youkeles L. Irritable bowel syndrome in women having diagnostic laparoscopy or hysterectomy. Relation to gynecologic features and outcome. Dig Dis Sci 1990; 35: 1285–1290
44 Camilleri M, Neri M. Motility disorders and stress. Dig Dis Sci 1989; 34: 1777–1786
45 Sarna SK. Physiology and pathophysiology of colonic motor activity. Dig Dis Sci 1991; 36: 827–862, 998–1018
46 Rogers J, Henry MM, Misiewicz JJ. Increased segmental activity and intraluminal pressures in the sigmoid colon of patients with the irritable bowel syndrome. Gut 1989; 30: 634–641
47 Welgan P, Meshkinpour H, Beelar M. Effect of anger on colon motor and myoelectric activity in irritable bowel syndrome. Gastroenterology 1988; 94: 1150–1156
48 Mayer EA, Raybould HE. Role of visceral afferent mechanisms in functional bowel disorders. Gastroenterology 1990; 99: 1688–1704
49 Lémann M, Dederling JP, Flourié B, Franchisseur C, Rambaud JC, Jian R. Abnormal perception of visceral pain in response to gastric distension in chronic idiopathic dyspepsia. The irritable stomach syndrome. Dig Dis Sci 1991; 36: 1249–1254
50 Greydanus MP, Vassallo M, Camilleri M, Nelson DK, Hanson RB, Thomforde GM. Neurohormonal factors in functional dyspepsia: insights on pathophysiological mechanisms. Gastroenterology 1991; 100: 1311–1318
51 Bradette M, Pare P, Douville P, Morin A. Visceral perception in health and functional dyspepsia. Crossover study of gastric distension with placebo and domperidone. Dig Dis Sci 1991; 36: 52–58
52 Mearin F, Cucala M, Azpiroz F, Malagelada J-R. The origin of symptoms on the brain-gut axis in functional dyspepsia. Gastroenterology 1991; 101: 999–1006
53 Kellow JE, Eckersley GM, Jones MP. Enhanced perception of physiological intestinal motility in the irritable bowel syndrome. Gastroenterology 1991; 101: 1621–1627
54 Read NW, ed. Irritable bowel syndrome. Oxford: Blackwell. 1991
55 White AM, Stevens WH, Upton AR, O'Byrne PM, Collins SM. Airway responsiveness to inhaled methocholine in patients with irritable bowel syndrome. Gastroenterology 1991; 100: 68–74
56 Erkenbrecht JF. Noise and intestinal motor alterations. In: Bueno L, Collins C, Junien JL, eds. Stress and digestive motility. Paris: John Libbey. 1989: pp 93–96
57 Andrews PLR. Modulation of visceral afferent activity as a therapeutic possibility for gastrointestinal disorders. In: Read NW, ed. Irritable bowel syndrome. Oxford: Blackwell. 1991: pp 91–121

58 Cervero F. Gut sensitivity. In: Read NW, ed. Irritable bowel syndrome. Oxford: Blackwell, 1991: pp 83–90
59 Maxton DG, Martin DF, Whorwell PJ, Godfrey M. Abdominal distension in female patients with irritable bowel syndrome: exploration of possible mechanisms. Gut 1991; 32: 662–664
60 Catnach SM, Dewsnap P, Herdman M, Libby G, Farthing MJG, Fairclough PD. Abdominal bloating in the irritable bowel syndrome. Gut 1990; 31: A1171–1172
61 Chami TN, Schuster MM, Bohlman ME, Pulliam TJ, Kamal N, Whitehead WE. A simple radiologic method to estimate the quantity of bowel gas. Gastroenterology 1990; A163
62 Cook IJ, Irvine EJ, Campbell D, Shannon S, Reddy SN, Collins SM. Effect of dietary fiber on symptoms and rectosigmoid motility in patients with irritable bowel syndrome. A controlled crossover study. Gastroenterology 1990; 98: 66–72
63 Misra SP, Thorat VK, Sachdev GK, Anand BS. Long-term treatment of irritable bowel syndrome: results of a randomised controlled trial. Quart J Med 1989; 73: 931–939
64 Jalihal A, Kurian G. Ispaghula therapy in irritable bowel syndrome: improvement in overall well-being is related to reduction in bowel dissatisfaction. J Gastroenterol Hepatol 1990; 5: 507–513
65 Dobrilla G, Imbimbo BP, Piazzi L, Bensi G. Long-term treatment of irritable bowel syndrome with cimetropium bromide. Gut 1990; 31: 355–358
66 Klein KB. Controlled treatment trials in the irritable bowel syndrome: a critique. Gastroenterology 1988; 95: 232–241
67 Prior A, Read NW. Reduction of rectal sensitivity and postprandial motility by granisetron, a 5-HT_3 receptor antagonist, in patients with irritable bowel syndrome (IBS). Gut 1990; 31: A1174
68 Maxton DG, Haigh CG, Whorwell PJ. 5-HT_3 antagonists: a role in irritable bowel syndrome and non-ulcer dyspepsia? Gut 1991; 32: A1228
69 Nanda R, James R, Smith H, Dudley CRK, Jewell DP. Food intolerance and the irritable bowel syndrome. Gut 1989; 30: 1099–1104
70 Creed F, Guthrie E. Psychological treatments of the irritable bowel syndrome. Gut 1989; 30: 1601–1609
71 Guthrie E, Creed F, Dawson D, Tomenson B. A controlled trial of psychological treatment for the irritable bowel syndrome. Gastroenterology 1991; 100: 450–457
72 Harvey RF, Hinton RA, Gunary RM, Barry RE. Individual and group hypnotherapy in treatment of refractory irritable bowel syndrome. Lancet 1989; 1: 424–425
73 Prior A, Colgan SM, Whorwell PJ. Changes in rectal sensitivity after hypnotherapy in patients with irritable bowel syndrome. Gut 1990; 31: 896–898
74 Thompson WG. Gut reactions: understanding symptoms of the digestive tract. New York: Plenum Press. 1989
75 Watts G. Irritable bowel syndrome: a practical guide. London: Mandarin, 1990

4

Functional gastrointestinal disorders: psychological factors in aetiology and management

G. G. Lloyd

The concept of a functional medical disorder is a controversial topic, open to a wide range of interpretations. In gastroenterology it has come to be used to describe 'a variable combination of chronic or recurrent gastrointestinal symptoms which cannot be explained by structural or chemical abnormalities'.[1] The individual syndromes include oesophageal spasm, psychogenic vomiting, non-ulcer dyspepsia, irritable bowel, and proctalgia fugax. Although they are diagnosed separately, there is a considerable degree of overlap between them. Irritable bowel syndrome (IBS) has been shown to be associated with disturbance of oesophageal motility.[2] Several non-colonic gastrointestinal symptoms are more frequent in patients with this condition than in controls; these include nausea, vomiting, dysphagia, and early satiety. Symptoms arising from outside the gut are also commoner, notably nocturia, frequency and urgency of micturition, fatigue, and dyspareunia,[3] giving rise to the suggestion that the irritable bowel syndrome involves a generalized smooth muscle disorder. These observations have been confirmed by Jones & Lydeard,[4] who also found an increased prevalence of autonomic symptoms such as flushing and sweating, migraine, and previous hysterectomy.

Psychological factors have been linked with IBS since the condition was first defined. The proportion of patients diagnosed as having a psychiatric disorder varies according to the criteria used. In a previous review Creed & Guthrie[5] concluded that, when reliable and valid measures have been employed, approximately 50% of hospital clinic attenders have a psychiatric disorder. This usually takes the form of a neurotic illness with a mixture of depressive and anxiety symptoms. However, the Tenth Edition of the International Classification of Disease (ICD-10) has included in its section on mental and behavioural disorders a category of somatoform autonomic dysfunction (F45.3). The symptoms are presented by the patient as if they were due to a physical disorder of a system or organ that is largely or completely under control of the autonomic nervous system. The category is further subdivided according to the organ or system regarded as the origin of the symptoms (Table 4.1).

The symptoms of these diagnostic categories are of two types. The first type is characterized by objective signs of autonomic arousal, such as

Table 4.1   Somatoform autonomic dysfunction

F45.30	The heart and cardiovascular system
F45.31	The upper gastrointestinal tract (includes 'gastric neurosis')
F45.32	The lower gastrointestinal tract (includes irritable bowel syndrome)
F45.33	The respiratory system
F45.34	The urogenital system
F45.38	Other

palpitations, sweating, flushing, and tremor. The second type consists of subjective and non-specific symptoms, such as aches and pains, burning, heaviness, tightness, or distension. The combination of autonomic arousal, additional subjective symptoms, and consistent referral to a particular organ gives the characteristic clinical picture. Many patients have evidence of psychological stress or current social problems which appear to be related to the disorder, but this is not the case in a substantial proportion. It thus appears that IBS, non-ulcer dyspepsia, and the other functional gut disorders are regarded by ICD-10 as behavioural disorders, even if there is no associated psychopathology or major external stress.

AETIOLOGICAL CONSIDERATIONS

Irritable bowel syndrome

It has been repeatedly shown that there is a high prevalence of psychiatric illness in patients with IBS attending hospital clinics.[5] Recent studies have confirmed these observations. Walker et al[6] compared 28 patients with IBS with 19 patients with inflammatory bowel disease. The patients were assessed with a standardized psychiatric interview, the Diagnostic Interview Schedule (DIS), and diagnoses were made according to operational criteria (DSM-III-R). They also completed psychological self-reports. The IBS patients had significantly more lifetime diagnoses of major depression, somatization disorder, generalized anxiety disorder, panic disorder, and phobic disorder. Indeed, 93% of IBS patients had at least one lifetime psychiatric diagnosis as compared with 21% of patients with inflammatory disease. Some of these were concurrent disorders, but in other cases the time of onset of the psychiatric diagnosis ranged from a few weeks to several years before the onset of bowel symptoms. The IBS group also had significantly more medically-unexplained somatic symptoms localized outside the digestive tract. It should be noted here that a review paper[7] has concluded that no systematically conducted studies show an association between psychiatric illness and ulcerative colitis, nor, according to a second paper, do stressful life events precipitate exacerbations of inflammatory bowel disease.[8] The same psychiatric interview, the DIS, was used by

Toner et al,[9] who compared 44 IBS patients with 28 non-clinical controls. The IBS patients had significantly more psychiatric disorders in general, and more anxiety and affective disorders in particular, than did the controls. This applied to diagnoses made throughout the patient's lifetime and during the last year. However, the lifetime prevalence (61%) was considerably lower than that reported by Walker et al.[6] Toner et al[9] also found that IBS was associated with higher scores on the Lie scale of the Eysenck Personality Inventory. On the basis of their findings, they proposed that IBS patients have a great need for social acceptance, and that this explains their presentation with organic rather than psychological symptoms.

Blanchard et al,[10] using different methods of assessment, also found higher levels of anxiety and depression among IBS patients than among patients with inflammatory bowel disease, who were no more depressed than healthy control subjects. Kumar et al[11] reported higher levels of neurotic symptoms in 18 IBS patients, as compared with 10 healthy volunteers and 12 patients with benign gastrointestinal disease. The differences were mainly due to high levels of anxiety and obsessional traits; the scores for depression were similar in all three groups. The authors proposed that the neurotic symptoms are secondary effects of IBS and that IBS is not a manifestation of depression. An uncontrolled psychodynamic assessment of 60 female patients by Brook[12] observed that most were trapped in severe emotional conflicts with which they were unable to cope. These conflicts often had their roots in infancy, and in this context it may be relevant that a history of childhood sexual and physical abuse is commoner in women with functional gastrointestinal disorders than in those with organic disease.[13]

One recent study found no differences between patients with IBS, non-ulcer dyspepsia, and organic bowel disease on the Minnesota Multiphasic Personality Inventory (MMPI).[14] However, the MMPI is not a satisfactory instrument for use with physically ill patients because it contains several 'disease-related' items.[15]

Influence of psychological factors on referral

The high prevalence of psychiatric illness among IBS patients has contributed to the widely held view that IBS is a psychophysiological disorder. But this view is coming under increasing scrutiny. Whitehead & Crowell[16] have argued that the psychological symptoms associated with IBS have nothing to do with the development of bowel symptoms, but do influence the patient's decision to seek medical treatment. This conclusion derives from their observation that people who have IBS symptoms but who do not consult a doctor have no higher levels of psychological distress than asymptomatic control subjects.[17] Support for this hypothesis has been provided by Smith et al,[18] who found that psychosocial criteria were of limited value in distinguishing IBS from organic disease but were likely to have determined the decision to seek health care.

In a postal survey of patients registered with eight general practitioners, Jones & Lydeard[4] found that 22% reported symptoms consistent with the diagnosis of IBS. However only one-third of these had sought medical advice for their symptoms during the previous 2 years. Consultation rates varied widely between the eight general practices. These differences could not be explained by demographic factors nor by the severity of IBS symptoms. The authors concluded that the relationship between patient and doctor, and the patient's expectations of this relationship, are important determinants of the decision to seek medical attention.

Non-ulcer dyspepsia

This is the latest in a succession of terms used to describe unexplained upper abdominal pain. The preferred definition is 'dyspepsia lasting for more than four months, unrelated to exercise and for which no focal lesion or systemic disease can be found responsible'.[19] Not surprisingly, psychological factors have been invoked in its aetiology. In a recent review, Morris[20] concluded that a significant proportion of patients have a psychiatric disorder, usually anxiety or depression, or personality traits which influence their presentation with dyspeptic symptoms. Severe life stresses may also have an important role. Three recent controlled studies have shed further light on this issue. Langeluddecke et al[21] compared 59 patients with non-ulcer dyspepsia with 83 who had peptic ulcer disease proven endoscopically. On a series of psychological tests the non-ulcer group had significantly higher levels of tension, hostility, and anxiety, but there were no differences in levels of depression or the tendency to suppress anger.

Stressful life events, particularly if they were severe, threatening, and prolonged, were much more frequent in non-ulcer dyspeptics than in healthy controls.[22] Acute stress was also more common in the non-ulcer group, as were anxiety and depressive symptoms and neurotic personality traits. Severely threatening life events also appear to be associated with the onset of non-organic abdominal pain which simulates acute appendicitis.[23] Hui et al[24] found no differences in the rate of negative or positive major life events when they compared 33 non-ulcer dyspeptics with 33 controls matched for age, sex, and social class. However, the dyspeptic patients perceived their life events as having had a greater negative effect on their lives. It was concluded that the way life events are perceived is more important than their rate of occurrence in the onset of dyspeptic symptoms. When the individual life events were analysed, the dyspeptic patients had significantly higher scores than controls on items of minor law violation, changes in closeness of family relationships, and major personal illness or injury.

The significance of these findings must be treated with the same degree of caution as applied to observations on patients with IBS. Life stresses, psychological symptoms, and psychiatric illness may influence medical consultation and patterns of referral in non-ulcer dyspepsia or non-organic abdominal pain, but they may not have much influence in bringing on these symptoms.

PSYCHOLOGICAL TREATMENTS

Further studies have clarified the role of various psychological treatments in functional bowel disorders. These have focused on IBS, but they could be readily modified for use with patients with other disorders.

In the broadest sense, psychological treatment is necessary for all patients with functional disorders. Many respond to explanation, re-assurance, and support, although it is important that these be based on a thorough physical examination and appropriate investigations. Patients are unlikely to be reassured if they are merely told there is nothing seriously wrong with their bowels. This should be regarded only as a preliminary step. The nature of the symptoms should then be explained in terms of increased sensitivity and motility of the gut, using appropriate diagrams if these are available.

Specific psychological treatments are usually reserved for those who do not respond to the first-line medical treatment of reassurance and explan-ation, supplemented by a bulking agent or antispasmodic drug. They may also be used for patients who relapse regularly after an initial response to treatment. Before discussing individual psychological treatments, we should mention tricyclic antidepressant drugs. These are widely used by gastroenterologists, and there is evidence that they are effective in improv-ing bowel symptoms, particularly diarrhoea.[25] They may work by altering bowel motility through their anticholinergic effect and also by virtue of their analgesic properties. It is not established that they improve bowel symptoms as a result of their effect on elevating a depressed mood or reducing anxiety.

Hypnotherapy

This approach has been pioneered by Whorwell,[26] who has summarized the essentials of the technique, which he describes as gut-directed hyp-nosis. Patients are first given a simple explanation of gut physiology, which they will be asked to modify during subsequent hypnotherapy sessions. After the induction of the hypnotic state, patients are asked to place a hand on their abdomen and to relate the sensation of warmth to the relief of pain, spasm, and bloating. They are then asked to visualize a flowing river and imagine it as their gut. Next they are asked to modify the flow to achieve a more satisfactory bowel habit. Some patients take many weeks to respond, and this delay can be a testing time for both patient and doctor. However, the efficacy of this approach is becoming established. In addition to Whorwell's controlled studies,[27, 28] an independent group has now reported beneficial results. Harvey et al[29] used a similar hypnotic technique for four sessions, although the patients were also encouraged to use autohypnosis at home for at least two 10-minute sessions daily. Twenty patients out of 33 improved, and 11 lost almost all their symptoms. Short-term improvement was maintained at 3 months. There were no differences in rates of improvement between those treated individually and those treated in groups. Patients whose General Health Questionnaire scores suggested probable psychiatric morbidity were less likely to improve than those whose scores were in the normal range. Unfortunately, there was no control group, but all these patients were refractory to other medical treatments, so spontaneous improvement was unlikely.

Whorwell[26] acknowledges that conventionally trained doctors may feel uneasy with the language and jargon used in hypnosis. But he emphasizes that the technique is easy to acquire and can be modified to suit the doctor's own personality. Deep levels of hypnosis are not necessary, nor is this technique used to treat severe psychological problems. Hypnosis may be effective by influencing gut physiology directly. Patients with IBS may have increased or decreased rectal sensitivity, and hypnosis appears to modify sensitivity towards normal whether the rectum is hypersensitive or hyposensitive.[30, 31] Hypnotherapy also appears to reduce the relapse rate in patients who had been treated for duodenal ulceration, although the results were not as impressive as those for IBS.[32] There may also be a place for using hypnotherapy in patients with inflammatory bowel disease.

Behaviour therapy

Schwarz et al[33] have reported a 4-year follow-up of an uncontrolled study of behaviour therapy. This consisted of a multicomponent treatment package including training in both progressive muscle relaxation and thermal bio-feedback, instruction in cognitive coping strategies, and education about IBS. Nineteen of 27 patients who had completed the treatment were contacted 4 years later, and 17 of these rated themselves as more than 50% improved. The fluctuating course of IBS makes these figures difficult to interpret, and controlled treatment studies are essential in a condition of this type.

A better-designed study has been described by Corney et al.[34] Forty-two patients with IBS were allocated to either conventional medical treatment or behavioural psychotherapy with a nurse therapist. The medical treatment consisted of explanation, dietary advice, bulk laxatives, antispasmodics, and a variety of other medications. The behaviour therapy comprised advice on pain management and bowel retraining, and rehearsing coping with situations or activities which had previously been avoided. When assessed 9 months after entry into the trial, both groups had improved on several measures, but there were no differences between the groups with regard to bowel or psychological symptoms, with the exception of two avoidance scores. These were for the avoidance of certain foods and avoidance of domestic activities, both of which were reduced to a significantly greater extent in the behaviour therapy group. The authors pointed out that considerably more therapeutic time had been devoted to the behaviour therapy group, and they concluded that this form of treatment is no more effective than conventional medical management.

A newer form of treatment, cognitive behaviour therapy, is also appropriate for IBS.[35] This treatment is based on the hypothesis that many symptoms of an illness result from the patient's distorted pattern of thinking and maladaptive behaviour. Treatment aims to help patients identify their dysfunctional beliefs, particularly those which convince them they are suffering from serious physical illness. The assessment should also identify patterns of avoidance which anticipate bowel symptoms. The next step is to change the patient's beliefs about the symptoms by identifying negative thoughts and the evidence upon which they are based.

Psychotherapy

The most impressive study of psychological treatment yet reported was conducted by Guthrie et al.[36] It included 102 patients whose IBS symptoms had not responded to standard medical treatment over the previous 6 months, and it compared psychological treatment and standard medical treatment with standard medical treatment alone. The psychological treatment was based on the principles of dynamic psychotherapy. During an initial assessment of 2 hours or more, the patients' feelings about their illness and any emotional problems were explored. Therapy was aimed specifically at those emotional problems frequently associated with IBS, particularly marital and other relationship problems. It continued during a further six interviews. Patients were also given a relaxation tape to use at home; no psychotropic medication was prescribed. After 3 months the patients who had received psychological treatment showed greater improvement than the controls on several measures. Ratings of abdominal pain, diarrhoea, anxiety, and depression all showed improvement, but constipation changed little. Favourable prognostic indicators were the presence of overt psychiatric symptoms at the initial assessment and intermittent pain which was exacerbated by stress. The treatment did not appear to help those with constant abdominal pain.

SUMMARY AND CONCLUSIONS

Psychiatric illness and a history of specific life events are commonly observed in patients with functional bowel disorders attending hospital clinics. Many specialists regard these conditions as psychophysiological disorders, a view which is sanctioned by their inclusion in ICD-10 in the separate category of somatoform autonomic dysfunction. But the significance of psychosocial factors is not clearly established. Recent studies question their aetiological importance and suggest that they are more significant in determining the patient's decision to seek medical attention. More research is required to compare patients with community subjects who experience symptoms of functional bowel disease but who do not consult doctors. Particular attention needs to be given to the role of major stress, personality, and the pattern of psychological symptoms associated with consulting behaviour.

Psychological treatment, particularly hypnotherapy and dynamic psychotherapy, has a definite part to play in the management of patients with refractory symptoms. The disadvantage of such treatments is that they are time-consuming to administer. Attention needs to be given to the development of briefer, focused treatments, especially those which can be readily acquired by physicians who do not have specialist psychiatric experience.

REFERENCES

1 IBS Working Team Report. Handbook of International Congress of Gastroenterology. Rome. 1988
2 Whorwell PJ, Clouter C, Smith CL. Oesophageal motility in the irritable bowel syndrome. BMJ 1981; 282: 1101–1102
3 Whorwell PJ, McCallum M, Creed FH, Roberts CT. Non-colonic features of irritable bowel syndrome. Gut 1986; 27: 37–40
4 Jones R, Lydeard S. Irritable bowel syndrome in the general population. Br Med J 1992; 304: 87–90
5 Creed F, Guthrie E. Psychological factors in the irritable bowel syndrome. Gut 1987; 28: 1307–1318
6 Walker EA, Roy-Byrne PP, Katon WJ, Li L, Amos D, Jiranek G. Psychiatric illness and irritable bowel syndrome: a comparison with inflammatory bowel disease. Am J Psychiatry 1990; 147: 1656–1661
7 North CS, Clouse RE, Spitznagel EL, Alpers DH. The relation of ulcerative colitis to psychiatric factors: a review of findings and methods. Am J Psychiatry 1990; 147: 974–981
8 North CS, Alpers DH, Helzer JE, Spitznagel EL, Clouse RE. Do life events or depression exacerbate inflammatory bowel disease? A prospective study. Ann Intern Med 1991; 114: 381–386
9 Toner BB, Garfinkel PE, Jeejeebhoy KN. Psychological factors in irritable bowel syndrome. Can J Psychiatry 1990; 35: 158–161
10 Blanchard EB, Scharff L, Schwarz SP, Suls JM, Barlow DH. The role of anxiety and depression in the irritable bowel syndrome. Behav Res Ther 1990; 28: 401–405
11 Kumar D, Pfeffer J, Wingate DL. Role of psychological factors in the irritable bowel syndrome. Digestion 1990; 45: 80–87
12 Brook A. Bowel distress and emotional conflict. J R Soc Med 1991; 84: 39–42
13 Drossman DA, Leserman J, Nachman G et al. Sexual and physical abuse in women with functional or organic gastrointestinal disorders. Ann Intern Med 1990; 113: 828–833
14 Talley NJ, Phillips SF, Bruce B, Twomey CK, Zinsmeister AR, Melton LJ. Relation among personality and symptoms in non-ulcer dyspepsia and the irritable bowel syndrome. Gastroenterology 1990; 99: 327–333
15 Creed F, Guthrie E. Relation among personality and symptoms in non-ulcer dyspepsia and irritable bowel syndrome (Correspondence). Gastroenterology 1991; 100: 1154–1155

16 Whitehead WE, Crowell MD. Psychologic considerations in the irritable bowel
    syndrome. Gastroenterol Clin N Am 1991; 20: 249–267
17 Whitehead WE, Bosmajian L, Zonderman AB, Costa PT, Schuster MM. Symptoms of
    psychologic distress associated with irritable bowel syndrome: comparison of community
    and medical clinic samples. Gastroenterology 1988; 95: 709–714
18 Smith RC, Greenbaum DS, Vancouver JB et al. Psychosocial factors are associated with
    health care seeking rather than diagnosis in irritable bowel syndrome. Gastroenterology
    1990; 98: 293–301
19 Colin-Jones DG. Management of dyspepsia: report of a working party. Lancet 1988; 1:
    576–579
20 Morris C. Non-ulcer dyspepsia. J Psychosom Res 1991; 35: 129–140
21 Langeluddecke P, Goulston K, Tennant C. Psychological factors in dyspepsia of
    unknown cause: a comparison with peptic ulcer disease. J Psychosom Res 1990; 34:
    215–222
22 Bennett E, Beaurepaire J, Langeluddecke P, Kellow J, Tennant C. Life stress and non-
    ulcer dyspepsia: a case-control study. J Psychosom Res 1991; 35: 579–590
23 Beaurepaire JE, Jones M, Eckstein RP, Smith RC, Piper DW, Tennant C. The acute
    appendicitis syndrome: psychological aspects of the inflamed and non-inflamed appendix.
    J Psychosom Res 1992 (in press)
24 Hui WM, Shiu LP, Lam SK. The perception of life events and daily stress in non-ulcer
    dyspepsia. Am J Gastroenterol 1991; 86: 292–296
25 Creed F, Guthrie E. Psychological treatments of the irritable bowel syndrome: a review.
    Gut 1989; 30: 1601–1609
26 Whorwell PJ. Use of hypnotherapy in gastrointestinal disease. Br J Hosp Med 1991; 45:
    27–29
27 Whorwell PJ, Prior A, Faragher EB. Controlled trial of hypnotherapy in the treatment of
    severe refractory irritable bowel syndrome. Lancet 1984; 2: 1232–1234
28 Whorwell PJ, Prior A, Colgan SM. Hypnotherapy in severe irritable bowel syndrome:
    further experience. Gut 1987; 28: 423–425
29 Harvey RF, Hinton RA, Gunary RM, Barry RE. Individual and group hypnotherapy in
    treatment of refractory irritable bowel syndrome. Lancet 1989; 1: 424–425
30 Prior A, Maxton DG, Whorwell PJ. 1990 Anorectal manometry in irritable bowel
    syndrome: differences between diarrhoea and constipation predominant subjects. Gut
    1990; 31: 458–462
31 Prior A, Colgan SM, Whorwell PJ. Changes in rectal sensitivity following hypnotherapy
    for irritable bowel syndrome. Gut 1990; 31: 896–898
32 Colgan SM, Faragher ER, Whorwell PJ. A controlled trial of hypnotherapy in relapse
    prevention of duodenal ulceration. Lancet 1988; 1: 1229–1300
33 Schwarz SP, Taylor AE, Scharf L, Blanchard EB. Behaviourally treated irritable bowel
    syndrome patients: a four-year follow-up. Behav Res Ther 1990; 28: 331–335
34 Corney RH, Stanton R, Newell R, Clare A, Fairclough P. 1991; Behavioural
    psychotherapy in the treatment of irritable bowel syndrome. J Psychosom Res 1991; 35:
    461–469
35 Hawton K, Salkovskis PM, Kirk J, Clark DM. Cognitive behaviour therapy for
    psychiatric problems: a practical guide. Oxford: Oxford University Press. 1989
36 Guthrie E, Creed F, Dawson D, Tomensen B. A controlled trial of psychological
    treatment for the irritable bowel syndrome. Gastroenterology 1991; 100: 450–457

5

Molecular gastroenterology

J. A. Summerfield

Molecular biology is having the same profound effect on gastroenterology that it has had on other specialities. Furthermore, because of the breadth that gastroenterology embraces, the ultimate impact will probably be greater than in any other area except the neurosciences. In this chapter I shall review some of the areas where the application of molecular biological techniques has provided new insights into the functions of the liver and alimentary tract. In practical terms for the gastroenterologist doing clinical research, the cloned genes described here mean that probes for these genes are available for research, usually just by asking the authors of the papers. And such is the power of molecular biology, it is not even necessary to have the gene! With the published nucleotide sequence you can easily and cheaply get your own specific oligonucleotides made to use as probes or, if you want to isolate the gene, as primers for the polymerase chain reaction! This now permits gastroenterologists with very modest laboratory facilities and a manual[1] to ask basic genetic questions about gene structure and the level of gene expression in their clinical material, be it blood or biopsies.

STOMACH

Gastric proteases and receptors

Pepsinogens

Pepsins play a major role in acid-dependent protein digestion, the products of which cause gastrin release from antral G cells, which in turn mediates food-dependent gastric acid and pepsin secretion. Pepsins are made up of three closely related groups of enzymes, classified as I, II, and III. Clinical interest in pepsins has been renewed by evidence that they may be import- ant pathogenic factors in peptic ulcers and especially oesophagitis.[2] The genes for rabbit pepsinogens have now been cloned.[3] Five pepsinogen genes were isolated which encode similar, but not identical proteins. The deduced amino acid sequence showed that pepsinogens all bear a signal sequence (typical in secreted proteins) of 15 amino acids, a proregion (the activation segment) of 44 amino acids, and a pepsin region of 328 amino acids. The exception to this rule is pepsinogen F, which has a proregion of

43 and a pepsin region of 330 amino acids. Pepsinogen F appears to be a new type of pepsinogen.

It is also of interest that expression of pepsinogen genes is developmentally regulated. RNA analysis showed that pepsinogen F was expressed only in the early postnatal period and that then pepsinogens II and III were expressed, indicating a switch from fetal to adult pepsinogens during development. The reason for this switch is unknown. However, the availability of cloned pepsinogen genes now permits detailed studies of pepsin physiology in health and peptic ulcer disease.

Histamine H₂-receptor

Histamine H$_2$-receptor

The cloning of the histamine H_2-receptor was announced in 1991.[4] Histamine binds to an H_2-receptor on the basolateral membrane of the parietal cell, which is linked to a guanine nucleotide-binding protein (G_S). G_S then binds to guanosine triphosphate, which in turn induces the transfer of an adenosine diphosphate-ribose moiety to G_S, which locks G_S in the 'on' position. G_S is also linked to the catalytic subunit of adenylate cyclase, which, when stimulated, catalyses the production of cAMP, which in turn activates specific protein kinases, resulting in the generation of hydrogen ions.

The H_2-receptor belongs to a family of G protein-linked receptors that are known to share marked structural homology, which includes having seven transmembrane domains. Exploiting the homology between the G protein-linked receptors was the basis of the strategy used to clone the H_2-receptor. Using degenerate oligonucleotide primers to transmembrane domains of G protein-linked receptors, researchers obtained a partial length clone by polymerase chain reaction (PCR) from cDNA prepared from purified canine parietal cells. Screening a canine genomic library with this clone yielded a clone containing the entire H_2-receptor gene. The deduced amino acid sequence of the clone confirmed the homology between the H_2-receptor and other G protein-linked receptors. RNA analyses showed that the H_2-receptor gene is expressed by the parietal cells in the fundus of the stomach and to a lesser extent by the brain.

The coding regions of the H_2-receptor gene were inserted into an expression vector, and this construct was transfected into L cells to allow functional studies of the expressed H_2-receptor. The transfected L cells showed an increase in cAMP concentrations when stimulated by histamine, and the response was abolished by the addition of the H_2-antagonist cimetidine. Furthermore, the ligand [methyl-^{3}H] tiotidine bound to transfected L cells, and this binding was inhibited by cimetidine, but not by the H_1-antagonist, diphenylhydramine. These studies confirmed that the isolated gene did indeed encode the H_2-receptor. This information about the precise structure of the H_2-receptor not only will be valuable in clinical studies but should also lead to the design of even more specific drugs for patients with peptic ulcer disease.

H^+K^+-ATPase

The gastric H^+K^+-ATPase, or proton pump, is located in intracellular tubulovesicles which fuse with the apical membrane when parietal cells are stimulated to secrete hydrochloric acid. H^+K^+-ATPase consists of an α- and a β-subunit, both of which have now been cloned. Omeprazole inhibits acid secretion by binding covalently to the α-subunit; the function of the β-subunit is unknown. The gene encoding the human H^+K^+-ATPase α-subunit is large, having 22 exons, and encodes a protein of 114 kDa.[5] The protein has a phosphorylation site and binding sites for pyridoxil 5′-phosphate and fluorescein isothiocyanate. The primary structures of the H^+K^+-ATPase and Na^+K^+-ATPase α-subunits show about 60% homology, but their 5′ flanking sequences are different, indicating (not surprisingly) that different factors control the expression of these genes.

Recently the carbohydrate-rich β-subunit has been cloned.[6-8] RNA analysis has shown that expression of this gene is restricted to the stomach, and in the rat the gene has been localized to chromosome 8. The β-subunits of H^+K^+-ATPase gene and Na^+K^+-ATPase share a 41% amino-acid homology and a number of other structural features, suggesting that the β-subunits evolved from a common ancestral gene.

Finally, the sera of patients with pernicious anaemia have long been known to contain autoantibodies directed against parietal cells. The auto-antigens have now been shown to be the α- and β-subunits of H^+K^+-ATPase.[9] It remains to be seen whether these autoantibodies against the subunits of H^+K^+-ATPase ('endogenous omeprazole') are causally related to the development of autoimmune gastritis.

PANCREAS

Regulation of pancreatic enzyme genes

Pancreatic lipase hydrolyses dietary triglycerides to monoglycerides and fatty acids. In the presence of bile salts the activity of pancreatic lipase is markedly decreased. The activity of pancreatic lipase can be restored by the addition of another pancreatic protein, colipase. Colipase anchors pancreatic lipase non-covalently to the surface of lipid micelles to counteract the destabilizing detergent effect of bile acids.

The gene encoding pancreatic lipase has been cloned, and it has been shown that the expression of this gene is regulated by the amount of fat in the diet.[10] In passing, it is worth recording that the human hepatic lipase gene has also been shown to be closely related to the pancreatic lipase gene; these genes have evolved by duplication of a common ancestral gene.[11]

Human colipase cDNA has been isolated and shown to originate from one gene located on chromosome 6, and that gene expression is limited to the pancreas. The gene encodes a 112-amino-acid procolipase which includes a 17-amino-acid signal sequence.[12,13]

Related to the pancreas, it is of interest that the genes for cholecystokinin (CCK) and secretin have also been cloned. Experiments with the cloned mouse CCK gene have shown that the gene uses the same cap site and splice sites to encode identical CCK molecules in intestine, brain, and kidney.[14] Secretin, which stimulates the secretion of bicarbonate-rich pancreatic fluid, is a small (27-amino-acid) gut hormone whose sequence was long ago elucidated by chemical methods. Secretin cDNA has been difficult to isolate using oligonucleotides because it contains an unusually high number of serine, leucine, and arginine residues. However, through the use of a combination of highly degenerate oligonucleotide primers and PCR, rat and porcine secretin cDNAs have now been isolated.[15] The secretin precursor produced from secretin mRNA consists of a signal sequence, an N-terminal peptide, secretin, and a 72-amino-acid C-terminal peptide. RNA analysis has shown that the secretin gene is expressed throughout the small intestine, but (contrary to earlier reports) secretin is not found in the brain.

LIVER

Hepatocyte growth factor

Hepatocyte growth factor (HGF) was first found in the serum of patients with fulminant hepatic failure[16] and of partially hepatectomized rats[17] and has been shown to be a potent mitogen of hepatocytes in culture. The latest twist in this story is that HGF has now been shown by a variety of criteria to be identical to another protein, scatter factor (SF).[18]

Scatter factor was first identified as a protein secreted by fibroblasts which disperse epithelial cell colonies of various cell types in culture.[19] It was later shown that smooth-muscle cells also secrete SF and that endothelial cells are scattered by it.[20] Scattered cells are highly motile, continuously extending and retracting cell processes; however, SF was not observed to be mitogenic, at least not in one kidney epithelial cell line.[21]

Thus, HGF-SF (the name proposed for this molecule which acts as both a hepatocyte growth factor and a scatter factor) is a mitogen for hepatocytes but stimulates the motility of other cell types. HGF-SF is a heterodimer consisting of large (54–65 kDa) and small (31–35 kDa) subunits. The large subunit contains four kringle domains, which are found in a variety of proteins, such as plasminogen, and which are believed to mediate protein–protein interactions. The small subunit resembles the catalytic subunit of serine proteases. However, the HGF-SF molecule has no protease activity, probably because the histidine and serine residues of the active site are replaced.[22]

Recently the receptor for HGF-SF has also been identified. The receptor turns out to be the product of the c-*met* proto-oncogene.[23, 24] c-*met* is a membrane-bound tyrosine kinase of relative molecular mass 190 kDa which has structural and functional similarities to other growth factors, including platelet-derived and epidermal growth factors.

Clearly, these discoveries, not only of the origin and structure of the growth factor that mediates liver regeneration but also of the membrane receptor that this growth factor binds to, are going to have far-reaching implications for clinical research into liver regeneration in fulminant hepatic failure and cirrhosis. But there are also some tantalizing clues that HGF-SF may play a role in tumour growth and metastasis. HGF-SF is a growth factor for hepatocytes but stimulates the motility of other cell types. It promotes the migration of cells into collagen matrices, mimicking the properties of invasive tumours.[25] Thus, mutations which lead to over-expression of the c-*met* receptor and therefore responsiveness to HGF-SF might confer on tumours the qualities of invasiveness and metastasis.

Role of hepatic lectin in opsonic defect in immunodeficient children

Infants with this immunodeficiency syndrome suffer repeated bacterial and fungal infections between 6 and 18 months of age.[26, 27] The infections may be severe; five deaths have been reported. In these families there are usually relatives who also suffered repeated infections while infants. This immuno-deficiency is common; the estimated frequency is 5–7%.[28, 29] The sites of infection are varied. Otitis media, chronic diarrhoea, and meningitis are the most common diseases, but infected eczema, septicaemia, pneumonia, osteomyelitis, and oral infections are also reported.

The laboratory findings in this immunodeficiency syndrome are charac-teristic. In vitro, normal polymorphonuclear leucocytes, when incubated with serum from patients, do not phagocytose bacteria or yeasts. The defect can be corrected by the addition of heterologous serum, indicating that the patient's serum lacks an opsonin which is essential to prepare the micro-organisms for phagocytosis. Turner et al[30] first showed an association between the opsonic defect and the deposition of low amounts of the complement components C3b/C3bi on the surface of yeast. They then showed that antibody-independent cleavage of C4 occurred when serum was incubated with mannan, a component of the yeast cell wall and that the opsonin mediating this complement cleavage was mannose-binding protein (MBP).[31] Furthermore, they found that children with the opsonic defect had very low serum-MBP levels and that the opsonic defect could be corrected in vitro by the addition of purified MBP to their serum.[32]

MBP is a calcium-dependent lectin secreted by hepatocytes which binds glycoproteins terminating in mannose or N-acetylglucosamine. MBP occurs in serum as a mixture of oligomers of from 9 to 18 identical polypeptide chains of 32 kDa.[33–36] On binding to a mannose-rich surface, MBP activates complement through the classical pathway.[37]

The gene encoding MBP has been cloned.[38, 39] The MBP comprises four exons which each code for different functional domains of the molecule. Exon 1 encodes the signal sequence of a secreted protein, a cysteine-rich domain, and seven copies of the motif Gly-Xaa-Yaa, which is typical of a collagen domain. The junction between exon 1 and exon 2 encodes the sequence Gly-Gln-Gly. Exon 2 encodes a further 12 Gly-Xaa-Yaa collagen repeats. Exon 3 encodes a short 'neck' domain, and exon 4, the largest exon, encodes the carbohydrate-binding domain.

The structure of the high-molecular-weight oligomers of MBP found in serum can be inferred from the organization of the MBP gene. Trimers of the MBP subunit, translated by the MBP gene, associate by the formation of a triplex helix between their collagen domains. The interruption of the collagen motif by the sequence Gly-Gln-Gly between exons 1 and 2, by analogy with C1q, is probably the site where the triple helical chains of MBP appear to bend on electronmicroscopy.[40] The triple helices are stabilized by disulphide bridges between the cysteine-rich domains. These trimers then associate, again by disulphide bridges, into oligomers of from 9 to 18 identical MBP polypeptide chains. This gives the final MBP oligomer the appearance of a bunch of flowers where the flower-heads are the carbohydrate-binding domains and the stalks are the collagen domains.

To determine the molecular basis of this opsonization defect associated with low serum-MBP levels, researchers studied the MBP gene structure in three families with affected children.[41] The data showed that the trans-mission of low serum-MBP levels in the three families fitted best with autosomal dominant inheritance. In probands the sequence showed a point mutation, at base 230 of exon 1, causing a change of codon 54 from G*G*C to G*A*C, resulting in the substitution of aspartic acid for glycine in the translated protein. All 14 family members with low serum-MBP levels were either heterozygous or homozygous for the aspartic acid substitution at codon 54.

This mutation in exon 1 of the MBP gene, by encoding aspartic acid instead of glycine, disrupts the fifth Gly-Xaa-Yaa repeat in the collagen domain of the MBP subunit. The mechanism whereby such a mutation in the collagen domain reduces serum-MBP levels is probably analogous to the mechanism in osteogenesis imperfecta. In osteogenesis imperfecta, mutations of homologous axial glycine residues result in failure of collagen polymerization.[42] This is because in the tightly wound helical coils of collagen only the glycine residues are small enough to pack into the axial (central) positions which occur every third amino acid. Substitution of a glycine by aspartic acid, which is much larger and electrically charged, prevents the collagen chains from winding into a triple helix. Thus, the mutation in the MBP gene appears to result in low serum-MBP levels because of failure of the abnormal MBP subunits to polymerize into functional oligomers.

MBP deficiency appears to be the first example of a lectin deficiency being associated with human disease. The pathology observed in infants with this defect suggests that MBP is a major antigen non-specific defence mechanism in early life. The relevance of MBP in adult infections remains to be determined.

Different proteins from the same gene – RNA editing of apolipoprotein B

At first sight, RNA editing may seem a recherché topic to include in a review of the impact of molecular biology in gastroenterology. However, it seems that this phenomenon accounts for some otherwise inexplicable events. Received wisdom (the 'Central Dogma' in a molecular biologist's terms) states that the sequence of a protein is determined by the DNA structure of its gene and that this is faithfully transcribed into RNA. This primary RNA transcript is spliced to remove the intron sequences, and the exon (coding) sequences rejoin to form mRNA. In the ribosomes, mRNA is translated into the protein sequence. Perhaps predictably, this view is not always correct! RNA editing is the phenomenon whereby an RNA transcript is altered by mechanisms other than splicing.

The first description of RNA editing in mammals involved the alteration of apolipoprotein (apo) B mRNA in the small intestine.[43, 44] ApoB is a major protein constituent of plasma lipoproteins and exists in two forms, apoB-100, which is made by the liver, and apoB-48, which is made by the small intestine. ApoB-100 consists of 4536 amino acids; apoB-48 of 2152 amino acids. However, both apoB-100 and apoB-48 are encoded by an identical gene. In human beings, apoB-100 is the product of a 14-kb mRNA in the liver. ApoB-48 is the product of an intestinal mRNA which is identical to apoB-100 mRNA except for a single base substitution (C to U) at C-6666. This substitution changes the codon CAA (which encodes glutamine) to UAA, a premature stop codon. The mechanism causing this base substitution in the RNA transcript is probably enzymatic conversion of cytosine to uracil by a nucleotide-specific cytosine deaminase.[45] However, why this particular cytosine is selected for modification and not others is unknown. It is possible that a particular flanking sequence specifies which cytosine is modified.[46] Furthermore, when the apoB gene is introduced into cell lines that do not normally synthesize lipoproteins, apoB mRNA editing still occurs, suggesting that RNA editing may be a common phenomenon in mammalian cells. Finally, apoB RNA editing appears to be under metabolic control, since fasting will halve the amount of apoB mRNA edited to possess a premature stop codon and consequently the amount of low-molecular-weight apoB (apoB-48) that is secreted.[47]

Bile acid enzymes cloned

Cholesterol is disposed of from the body either by conversion into bile acids or in association with bile acids in bile. Since two of the major diseases of the West, atheroma and gallstones, are related to defective elimination of cholesterol, the importance of understanding the metabolism of bile acids can readily be seen. 1990 was a bumper year for the relentless onslaught of molecular biology on bile acid metabolism. The rate-limiting enzyme in bile acid synthesis, cholesterol 7α-hydroxylase, was cloned, and the message (mRNA) for the transporter of bile acids into hepatocytes was isolated.

The addition of an hydroxyl group to carbon-7 of the cholesterol nucleus is the first and rate-limiting step in the conversion of cholesterol to a bile acid. This reaction is catalysed by cholesterol 7α-hydroxylase, an enzyme restricted to the endoplasmic reticulum of the hepatocyte. Despite the clinical importance of this enzyme in regulating cholesterol metabolism, there are still large gaps in our understanding of how it is regulated. Crucial questions, of possible therapeutic impact, remain unanswered. For instance, is the rate of bile acid synthesis determined by the amount of enzyme or the amount of its substrate, cholesterol, that is present, and how do bile acids, returning by the entero-hepatic circulation, inhibit bile acid synthesis?

The first advance was the cloning of cDNA for rat cholesterol 7α-hydroxylase by two groups. Using the cDNA as a probe to measure levels of cholesterol 7α-hydroxylase mRNA in the liver, these experiments showed that depleting the bile acid pool with cholestyramine increases expression of the cholesterol 7α-hydroxylase gene, whereas increasing the bile acid pool by feeding bile acids reduces expression of the gene. Furthermore, cholesterol feeding dramatically increases expression of the cholesterol 7α-hydroxylase gene.[48] This observation explains an earlier observation that the rat (but not man) can respond to increased dietary cholesterol by increasing bile acid synthesis.[49]

The phenomenon of the circadian rhythm of bile acid synthesis has also yielded to molecular biology. It was known that in the rat bile acid synthesis is highest at night when the animals feed, but it was not known whether this was due to increased supply of dietary cholesterol, activation of existing enzyme, or synthesis of new cholesterol 7α-hydroxylase. It has now been shown that there is a close correlation, throughout the diurnal cycle, between the amount of cholesterol 7α-hydroxylase, its activity, and the mRNA that encodes it.[50, 51] This confirms that the circadian rhythm of bile acid synthesis is due not to variations in the supply of cholesterol but to a diurnal variation in expression of the cholesterol 7α-hydroxylase gene and hence the supply of new enzyme.

Since then, the cDNA encoding human cholesterol 7α-hydroxylase has been cloned,[52] and the rat cholesterol 7α-hydroxylase gene has been characterized.[53] Soon we shall have the human gene and by study of its control elements shall understand why expression of the rat gene, but not the human gene, is stimulated by cholesterol feeding.

The other area of progress in this field is the work that will lead to cloning the cell membrane transporter that moves bile acids from blood into the hepatocyte. Bile acids uptake by hepatocytes is mediated by a Na^+-bile acid cotransporter on the basolateral membranes of the hepatocyte. The method used to identify the mRNA encoding the Na^+-bile acid cotransporter was expression in *Xenopus laevis* oocytes (frog's eggs). mRNA from rat hepatocytes was injected into the oocytes, and after a few days the oocytes were shown to be able to take up the bile acid taurocholate. The taurocholate uptake was sodium-dependent and saturable, and showed other features characteristic of the Na^+-bile acid cotransporter.[54] With these results it will be relatively straightforward to isolate cDNA for the Na^+-bile acid cotransporter by the technique of 'expression cloning'.

The characterization of these critical genes will undoubtedly revitalize clinical research in bile acid metabolism and gallstone formation.

SUMMARY

This has been just a brief look at the enormous amount of molecular biological work now going on in gastroenterology. Large areas have been left out of this review, including the genetics of cancer, genetic gastrointestinal disease, and molecular virology. One thing is certain – that molecular biology is going to have a steadily increasing impact on all gastroenterologists, ranging from their diagnostic tests, medicines, and vaccines to their clinical research.

REFERENCES

1 Sambrook J, Fritsch EF, Maniatis T. Molecular cloning, a laboratory manual. 2nd ed. Cold Spring Harbor: Cold Spring Harbor Laboratory Press. 1989
2 Hirschowitz BI. Pepsin in the pathogenesis of peptic ulceration. In: Halter F, Garner A, Tytgat GNJ, eds. Mechanisms of peptic ulcer healing. Norwell MA: Kluwer. 1990: pp 183–194
3 Kageyama T, Tanabe K, Koiwai O. Structure and development of rabbit pepsinogens. Stage specific zymogens, nucleotide sequences of cDNAs, molecular evolution and gene expression during development. J Biol Chem 1990; 265: 17 031–17 038
4 Gantz I, Schaffer M, DelValle J et al. Molecular cloning of a gene encoding the histamine H_2 receptor. Proc Natl Acad Sci USA 1991; 88: 429–433
5 Maeda M, Oshiman K, Tamura S, Futai M. Human gastric $(H^+ + K^+)$-ATPase gene. Similarity to $(Na^+ + K^+)$-ATPase genes in exon/intron organisation but difference in control regions. J Biol Chem 1990; 265: 9027–9032
6 Shull GE. cDNA cloning of the beta subunit of the rat gastric H,K ATPase. J Biol Chem 1990; 265: 12 123–12 126
7 Reuben MA, Lasater LS, Sachs G. Characterisation of a beta subunit of the gastric H^+/K^+-transporting ATPase. Proc Natl Acad Sci USA 1990; 87: 6767–6771
8 Canfield VA, Okamoto CT, Chow D et al. Cloning of the H,K-ATPase beta subunit. Tissue specific expression, chromosomal assignment and relationship to NA,K-ATPase beta subunits. J Biol Chem 1990; 265: 19 878–19 884
9 Toh BH, Gleeson PA, Simpson RJ et al. The 60–90 kDa parietal cell autoantigen

associated with autoimmune gastritis is a beta subunit of the gastric H^+/K^+-ATPase (proton pump). Proc Natl Acad Sci USA 1990; 87: 6418–6422

10 Wicker C, Puigserver A. Expression of rat pancreatic lipase gene is modulated by a lipid-rich diet at a transcriptional level. Biochem Biophys Res Commun 1990; 166: 358–364

11 Ameis D, Stahnke G, Kobayashi J et al. Isolation and characterization of the human hepatic lipase gene. J Biol Chem 1990; 265: 6552–6555

12 Lowe ME, Rosenblum JL, McEwen P, Strauss AW. Cloning and characterization of the human colipase cDNA. Biochemistry 1990; 29: 823–828

13 Davis RC, Xia YR, Mohandas T, Schotz MC, Lusis AJ. Assignment of the human pancreatic colipase gene to chromosome 6p21.1 to pter. Genomics 1991; 10: 262–265

14 Vitale M, Vashishtha A, Linzer E, Powell DJ, Friedman JM. Molecular cloning of the mouse CCK gene: expression in different brain regions and during cortical development. Nucleic Acids Res 1991; 19: 169–177

15 Kopin AS, Wheeler MB, Leiter AB. Secretin: structure of the precursor and tissue distribution of the mRNA. Proc Natl Acad Sci USA 1990; 87: 2299–2303

16 Gohda E, Tsubouchi H, Nakayama H et al. Purification and partial characterization of hepatocyte growth factor from plasma of a patient with fulminant hepatic failure. J Clin Invest 1988; 81: 414–419

17 Nakamura T, Nawa K, Ichihara A, Kaise N, Nishino T. Purification and subunit structure of hepatocyte growth factor from rat platelets. FEBS Lett 1987; 224: 311–316

18 Weidner KM, Arakaki N, Hartmann GL et al. Evidence for the identity of human scatter factor and human hepatocyte growth factor. Proc Natl Acad Sci USA 1991; 88: 7001–7005

19 Stoker M, Gherardi E, Perryman M, Gray J. Scatter factor is a fibroblast derived of epithelial cell mobility. Nature 1987; 327: 239–242

20 Rosen EM, Carley W, Goldberg ID. Scatter factor regulates vascular endothelial cell motility. Cancer Invest 1990; 8: 647–650

21 Gherardi E, Gray J, Stoker M, Perryman M, Furlong R. Purification of scatter factor, a fibroblast-derived basic protein that modulates epithelial interactions and movement. Proc Natl Acad Sci USA 1989; 86: 5844–5848

22 Nakamura T, Nishizawa T, Hagiya M et al. Molecular cloning and expression of human hepatocyte growth factor. Nature 1989; 342: 440–443

23 Naldini L, Vigna E, Narsimahn RP et al. Hepatocyte growth factor (HGF) stimulates the tyrosine kinase activity of the receptor encoded by the proto-oncogene *c-met*. Oncogene 1991; 6: 501–504.

24 Bottaro DP, Rubin JS, Faletto DL et al. Identification of the hepatocyte growth factor receptor as the *c-met* proto-oncogene product. Science 1991; 251: 802–804

25 Weidner KM, Behrens J, Vandekerckhove J, Birchmeier W. Scatter factor: molecular characteristics and effect on the invasiveness of epithelial cells. J Cell Biol 1990; 111: 2097–2108

26 Miller ME, Seals J, Kaye R, Levitsky LC. A familial, plasma associated defect of phagocytosis. Lancet 1968; 2: 60–63

27 Soothill JF, Harvey BAM. Defective opsonization: a common immunity deficiency. Arch Dis Child 1976; 51: 91–99

28 Levinsky RJ, Harvey BAM, Paleja A. A rapid objective method for measuring the yeast opsonization activity of serum. J Immunol Method 1978; 24: 251–256

29 Kerr MA, Falconer JS, Bashey A, Swanson Beck J. The effect on C3 levels of yeast opsonization by normal and pathological sera: identification of a complement independent opsonin. Clin Exp Immunol 1983; 54: 793–800

30 Turner MW, Mowbray JF, Robertson DR. A study of C3b deposition on yeast surfaces by sera of known opsonic potential. Clin Exp Immunol 1981; 46: 412–419

31 Super M, Levinsky RJ, Turner MW. The level of mannan binding protein regulates the binding of complement-derived opsonins to mannan and zymosan at low serum concentrations. Clin Exp Immunol 1990; 79: 144–150

32 Super M, Thiel S, Lu J, Levinsky RJ, Turner MW. Association of low levels of mannan-binding proteins with a common defect of opsonisation. Lancet 1989; 2: 1236–1239

33 Wild J, Robinson D, Winchester B. Isolation of mannose-binding proteins from human and rat liver. Biochem J 1983; 210: 167–174

34 Kawasaki N, Kawasaki T, Yamashina I. Isolation and characterization of a mannan-binding protein from human serum. J Biochem (Tokyo) 1983; 94: 937–947

35 Summerfield JA, Taylor ME. Mannose-binding proteins in human serum: identification of mannose specific immunoglobulins and a calcium-dependent lectin, of broader carbohydrate specificity, secreted by hepatocytes. Biochim Biophys Acta 1986; 883: 197–206

36 Taylor ME, Summerfield JA. Carbohydrate binding proteins of human serum: isolation of two mannose/fucose-specific lectins. Biochim Biophys Acta 1987; 915: 60–67

37 Lu J, Thiel S, Wiedemann H, Timpl R, Reid KBM. Binding of the pentamer/hexamer forms of mannan binding protein to zymosan activates the proenzyme C1r2C1s2 complex of the classical pathway of complement without involvement of C1q. J Immunol 1990; 144: 2287–2294

38 Taylor ME, Brickell PM, Craig RK, Summerfield JA. Structure and evolutionary origin of the gene encoding a human serum mannose-binding protein. Biochem J 1989; 262: 763–771

39 Sastry K, Herman GA, Day L et al. The human mannose-binding protein gene. J Exp Med 1989; 170: 1175–1189

40 Thiel S, Reid KBM. Structures and functions associated with the group of mammalian lectins containing collagen-like sequences. FEBS Lett 1989; 250: 78–84

41 Sumiya M, Super M, Tabona T et al. Molecular basis of opsonic defect in immunodeficient children. Lancet 1991; 337: 1569–1570

42 Sykes B. Inherited collagen disorders. Mol Biol Med 1989; 6: 19–26

43 Powell LM, Wallis SC, Pease RJ, Edwards YH, Knott TJ, Scott J. A novel form of tissue specific RNA processing produces apolipoprotein B48 in intestine. Cell 1987; 50: 831–840

44 Chen SH, Habib G, Yang CY et al. Apolipoprotein B48 is the product of a messenger RNA with an organ-specific in frame stop codon. Science 1987; 238: 363–366

45 Bostrom K, Garcia Z, Poksay KS, Johnson DF, Lusis AJ, Innerarity TL. Apolipoprotein B mRNA editing. Direct determination of the edited base and occurrence in non-apolipoprotein B-producing cell lines. J Biol Chem 1990; 265: 22 446–22 452

46 Chen SH, Li X, Liao WSL, Wu JH, Chan L. RNA editing of apolipoprotein B. Sequence specificity determined by in vitro coupled transcription editing. J Biol Chem 1990; 265: 6811–6816

47 Leighton JK, Joyner J, Zamarripa J, Deines M, Davis RA. Fasting decreases apolipoprotein B mRNA editing and the secretion of small molecular weight apoB by rat hepatocytes: evidence that the total amount of apoB secreted is regulated post-transcriptionally. J Lipid Res 1990; 31: 1663–1668

48 Jelinek DF, Anderson S, Slaughter CA, Russell DW. Cloning and regulation of cholesterol 7α-hydroxylase, the rate limiting enzyme in bile acid synthesis. J Biol Chem 1990; 265: 8190–8197

49 Wilson JD. The quantification of cholesterol excretion and degradation in the isotopic steady state in the rat: the influence of dietary cholesterol. J Lipid Res 1964; 5: 409–417

50 Noshiro M, Nishimoto M, Morohashi K, Okuda K. Molecular cloning of cDNA for cholesterol 7α-hydroxylase from rat liver microsomes. FEBS Lett 1989; 257: 97–100

51 Noshiro M, Nishimoto M, Okuda K. Rat liver cholesterol 7α-hydroxylase: pretranslational regulation for circadian rhythm. J Biol Chem 1990; 265: 10 036–10 041

52 Noshiro M, Okuda K. Molecular cloning and sequence analysis of cDNA encoding human cholesterol 7α-hydroxylase. FEBS Lett 1990; 268: 137–140

53 Jelinek DF, Russell DW. Structure of the rat gene encoding cholesterol 7α-hydroxylase. Biochemistry 1990; 29: 7781–7785

54 Hagenbuch B, Lubbert H, Stieger B, Meier PJ. Expression of the hepatocyte Na$^+$-bile acid cotransporter in *Xenopus laevis* oocytes. J Biol Chem 1990; 265: 5357–5360

6

Pancreatic disease

J. P. Neoptolemos

Diseases of the pancreas are being studied intensively at present, and particularly fruitful results have emerged when epidemiologists, clinicians, and basic scientists have collaborated. In this chapter, exciting developments in selected areas relating to pancreatic cancer, chronic pancreatitis, acute pancreatitis, pancreas divisum, and cystic fibrosis are highlighted.

PANCREATIC CANCER

Epidemiology and aetiology

This has been well-reviewed recently.[1, 2] The only factor to emerge from epidemiological studies showing a causative link with pancreatic cancer is tobacco smoking;[3] this has recently been confirmed in experimental studies.[4] The odds ratio (relative risk) is only about 2.0, indicating other, perhaps more important, aetiological factors. For example, epidemiological and case-control studies suggest that diets which are high in fat are tumour-promoting; this has also been demonstrated in experimental studies.[5] The increased incidence of pancreatic cancer observed over the last 60 years could be related to the consumption of polyunsaturated (N-6) fats, since these cause maximum release of CCK-PZ,[6] which has been found to be tumour-promoting in experimental models.[7]

Molecular and cell biology

A genetic basis for the development of pancreatic cancer is suggested by reports of familial clustering of the disease and by the growing list of autosomal dominant disorders associated with pancreatic cancer, including Gardner's syndrome, Lynch type II syndrome, hereditary pancreatitis, MEN-1, and glucagonoma syndrome.[8] Falk et al[9] have reported an odds ratio of 5.25 for pancreatic cancer in those with a close relative who has the disease. The genetic basis is not fully understood, but an identical allelic loss (INT-2 (SS6) locus of chromosome 11_q13) has been described in sporadic and familial pancreatic endocrine tumours.[10]

The role of growth factors and oncogenes has been reviewed extensively.[11, 13] Pancreatic cancer may be under autocrine control, particularly involving TGF-α as the ligand for EGFr and hormonal or paracrine control by CCK-PZ, bombesin, VIP, and somatostatin. The role of steroid sex hormones in pancreatic oncogenes is less certain.[13] A striking feature of pancreatic cancer is that well over 75% of these tumours have point mutations of the Kis-*ras* oncogene (G protein) exclusively affecting codon 12 (mainly G-T transversions) at the first or second codon. Moreover, 60% of cancers have been shown to overexpress mutant forms of the tumour-suppressor gene p53.[14] These observations are important since *ras* oncogenes are known to upregulate TGF-α expression and there is co-operation between *ras* and (mutant) p 53 in malignant transformation in vitro. DNA analysis following polymerase chain reaction (PCR) or immunohisto-chemical techniques to detect these abnormalities may be applied to cyto-logical aspirates and may permit the precise differential diagnosis between cancer and chronic pancreatitis.[14, 15]

Diagnosis and staging

Despite the development of newer serum markers for pancreatic cancer, their sensitivity and specificity remain insufficient for use either in popula-tion screening or primary diagnosis.[16] Similarly, radioimmunolocalization is insufficiently accurate for routine diagnosis.[17] The important diagnostic modalities remain ultrasound, ERCP,[18] and contrast-enhanced CT scan-ning.[19] Endoluminal (endoscopic) ultrasonography has been shown to have a near 100% detection rate for pancreatic cancer, including tumours smaller than 2 cm.[20] Endoluminal ultrasound may have a particular place in

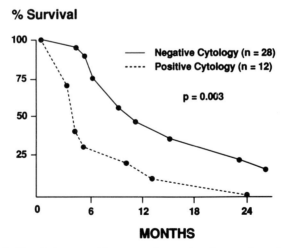

Fig. 6.1   Survival in relation to positive or negative cytology from peritoneal washings prior to surgery in patients' potentially curative resections. (Adapted with permission from Warshaw[23].)

staging: its overall accuracy is 80–90% and its detection of lymph nodes is around 75%. Particular difficulties remain in distinguishing inflammatory pseudotumours of the pancreas and in differentiating between metastatic and reactive lymphadenopathy. Contrast-enhanced CT has developed to become the main staging tool for surgeons;[19] laparoscopy may have a role in detecting peritoneal seedlings and small surface liver metastases not detected by other means.[21]

Ultrasound-guided core-biopsy is probably the best available technique for obtaining a tissue diagnosis, yielding an overall accuracy of 93% for pancreatic cancer.[22] Its routine use, however, should now be questioned, since Warshaw[23] has reported positive cytology by peritoneal washing in 75% of patients who had percutaneous biopsy, as compared to only 19% without biopsy ($P < 0.01$). Moreover, long-term survival was significantly related to positive cytology on peritoneal washings (Fig. 6.1). Thus, percutaneous biopsies should be considered only in certain patients, notably those in whom resection is precluded because of advanced disease or suspected lymphoma.

Palliative treatment: endoscopic stenting vs. surgical bypass

These techniques have been compared in three prospective randomized trials.[24–26] The data indicate reduced hospital mortality in favour of the endoscopic route, but this is accompanied by a greater risk of duodenal stenosis and recurrent jaundice (Table 6.1). Uncontrolled data suggest a trend for longer survival in patients who have undergone surgical bypass.[27] Taken together, these studies indicate that elderly, relatively unfit patients should be stented in comparison to surgical bypass for younger patients.

Curative resection and adjuvant therapy

Attitudes to surgical resection are beginning to change for two main reasons. Firstly, in the hands of experienced surgeons, the mortality of resectional surgery is less than 10%.[28] For example, Trede et al[29] have reported no deaths in a consecutive series of 91 pancreatoduodenectomies, and Spencer et al[30] reported a 9% mortality in 42 patients aged 70 years or older. Secondly, it is now appreciated that the poor long-term survival rate may be improved by using adjuvant therapy, radiotherapy, chemotherapy, or a combination of these.[31] Thus, the GITSG study[32] reported a 2-year survival rate of 43% following resection with 40 Gy external beam radiotherapy and intravenous 5-FU. Total pancreatectomy offers no advantage over the standard Kausch–Whipple procedure and produces a worse physiological outcome;[28] indeed, the more conservative pylorus-preserving pancreaticoduodenectomy results in an even more pleasing long-term

Table 6.1   Results of three randomized trials of endoscopic stenting vs. operative biliary bypass for pancreatic cancer

Variable	Shepherd et al 1988[26]		Dowsett et al 1989[25]		Anderson et al 1989[24]	
	Stent	Surgery	Stent	Surgery	Stent	Surgery
Number of patients	23	23	101	103	25	19
Successful drainage	91%	92%	94%	91%	96%	84%
30-day mortality	9%	20%	7%[a]	17%	0%	0%
Recurrent jaundice	17%	2%	18%[a]	3%	28%	16%
Duodenal stenosis	0%	0%	6%[a]	1%	0%	0%
Survival	152 days[b]	125 days[b]	5 mths[c]	5 mths[c]	84 days[b]	100 days[b]

[a] significant difference; [b] median; [c] mean.

physiological outcome without compromising survival.[33] For these reasons it is not tenable to stent patients without first giving most patients the benefit of a specialist surgical opinion.

In the future it may be possible to select patients for adjuvant treatment based on predictors such as preoperative cytology of peritoneal washings,[23] tumour DNA ploidy status,[34] and postresection levels of CA 19–9.[35]

CHRONIC PANCREATITIS

Classification and aetiology

The earlier classifications of Cambridge and Marseilles have undergone some useful refinements.[36, 37] Included now are obstructive pancreatopathy characterized by peri-lobular fibrosis,[38] and hypertensive pancreatopathy associated with stenosis or hyperkinesia of the sphincter of Oddi.[39] In these types, symptomatic improvement usually follows relief of the physical or functional obstruction by surgery or endoscopy. The connection between imaging procedures and function has been examined with an excellent correlation for the later stages of the disease but not the earlier ones.[40]

While the link between chronic alcohol abuse and chronic pancreatitis is beyond doubt, the mechanisms involved are not.[41] The acinar cells show a state of chronic stimulation; the pancreatic juice is viscid, showing low bicarbonate; increased amounts of calcium, protein, and lactoferrin; an increased ratio of lysosomal to digestive hydrolases; and reduced pancreatic trypsin inhibitor. Considerable interest has been shown in the composition of the protein plugs found with a high frequency in the pancreatic juice of patients with chronic calcific pancreatitis. According to Sarles et al,[37] the major component of these plugs is a degraded form of pancreatic stone protein (PSP), and other degraded varieties are found with calcium and salt precipitates in pancreatic stones. How all these observations fit into the aetiology of chronic pancreatitis is still a matter of speculation.

A powerful hypothesis has been developed round PSP (lithostathine) which states that the initial common pathway for all types of chronic pancreatitis is decreased secretion of PSP. Evidence in support of this hypothesis includes the following observations:

1. There is impaired acinar cell secretion of PSP by ethanol.
2. PSP prevents calcium precipitation in saturated solutions.
3. mRNA for PSP is reduced in chronic pancreatitis, irrespective of aetiology.
4. PSP is decreased in the pancreatic juice of patients with chronic pancreatitis.
5. The pancreatic stone composition of patients with tropical pancreatitis is similar to that of Western pancreatitis.
6. Childhood hereditary dominant pancreatitis is also associated with reduced PSP in pancreatic juice.[37]

Recent work, however, has challenged important elements of this hypothesis. Schmiegel et al[42] have shown PSP to be secreted in similar amounts in patients with pancreatic cancer and chronic pancreatitis. Moreover, significantly increased levels of PSP were found in the sera of patients with acute as well as chronic pancreatitis.

A role for heightened free-radical activity in chronic pancreatitis is suggested by the finding of an increase in the serum molar ratio of octadeca-9,11-dienoic acid (18:2,n-7) to linoleic acid (18:2,n-6) in such patients.[43] An alternative explanation is that an increase in this ratio reflects the increased turnover of linoleic acid which occurs in relative malnutrition. Furthermore, this ratio was no different in duodenal juice obtained following secretin-pancreozymin stimulation, although there was an increase in diene conjugates as measured by absorbence in a (largely separate) group of patients with chronic pancreatitis. Since similar findings were obtained in patients following an attack of acute pancreatitis,[43] as well as increased pancreatic tissue lipid peroxidation in patients with acute pancreatitis,[44] it seems that free radicals are a common end-point of pancreatic inflammation but not necessarily the initiating aetiological factor, as suggested by Guyan et al.[43]

It has recently been proposed that induction of the pancreatic cytochrome $p450$ systems is the cause of excess free radicals; the failure to detect these in the pancreatic juice of patients with chronic pancreatitis is ascribed to methodological difficulties.[45]

Another hypothesis has been proposed by Figarella et al.[46] A critical aspect appears to be the intracellular activation of trypsinogen 1, which may be autoactivated at pH 5, or, alternatively, by cathepsin B following colocalization of digestive enzymes and lysosomes. This ultimately leads to the precipitation of protein X, which is identical to the pancreatic thread protein, and a form of pancreatic stone protein.[47] Finally, the role of colocalization may have to be modified in view of convincing evidence that this is not a pathological condition but a protective physiological mechanism.[48]

Medical treatment of chronic pancreatitis

In a recent review of the role of enzyme therapy, Ihse & Permerth concluded that enzyme supplements are worth trying in patients before steatorrhoea develops.[49] Patients' self-regulation of enzyme supplementation may provide optimum results.[50] The notion that the mechanism of action is due to feedback inhibition, however, is not supported by some work.[51]

Octreotide is a long-acting somatostatin analogue (half-life 113 mins after subcutaneous injection) which offers possibilities in the management of pain in chronic pancreatitis. Already it has been shown to be valuable in treating pancreatic fistulas[52] and to reduce this complication following pancreatic surgery.[53] Used in seven patients with painful pseudocysts, octreotide reduced the size of pseudocysts in four (by 29–52%) after only 2 weeks, resulting in complete relief of symptoms.[54]

Uden et al[55] have reported a placebo-controlled crossover trial of an antioxidant cocktail in 28 patients with recurrent/chronic pancreatitis. Although the data suggested a benefit from the new treatment, further studies will be required before this can be accepted as standard therapy.

Whereas coeliac plexus block with alcohol or phenol has some value in treating pain due to pancreatic cancer, this is not so in chronic pancreatitis. The use of a steroid coeliac plexus block deserves wider consideration. If the patient responds, treatment can be repeated if need be, and, unlike alcoholic coeliac plexus block, it does not further complicate resectional surgery if that should be required. Such treatment was effective in 4/5 cases that were not opiate dependent but worked in only 1/12 cases that were.[56] This again emphasizes the need for effective treatment *before* narcotic dependence and, in particular, for consideration of resection.

Endoscopic management

The cause of pain in chronic pancreatitis is likely to be multifactorial. Recently it has been possible to demonstrate a clear relationship between ductal and tissue pressure with pain and subsequent improvement by decompression.[57, 58] Endoscopic methods of draining the main pancreatic duct may be able to supplement those of surgery.

In a few patients with papillary stenosis, endoscopic sphincterotomy (ES) alone may suffice.[59] Fuji et al,[60] have also reported improvement in pain following ES in eight patients with an abnormal main pancreatic duct (MPD) but without papillary strictures or dysfunction. Strictures of the MPD may be treated by dilatation alone, but more commonly a stent is inserted with multiple side-holes, or a naso-pancreatic catheter is used. The latter is similar to a naso-biliary catheter but differs in having a straight tip and multiple side-holes extending further back.[59, 61] The technical success rate is high and although the technique is associated with a low complication rate, a death has been reported as caused by perforation following ES (Table 6.2). The stents may be left in situ for several months or longer, and clinical improvement may be sustained following removal. Patients may remain asymptomatic with stent clogging,[59] but there is concern that sepsis may develop, as sepsis can seriously complicate subsequent surgery. Stents may occasionally migrate into the MPD and can usually be retrieved endoscopically, although surgery may be required. Mild to moderate exacerbation of MPD stricturing, which can become severe, may follow stent insertion.[66, 67]

Complete stone clearance from the MPD by using ES and the Dormia basket has been achieved in 67 of 82 (82%) cases, although extra-corporeal shock-wave lithotripsy (ESWL) was also required in 17

Table 6.2   Results of endoscopic stenting in chronic pancreatitis (Adapted from Geenen & Rolny[65].)

Series	No. of patients	Success rate	Clinical improvement	Stent time (mths)	Follow-up (mths)	Complications
Huibregtse et al 1988[59]	11	8	7 (87%)	2–41	2–69	2 (18%)
McCarthy et al 1988[62]	5	5 (100%)	4 (80%)	6–36	6–36	2 (40%)
Grimm et al 1989[61]	NA	(31)	NA	2–36	1–36	NA (1†)
Kozarek et al 1989[63]	3	3 (100%)	3 (100%)	4–6	0–8	0
Siegel et al 1989[64]	44	44 (100%)	41 (93%)	2–18	0–72	NA
Geenen et al* 1991[65]	10	8 (80%)	5 (63%)	3–12	0–36	0
Total ≠	73	68 (93%)	60 (82%)	2–41	0–72	2 (7%) (1%†)

* quoted by Geenen & Rolny;[65] † death; ≠ only patients that could be evaluated; NA = not applicable.

patients.[59-61, 64, 68-70] Improvement in pain was noted in 25 of 42 (60%) cases that could be evaluated; complications occurred in up to 21%, but this was usually only mild pancreatitis, and there have been no deaths.

Percutaneous needle aspiration of pseudocysts is associated with a high recurrence rate (about 75%), but prolonged catheter drainage and pseudo-cystogastrostomy stenting are associated with success rates of 60–100%.[71, 72] Henrikssen & Hanck[73] have reported success in 31 (97%) patients treated by percutaneous pancreatic cystogastrostomy with five (17%) complications. Endoscopically, it is now possible to perform endo-cystogastrostomy or endocystoduodenostomy, depending upon the position of the pseudocyst.[74-79] In over 100 cases treated, there was a technical success rate of 98% with resolution of the pseudocysts in 84%, although 15% required additional surgery.[65] The complication rate was 12%, including perforation (3%), bleeding (5%), and infection (4%); there was a low mortality of 1.3%. With a follow-up period of 2–84 months, there was a recurrence rate of 14% and a need to undertake further surgery in 11%. Bleeding, when it occurs, can be massive, and adequate surgical support is necessary to avoid mortality.[75, 80] More recently, transpapillary drainage has been described for communicating pseudocysts,[59, 61, 79] but is no less hazardous than the puncture techniques, since pancreatitis, infection, and death have all been reported.

Successful endoscopic biliary drainage has been reported in 24 of 34 (79%) patients with jaundice or cholangitis caused by pancreatic head obstruction in chronic pancreatitis.[75, 81] In 14 patients with a follow-up of 7–42 months, two deaths occurred which were due to sepsis; stent migration ($n = 10$) or blockage ($n = 8$) resulted in recurrent jaundice in 12 patients and cholangitis in four.[75] In 25 patients with a mean follow-up of 14 months, initial success was 100%, but two patients died within 2 months.[81] Follow-up in 19 patients revealed a high incidence of stent blockage, stent migration, and cholangitis. Only three patients were asymptomatic following stent removal. Similarly, poor results were reported by Cheng et al[82] in 26 patients (mean follow-up 1.7 months). In contrast, the results of surgery were excellent with a success rate of 95–100% and virtually no mortality.[83]

New operations for chronic pancreatitis

Pancreatitis-associated neuritis is a new concept which has been proposed to account for pain in chronic pancreatitis. This is based on an ultrastructural analysis which has revealed preferential preservation of nerves while the parenchyma was replaced by fibrosis. The increase in mean diameters of the nerves argues against constriction from oedema or fibrosis as the mechanism. Disintegration of the perineurium makes the nerves susceptible to a variety of bioactive materials.[84] The sensory nature of the nerves involved is confirmed by finding increased substance P and calcitonin-gene related peptide.[85]

This concept gives strength to the idea that resection in dominant active disease is of value in certain patients with intractable pain. The problems with traditional left-sided resectional surgery are: (a) high incidence of recurrence with lesser procedures; (b) the development of diabetes mellitus (since the islets are predominantly in the tail); and (c) the loss of the spleen. Conversely, traditional resection of the head of the gland (Kausch–Whipple) has been associated with a high morbidity both short- and long-term. Surgical developments have recently overcome a number of these problems.

Distal pancreatectomy can now be safely performed while preserving an intact spleen.[86] The importance of preserving the pylorus during proximal resection for chronic pancreatitis, following pioneering work by Watson in 1944 and Klempa in 1978,[87] has recently been confirmed.[88] This concept has been further extended to preserving the duodenum. A 16-year experience involving 141 patients indicated a low mortality (0.7%); 77% were completely asymptomatic, 67% returned to employment, and glucose metabolism was unchanged or improved in 90%.[89] The success of Beger's operation (Fig. 6.2) has been confirmed in another series of 24 cases by Wilker et al.[90] Similarly, Russell's operation for end-stage disease involves a total pancreatectomy with duodenum preservation, providing good long-term results in the 28 patients so reported.[91]

Part of the value of Beger's operation is the improvement in ductal drainage of the relatively normal part of the gland. The long-term results indicate stability of the disease in most patients and even some improvement, a notion at some odds with traditional teaching. This is supported by another study of 68 patients of whom 30 had ductal drainage; excluding severe cases, we find that only 16% who had drainage developed progressive disease, as compared to 71% who did not.[92] Equally intriguing is the report by Amman et al[93] revealing regression of calcification in a third of patients with chronic pancreatitis, most of whom had ductal drainage. Such studies suggest that earlier intervention to improve drainage of the MPD, either endoscopically or surgically, may modify long-term outcome.

ACUTE PANCREATITIS

Diagnosis and treatment of necrotizing pancreatitis

It is only within the last 5–6 years that the importance of high-dose-bolus contrast-enhanced CT scanning has become recognized as an accurate indicator of the extent of pancreatic necrosis.[94] This is now a mandatory investigation allowing a rational approach for the indicaton and timing of surgical intervention. This has contributed to a relatively low mortality of 8–18% in patients treated by necrosectomy and closed peritoneal lavage.[95, 96] The need for surgery cannot be entirely dependent upon CT,[97] and other objective means of assessment are under scrutiny. These include clinical systems such as APACHE-II,[98] and serum markers such as C-reactive protein,[99] phospholipase A_2,[100] and granulocyte elastase.[101] The finding of a disrupted pancreatic duct by ERCP in the presence of CT-delineated necrosis may be another useful indication for intervention.[102] *On admission*, CT can effectively predict outcome, but overall it is no better than clinicobiochemical assessment.[103]

Bradley has proposed 'open packing' following debridement which has necessitated multiple repeat laparotomies. This approach has now been modified by using closed drainage and lavage, once granulation tissue appears in the retroperitoneum.[104] The technique appears comparable to closed lavage from the outset with a mortality of 14%. The success rate of percutaneous methods of treating pancreatic fluid collections is reported as 65–79%,[105, 106] but at present this approach is regarded as an adjunct to surgery rather than a complete alternative.

Improvements in medical therapy are much required. Increasing appreciation of the patho-biochemical nature of pancreatitis, in particular, the damaging role of leucocyte by-products, has led to several novel approaches, including the use of antioxidants; antagonists of TNF, leukotrienes, and plasminogen activation factor; urinary trypsin inhibitor; and recombinant pancreatic secretory trypsin inhibitor.[107, 108] Blanket anti-protease therapy with high-dose, fresh-frozen plasma, however, has proved to be disappointing.[109]

Severe gallstone pancreatitis

Although the evidence is largely indirect, it does appear that severe cases of acute pancreatitis caused by gallstones are associated with obstruction to the pancreatic duct.[110] Not only has ERCP been shown to be relatively safe in acute pancreatitis, but also two prospective randomized trials have shown that if ES is performed early in the attack, morbidity and mortality are reduced.[111, 112] In over 1000 patients so treated, the complication rate has been only 6% with a mortality of 2%, results which are superior to those of surgery[113] (Table 6.3). Although there is little effect by ES on mild cases, it may be useful in elderly patients with a gallbladder in situ, as it seems to prevent further attacks.[114] ES and stenting may also be successful in treating selected cases of pancreatic necrosis.[79]

PANCREAS DIVISUM

Epidemiological data continue to be produced either supporting[115] or not supporting[116] a role for divisum as an aetiological factor in pancreatitis. Nevertheless, the evidence that pancreas divisum is relevant when it is associated with a degree of sphincter obstruction (organic or functional) is

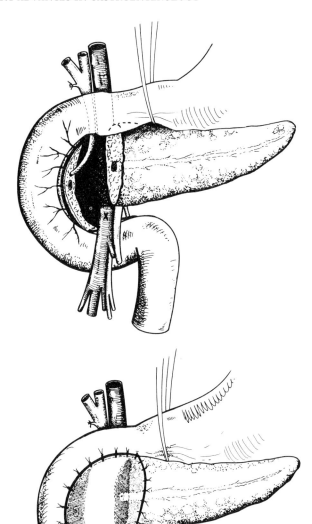

A

B

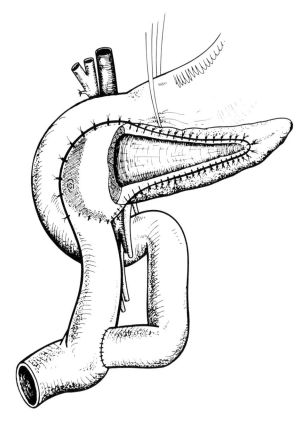

C

Fig. 6.2 Duodenum-preserving resection of the head of the pancreas for chronic pancreatitis, as described by Beger.[89] The extent of resection is shown in **A** and a standard reconstruction in **B**; this may be combined with a pancreatico-jejunostomy if there is a large irregular duct in the remnant, as shown in **C**.

now substantial; this evidence includes studies of exocrine and endocrine function,[117] manometry,[118] and secretion-provocation testing with pancreatic duct measurement by CT[119] or ultrasound.[120] Endoscopic treatment of the minor papilla is available either by ES[121] or stenting.[122] Major problems include the low symptomatic success rate, restenosis, and stent migration. Surgery appears to be much more effective than endoscopic treatment.[123] Indeed, Siegel et al[122] have indicated that stenting should be used only as a therapeutic predictor of eventual surgical outcome; this has been rejected by some surgeons because of the lack of evidence that it can predict outcome and because of the complications associated with endoprostheses. The results overall are best for those patients with documented recurrent attacks of acute pancreatitis (success rates 71–82%) rather than pancreatic pain syndrome (success rates 40–56%).

Table 6.3 Results of endoscopic sphincterotomy for acute pancreatitis in 17 series worldwide, 1978–1990 inclusive: multicentre studies[†]

Series	Number	Complications	Deaths
Classen et al 1978	17	0	0
Van Spuy 1981	10	1	0
Kautz et al 1982	21	1	1
Reimann & Lux 1984	15	0	0
Rosseland & Solhaug 1984	29	2	1
Van Hussen 1986	44	2	1
Escourrou et al 1987[†]	92	2	2
Leung et al 1987	15	0	1
Neoptolemos et al 1988	37	3	0
Farkas et al 1988[†]	284	15	5
Safrany 1989[*]	179	15	5
Uomo et al 1989	35	0	0
Lygren et al 1990	21	0	1
Nowak et al 1990	101	12	1
Dufek et al 1990	76	1	0
Shemesh et al 1990	18	1	0
Saowaros 1990	16	3	0
Total	1010	58 (5.7%)	18 (1.8%)

[*] Personal communication.
For references in this table, see Neoptolemos et al.[113]

CYSTIC FIBROSIS

The study of cystic fibrosis at the molecular level may have major implications for predictive diagnosis of this disease.[124] In addition, elucidation of the basic defect may enable the development of specific therapy. The cystic fibrosis gene product is called the cystic fibrosis transmembrane regulator (CFTR), and it resembles a family of membrane transporter proteins which includes the multidrug-resistance protein.[125] Point mutations leading to inactivation of CFTR may result in the closing of cell surface membrane chloride channels. Exactly how CFTR interacts with other key cell signal transducers and messengers, such as protein kinase C, phospholipase C and A_2, and arachidonic acid, is under intense investigation.[126] Such studies may ultimately give important clues as to the pathogenesis of other pancreatic diseases.

CONCLUSIONS

There have been great improvements in the diagnosis and treatment of pancreatic disease, but this has been possible only because of the formation of specialist clinical units. This trend must be continued since it is only in this manner that standards can be improved, and such units also enable us to evaluate the new forms of treatment that basic research is revealing.

ACKNOWLEDGEMENTS

I am very grateful to the Medical Illustration Department, Dudley Road Hospital, Birmingham, UK, for Figures 6.1 and 6.2, and to Fay Cox and Dilys Thomas for secretarial assistance.

REFERENCES

1 Boyle P, Hsieh C, Maisonneuve P et al. Epidemiology of pancreas cancer. Int J Pancreatol 1989; 5: 327–346
2 Haddock G, Carter DC. Aetiology of Pancreatic Cancer. Br J Surg 1990; 77: 1159–1166
3 International Agency for Research on Cancer. IARC monographs on the evaluation of carcinogenic risk of chemicals to man. Vol 38. Tobacco smoking. Lyon, France: IARC. 1986
4 Rivenson A, Hoffman D, Prokopczk B, Amin S, Hecht SS. Induction of long and exocrine pancreas tumours in F344 rats by tobacco-specific and Areca-derived N-nitrosamines. Cancer Res 1988; 48: 6912–6917
5 Birt DF, Julius AD, White LT, Pour PM. Enhancement of pancreatic carcinogenesis in hamsters fed a high fat diet ad libitum and at a controlled calorie intake. Cancer Res 1989; 49: 5848–5851
6 Beardshall K, Frost G, Morarji Y, Domin J, Bloom SR, Calam J. Saturation of fat and cholecystokinin release: implications for pancreatic carcinogenesis. Lancet 1989; 2: 1008–1010
7 Douglas BR, Woutersen RA, Jansen JBMJ, DeJong AJL, Rovati LC, Lamers CBHW. Modulation by CR-1409 (lorglymide), a cholecystokinin receptor antagonist of trypsin-enhanced growth of azaserine-induced putative neoplastic lesions in rat pancreas. Cancer Res 1989; 49: 2438–2441
8 Lynch HT, Fitzsimmons ML, Smyrk TC et al. Familial pancreatic cancer: clinicopathologic study of 18 nuclear families. Am J Gastroenterol 1989; 85: 54–70
9 Falk RT, Pickle LW, Fontham ET et al. Occupation and pancreatic cancer risk in Louisiana. Am J Ind Med 1990; 18: 565–576
10 Teh BT, Hayward NK, Wilkinson S, Woods GM, Cameron D, Shepherd JJ. Clonal loss of INT-2 alleles in sporadic and familial pancreatic endocrine tumours. Br J Cancer 1990; 62: 253–254
11 Lemoine NR, Hall PA. Growth factors and oncogenes in pancreatic cancer. Clin Gastroenterol 1990; 4: 815–832
12 Gillespie J, Poston GJ. The molecular biology of pancreatic adenocarcinoma. In: Johnson CD, Imrie CW, eds. Pancreatic disease: progress and prospects. London: Springer-Verlag, 1991: pp 47–64
13 Andren-Sandberg A, Backman PL. Sex hormones and pancreatic cancer. Clin Gastroenterol 1990; 4: 941–952
14 Barton CM, Staddon SL, Hughes CM et al. Abnormalities of the p53 tumour suppressor gene in human pancreatic cancer. Br J Cancer 1991; 64: 1076–1082
15 Tada M, Omata M, Ohto M. Clinical application of *ras* gene mutation for diagnosis of pancreatic adenocarcinoma. Gastroenterology 1991; 100: 233–238
16 Rhodes JM, Ching CK. Serum diagnostic tests for pancreatic cancer. Clin Gastroenterol 1990; 4: 833–854
17 Allum WH. Radioimmunolocalization of tumours of the pancreas and biliary tree. Clin Gastroenterol 1990; 4: 853–868
18 Shemesh E, Czerniak A, Nass S, Klein E. Role of endoscopic retrograde cholangiopancreatography in differentiating pancreatic cancer co-existing with chronic pancreatitis. Cancer 1990; 65: 893–896
19 Freeny PC, Marks WM, Ryan JA. Pancreatic ductal adenocarcinoma: diagnosis and staging with dynamic CT. Radiology 1888; 166: 125–133
20 Grimm H, Maydeo A, Soehendra N. Endoluminal ultrasound for the diagnosis and staging of pancreatic cancer. Clin Gastroenterol 1990; 4: 869–888
21 Warshaw AL, Gu Z, Wittenberg J, Waltman AC. Pre-operative staging and assessment of resectability of pancreatic cancer. Archiv Surg 1990; 125: 230–233

22 Jennings PE, Donald JJ, Coral A, Rode S, Lees WR. Ultrasound-guided cure biopsy. Lancet 1989; 2: 1369–1371

23 Warshaw AL. Implications of peritoneal cytology for staging of early pancreatic cancer. Am J Surg 1991; 161: 26–30

24 Anderson JR, Sorensen SM, Kruse A, Rokkjae R, Matzen P. Randomised trial of endoscopic endoprosthesis versus operative bypass in malignant obstructive jaundice. Gut 1989; 30: 1132–1135

25 Dowsett JF, Russell RCG, Hatfield ARW et al. Malignant obstructive jaundice: a prospective randomized trial of surgery versus endoscopic stenting. Gastroenterology 1989; 96: A128

26 Shepherd HA, Royle G, Ross APR, Diba A, Arthur M, Colin-Jones D. Endoscopic biliary endoprosthesis in the palliation of malignant obstruction of the distal common bile duct: a randomised trial. Br J Surg 1988 75: 1166–1168

27 Neoptolemos JP, Hendrickse C. Palliative biliary bypass for pancreatic cancer. In: Beger HG, Büchler M, eds. Standards of pancreatic surgery. Berlin: Springer-Verlag, 1992. (in press)

28 Russell RCG. Surgical resection for cancer of the pancreas. Clin Gastroenterol 1990; 4: 889–916

29 Trede M, Schwall G, Saeger HD. Survival after pancreatoduodenectomy. 118 consecutive resections without an operative mortality. Ann Surg 1990; 211: 447–458

30 Spencer MP, Sarr MG, Nagorney DM. Radical pancreatectomy for pancreatic cancer in the elderly. Ann Surg 1990 212; 140–143

31 Isgar B, Neoptolemos J. Adjuvant therapy after resection of pancreatic cancer. In: Johnson CD, Imrie CW, eds. Pancreatic disease: progress and prospects. London: Springer-Verlag, 1991: pp 103–113

32 Gastrointestinal Tumor Study Group (GITSG). Further evidence of effective adjuvant combined radiation and chemotherapy following curative resection of pancreatic cancer. Cancer 1987; 39: 2006–2010

33 Pitt HA, Grace PA. Pylorus-preserving resection of the pancreas. Clin Gastroenterol 1990; 4: 917–930

34 Weger AR, Glaser KS, Schwab G et al. Quantitative nuclear DNA content in fine needle aspirates of pancreatic cancer. Gut 1991; 32: 325–328

35 Schmiegel W. Tumour markers in pancreatic cancer – current concepts. Hepatogastroenterology 1989; 36: 446–449

36 Sarner M. Update in the classification of chronic pancreatitis. In: Beger H, Büchler M, Ditschuneit H, Malfertheiner P, eds. Chronic pancreatitis. Berlin: Springer-Verlag, 1990: pp 3–7

37 Sarles H, Bernard JP, Gullo L. Pathogenesis of chronic pancreatitis. Gut 1990; 31: 629–632

38 Lowes JR, Rode J, Lees WR, Russell RCG, Cotton PB. Obstructive pancreatitis: unusual causes of chronic pancreatitis. Br J Surg 1988; 75: 1129–1133

39 Venu RP, Greenen JL, Hogan W, Stone J, Johnson GK, Soergel K. Idiopathic recurrent pancreatitis. Dig Dis Sci 1989; 34: 56–60

40 Malfertheiner P, Büchler M. Correlation of imaging and function in chronic pancreatitis. Radiol Clin N Amer 1989; 27: 51–64

41 Singh M, Simsek H. Ethanol and the pancreas. Current status. Gastroenterology 1990; 98: 1051–1062

42 Schmiegel W, Burchert M, Kalthoff H et al. Immunochemical characterization and quantitative distribution of pancreatic stone protein in sera and pancreatic secretions in pancreatic disorders. Gastroenterology 1990; 99: 1421–1430

43 Guyan PM, Uden S, Braganza JM. Heightened free radical activity in pancreatitis. Free Radical Biol Med 1990; 8: 347–354

44 Schoenberg MH, Büchler M, Beger HG. Lipid peroxidation products in the pancreatic tissue of patients with acute pancreatitis (abstract). Br J Surg 1988; 75: 1254

45 Sandilands D, Jeffrey IJM, Haboubi NY, MacLennan IAM, Braganza JM. Abnormal drug metabolism in chronic pancreatitis. Gastroenterology 1990; 98: 766–772

46 Figarella C, Basso D, Guy-Grotto O. Lysosomal enzyme activation of digestive enzymes during chronic pancreatitis? In: Beger H, Büchler M, Ditschuneit H, Malfertheiner P, eds. Chronic pancreatitis. Berlin: Springer-Verlag, 1990: 134–139

47 DeCaro AM, Adrich Z, Fournet B et al. N-terminal sequence extension in the glycosylated form of human pancreatic stone protein. The 5-oxoproline N-terminal chain is O-glycosylated on the 5th amino acid residue. Biochem Biophys Acta 1989; 994: 281–284

48 Willemar S, Bialek R, Adler G. Localisation of lysosomal and digestive enzymes in cytoplasmic vacuoles in caerulein – pancreatitis. Histochemistry 1990; 94: 161–170

49 Ihse I, Permerth J. Enzyme and pancreatic pain. Acta Chir Scand 1990; 156: 281–283

50 Ramo OJ, Puolakkainen PA, Seppala K, Schroder TM. Self-administration of enzyme substitution in the treatment of exocrine pancreatic insufficiency. Scand J Gastroenterol 1989; 24: 688–692

51 Mossner J, Wresky HP, Kestel W, Zeeh J, Regner U, Fischbach W. Influence of treatment with pancreatic enzymes on pancreatic enzyme secretion. Gut 1989; 30: 1143–1149

52 Prinz RA, Pickleman J, Hoffman JP. Treatment of pancreatic cutaneous fistulas with a somatostatin analog. Am J Surg 1988; 155: 36–42

53 Büchler M, Freiss H, Klempa I et al. The role of the somatostatin analogue octreotide in the prevention of postoperative complications following pancreatic resection. The results of a multicenter controlled trial. Am J Surg 1992; 163: 125–131

54 Gullo L, Barbara L. Treatment of pancreatic pseudocysts with octreotide. Lancet 199; 338: 540–541

55 Uden S, Bilton D, Nathan L, Hunt LP, Main C, Braganza JM. Antioxidant therapy for recurrent pancreatitis: placebo-controlled trial. Aliment Pharmacol Therapy 1990; 4: 357–371

56 Busch EH, Atchison SR. Steroid celiac plexus block for chronic pancreatitis: results in 16 cases. J Clin Anesth 1989; 1: 431–433

57 Ebbehj N, Borly L, Madsen P, Matzen P. Comparison of regional pancreatic tissue fluid pressure and endoscopic retrograde pancreatographic morphology in chronic pancreatitis. Scand J Gastroenterol 1990; 25: 756–770

58 Okazaki K, Yamamoto Y, Kagiyama S et al. Pressure of papillary zone and pancreatic main duct in patients with chronic pancreatitis in the early state. Scand J Gastroenterol 1988; 23: 501–506

59 Huibregtse K, Schneider B, Vrij AA, Tytgat J. Endoscopic pancreatic drainage in chronic pancreatitis. Gastrointest Endosc 1988; 34: 9–15

60 Fuji T, Amano R, Ohmura T, Akiyama T, Aibe T. Endoscopic pancreatic sphincterotomy – technique and evaluation. Endoscopy 1989; 21: 27–30

61 Grimm H, Meyer WH, Nam VCH, Soehendra N. New modalities in treating chronic pancreatitis. Endoscopy 1989; 21: 70–74

62 McCarthy J, Geenen JE, Hogan WJ. Preliminary experience with endoscopic stent placement in benign pancreatic diseases. Gastrointest Endosc 1988; 34: 16–18

63 Kozarek RA, Patterson DJ, Ball TJ, Traverso LW. Endoscopic placement of pancreatic stents and drains in the management of pancreatitis. Ann Surg 1989; 209: 261–266

64 Siegel JH, Pullano WJ, Safrany L. Endoscopic sphincterotomy for acquired pancreatitis: effective long-term management. Gastrointest Endosc 1989; 35: 108–109

65 Geenen JE, Rolny P. Endoscopic management of pancreatic disease. Clin Gastroenterol 1991; 5: 155–182

66 Kozarek RA. Pancreatic stents can induce ductal changes consistent with chronic pancreatitis. Gastrointest Endosc 1990; 36: 93–95

67 Derfus GA, Geenen JE, Hogan WJ. Effect of endoscopic pancreatic duct stent replacement on pancreatic duct morphology (abstract). Gastrointest Endosc 1990; 36: 206

68 Cremer M, Vandermeeren A, Delhaye M. Extracorporeal shock wave lithotripsy (ESWL) for pancreatic stones (abstract). Gastroenterology 1988; 94: A80

69 Schneider MV, Lux G. Floating pancreatic duct stones in chronic pancreatitis. Endoscopy 1985; 17: 8–10

70 Sauerbruch T, Holl J, Sackmann M, Paumgartner G. Extracorporeal shock wave lithotripsy of pancreatic stones. Gut 1989; 30: 1406–1411

71 Grosso M, Gandini G, Cassinis ML, Regge D, Righi D, Rossi P. Percutaneous treatment (including pseudocystogastrostomy) of 74 pancreatic pseudocysts. Radiology 1989; 173: 493–497

72 Andersson R, Janzon M, Sundberg I, Bengmark S. Management of pancreatic pseudocysts. Br J Surg 1989; 76: 550–552
73 Henricksen FW, Hanck ES. Non-operative management of chronic pancreatic pseudocysts. In: Beger H, Büchler M, Ditschuneit H, Malfertheiner P, eds. Chronic pancreatitis. Berlin: Springer-Verlag, 1990: pp 389–391
74 Liguory CH, Lefebyre JF, Canard JM et al. Le pancréas divisum: étude clinique et thérapeutique chez l'homme. A propos des 87 cas. Gastroenterol Clin Biol 1986; 10: 820–825
75 Sahel J, Bastid C, Pellat B, Schurgers P, Sarles H. Endoscopic cystoduodenostomy of cysts of chronic calcifying pancreatitis. A report of 20 cases. Pancreas 1987; 2: 447–453
76 Sahel J, Bastid C, Sarles H. Dérivation endoscopique des pseudokytes et abcès au cours des pancréatites aiguës. Gastroenterol Clin Biol 1988; 12: 431–435
77 Sahel J. Letter to editor. Pancreas 1988; 3: 115–116
78 Cremer M, Deviere J, Engelholm L. Endoscopic management of cysts and pseudocysts in chronic pancreatitis: long-term follow-up after 7 years of experience. Gastrointest Endosc 1989; 35: 1–9
79 Kozarek RA, Ball TJ, Patterson DJ, Freeny PC, Ryan JA, Travers LW. Endoscopic transpapillary therapy for disrupted pancreatic duct and pancreatic fluid collection. Gastroenterology 1991; 100: 1362–1370
80 Donnelly PK, Lavelle J, Carr-Locke DL. Massive haemorrhage following endoscopic transgastric drainage of pancreatic pseudocyst. Br J Surg 1990; 77: 758–759
81 Deviere J, Devaere S, Baize M, Cremer M. Endoscopic biliary drainage in chronic pancreatitis. Gastrointest Endosc 1990; 36: 96–100
82 Cheng J, Gish B, Landiheer MH, Tytgat GNJ, Huibregtse K. Endoscopic biliary stenting in chronic pancreatitis. Abstracts of the World Congress of Gastroenterology. Sydney: 1990: p 1171
83 Huizinga WKJ et al. Chronic pancreatitis with biliary obstruction. Ann R Coll Surg Engl 1992; 74: 119–125
84 Bockman DE, Büchler M, Malfertheiner P, Beger HG. Analysis of nerves in chronic pancreatitis. Gastroenterology 1988; 94: 1459–1469
85 Weihe E, Büchler M, Muller S, Freiss H, Zentel HJ. Peptidergic innervation in chronic pancreatitis. In: Beger H, Büchler M, Ditschuneit H, Malfertheiner P, eds. Chronic pancreatis. Berlin: Springer-Verlag, 1990: pp 83–105
86 Aldridge MC, Williamson RCN. Distal pancreatectomy with and without splenectomy. Br J Surg 1991; 78: 976–979
87 Klempa I. Jejunumtransposition und selective proximate Vagotomie nach Duodeno-pankreatektomie. Chirurg 1978; 49: 556–560
88 Morel P, Mathey P, Corboud H, Huber O, Egeli RA, Rohner A. Pylorus-preserving duodenopancreatectomy: long-term complications and comparison with the Whipple procedure. World J Surg 1990; 14: 642–647
89 Beger HG, Büchler M. Duodenum-preserving resection of the head of the pancreas in chronic pancreatitis with inflammatory mass in the head. World J Surg 1990; 14: 83–87
90 Wilker DK, Izbicki JR, Knoefel WT, Geissler K, Schweiderer L. Duodenum-preserving resection of the head of the pancreas in treatment of chronic pancreatitis. Am J Gastroenterol 1990; 85: 1000–1004
91 Russell RCG. Preservation of the duodenum in total pancreatectomy for chronic pancreatitis. In: Beger H, Büchler M, Ditschuneit H, Malfertheiner P, eds. Chronic pancreatitis. Berlin: Springer-Verlag, 1990: pp 539–550
92 Nealon WH, Townsend CM, Thompson JC. Operative drainage of the pancreatic duct delays functional impairment in patients with chronic pancreatitis: a prospective analysis. Ann Surg 1988; 208: 321–329
93 Amman RW, Muench R, Otto R, Buehler H, Freiburghaus AU, Siegenthaler W. Evolution and regression of pancreatic calcification in chronic pancreatitis. A prospective long-term study of 107 patients. Gastroenterology 1988; 95: 1018–1028
94 Block S, Maier W, Bittner R, Büchler M, Malfertheiner P, Beger HG. Identification of pancreas necrosis in severe acute pancreatitis: imaging procedure versus clinical staging. Gut 1986; 27: 1035–1042
95 Beger HG, Büchler M, Bittner R, Block S, Nevalainen T, Roscher R. Necrosectomy and postoperative local lavage in necrotizing pancreatitis. Br J Surg 1988; 75: 207–212

96 Pederzoli P, Bassi C, Vesentini S et al. Necrosectomy by lavage in the surgical treatment of severe necrotizing pancreatitis. Acta Chir Scand 1990; 56: 775–780

97 London NJM, Leese T, Lavelle JM et al. Rapid-bolus contrast-enhanced dynamic computed tomography in acute pancreatitis: a prospective study. Br J Surg 1991; 78: 1452–1456

98 Larvin M, McMahon M. APACHE-II score for assessment and monitoring of acute pancreatitis. Lancet 1989; 2: 201–205

99 Wilson C, Heads A, Shenkin A, Imrie CW. C-reactive protein antiproteases and complement factors as objective markers of severity in acute pancreatitis. Br J Surg 1989; 76: 177–181

100 Büchler M, Malfertheiner P, Szchadlich H, Nevalainen TJ. Role of phospholipase A$_2$ in human acute pancreatitis. Gastroenterology 1989; 97: 1521–1526

101 Gross V, Scholmerich J, Leser HG et al. Granulocyte elastase in assessment of severity of acute pancreatitis. Dig Dis Sci 1990; 35: 97–105

102 Neoptolemos JP, London N, Carr-Locke DL. Endoscopic retrograde pancreatography (ERP): a possible diagnostic role in acute necrotising pancreatitis (abstract). Gut 1992 (in press)

103 London NJM, Neoptolemos JP, Lavelle J, Bailey I, James D. Contrast-enhanced abdominal computed tomography scanning and prediction of severity of acute pancreatitis: a prospective study. Br J Surg 1989; 76: 268–272

104 Bradley EL. Open packing for infected pancreatic necrosis. In: Beger H, Büchler M, eds. Standards of pancreatic surgery. Berlin: Springer-Verlag, 1992. (in press)

105 Freeny PC, Lewis GP, Traverso LW, Ryan JA. Infected pancreatic fluid collections: percutaneous catheter drainage. Radiology 1988; 167: 435–441

106 Adams DB, Harvey TS, Anderson MC. Percutaneous catheter drainage of infected pancreatic and peripancreatic fluid collections. Arch Surg 1990; 125: 1554–1557

107 Rinderknecht H. Acute necrotizing pancreatitis and its complications: an excessive reaction of natural defence mechanisms? In: Braganza JM, ed. The pathogenesis of pancreatitis. Manchester: Manchester University Press, 1991: pp 87–100

108 Ohlsson K, Genell S. Role of enzyme inhibitors in acute pancreatitis and rationale for their therapeutic use. In: Braganza JM, ed. The pathogenesis of pancreatitis. Manchester: Manchester University Press, 1991: pp 198–209

109 Leese T, Hall C, Holliday M et al. Multicentre prospective randomized trial of high volume fresh frozen plasma therapy in severe pancreatitis. Ann R Coll Surg Engl 1991; 73: 542–544

110 Neoptolemos JP. The theory of 'persisting' common bile duct stones in severe gallstone pancreatitis. Ann R Coll Surg Engl 1989; 71: 326–331

111 Neoptolemos JP, Carr-Locke DL, London NJ, Bailey IA, James D, Fossard DP. Controlled trial of urgent endoscopic retrograde cholangiopancreatography and endoscopic sphincterotomy versus conservative treatment for acute pancreatitis due to gallstones. Lancet 1989; 2: 979–983

112 Nowak A, Nowakowska-Duzawa E, Rybicka J. Urgent endoscopic sphincterotomy vs. conservative treatment in acute biliary pancreatitis – a prospective, controlled trial (abstract). Hepatogastroenterology 1990; 37 (suppl 2): A5

113 Neoptolemos JP, Stonelake P, Radley S. Endoscopic sphincterotomy in acute pancreatitis. Hepatogastroenterology 1992 (in press)

114 Neoptolemos JP, Carr-Locke DL. ERCP in acute cholangitis and pancreatitis. In: ERCP: techniques and therapeutic applications. New York: Elsevier, 1989; pp 93–128

115 Bernard JP, Sahel J, Giovannini M, Sarles H. Pancreas divisium is a probable cause of acute pancreatitis: a report of 137 cases. Pancreas 1990; 2: 248–254

116 Hayakawa T, Kondo T, Shibata T et al. Pancreas divisium. Int J Pancreatol 1989; 5: 317–326

117 Lindstrom E, von Schenck H, Ihse I. Pancreatic exocrine function in patients with pancreas divisum and abdominal pain. Int J Pancreatol 1990; 6: 17–24

118 Saterfield ST, McCarthy JH, Geenan JE et al. Clinical experience in 82 patients with pancreas divisum: preliminary results of manometry and endoscopic therapy. Pancreas 1988; 3: 248–253

119 Lindstrom E, Ihse I. Dynamic CT scanning of pancreatic duct after secretion provocation in pancreas divisum. Dig Dis Sci 1990; 11: 1371–1376

120 Warshaw AL, Simeone JF, Schapiro RH, Flavin-Warshaw B. Evaluation and treatment of the dominant dorsal duct syndrome (pancreas divisum redefined). Am J Surg 1990; 159: 59–66
121 Lehman G, O'Connor K, Troiano F, Benage D. Endoscopic papillotomy and stenting of the minor papilla in pancreas divisum. Gastrointest Endosc 1989; 35: 167
122 Siegel JH, Ben-zvi JS, Pullano W, Cooperman A. Effectiveness of endoscopic drainage for pancreas divisum: endoscopic and surgical results in 31 patients. Endoscopy 1990; 22: 129–133
123 Keith RG, Shapero TF, Saibil FG, Moore TL. Dorsal duct sphincterotomy is an effective long-term treatment of acute pancreatitis associated with pancreas divisum. Surgery 1989; 106: 4660–4666
124 Watson EK, Mayall E, Chapple J, Harrington K, Williams C, Williamson R. Screening for carriers of cystic fibrosis through primary health care services. Br Med J 1991; 303: 504–507
125 Hyde SC, Emsley P, Hartshorn MJ et al. Structural model of ATP-binding proteins associated with cystic fibrosis, multidrug resistance and bacterial transport. Nature 1990; 346: 362–365
126 Ringe D, Petsko GA. A transport problem? Nature 1990; 346: 372–373

7

Duodenal ulceration

R. Pounder   A. G. Fraser

The aetiology, diagnosis, and treatment of peptic ulceration have been reviewed in past editions of *Recent Advances in Gastroenterology*, and also more recently in a series of excellent in-depth review articles published by the *New England Journal of Medicine*.[1-5] The purpose of this chapter is to review publications about duodenal ulceration which have appeared in the last 2 years.

AETIOLOGY

Are duodenal ulcers caused by 'Hurry, worry, and curry'? Acute and chronic life-event stresses were assessed in a sample of duodenal ulcer patients and community controls: chronic stresses (those of 6 months' duration or more) involving high goal frustration were significantly and independently associated with the onset and relapse of duodenal ulcers.[6] So perhaps hurry and worry do matter, although most earlier studies had rejected these factors.[7]

Patients always want to blame their diet for their duodenal ulceration, but it has been difficult to prove any association. It has been suggested that the falling incidence of duodenal ulcer disease is related to an increase of dietary polyunsaturated essential fatty acid intake.[8] Some support for this hypothesis came from a study which found that the linoleic content of adipose tissue was lower in duodenal ulcer patients than healthy patients, suggesting that duodenal ulcer patients have a diet deficient in linoleic acid.[9] An association between duodenal ulceration and a low-fibre diet has been excluded in a study of 78 duodenal ulcer patients, who were compared with age-matched controls by logistic regression analysis.[10]

The theory of a genetic predisposition to duodenal ulceration had been based on the familial incidence of ulcers, and apparent genetic markers such as hyperpepsinogenaemia. The discovery of *Helicobacter pylori* has provided an alternative explanation for these observations. Studies using antibodies to *H. pylori* have shown a high incidence of positivity in parents and siblings of infected children,[11] but the best evidence for person-to-person spread of *H. pylori* within families comes from DNA fingerprinting of isolates. Each infected person usually has one unique strain type which can be characterized by the DNA fingerprint pattern.[12] Family studies with this technique are limited at present, but there is evidence of transmission of the same strain type through three generations of one family.[13] Hyperpepsinogenaemia was considered to be a genetic marker of the predisposition to develop duodenal ulceration, but the finding that eradication of *H. pylori* can lower to normal the 24-hour plasma concentration of pepsinogen I and II suggests that hyperpepsinogaemia may be due to *H. pylori* gastritis.[14]

The influence of age on the onset of symptoms was studied in a large personal series of duodenal ulcer patients: early onset was associated with male gender, a positive family history of dyspepsia, and a history of haemorrhage.[15] The incidence of duodenal ulceration was studied in two special circumstances: following open-heart surgery and in patients awaiting liver transplantation. Upper-gastrointestinal haemorrhage complicated open-heart surgery in 0.4% of patients and was almost always due to duodenal ulceration.[16] The prevalence of duodenal ulceration in 216 male cirrhotics awaiting liver transplantation was 7.8%: it was higher in alcoholics (12.2%) as compared to patients with autoimmune chronic active hepatitis (6.6%). The authors concluded that the estimated risk of a duodenal ulcer is increased 3.7-fold in cirrhotic males as compared to the general population, but there was no association with the degree of portal hypertension.[17] A major review confirmed that peptic ulceration hardly ever occurs during pregnancy.[18]

The understanding of mucosal events associated with duodenal ulceration remains elusive. Generation of platelet-activating factors, leukotriene B4 and leukotriene C4, were several times higher in the duodenal mucosa of patients with an ulcer as compared to normal patients, and they decreased to normal after treatment of the ulcer.[19] Some strains of *H. pylori* are capable of synthesizing platelet-activating factor,[20] and levels of leukotriene B4 correlate with the degree of *H. pylori*-related gastritis.[21] Interleukin 8, a potent attractant of neutrophils, is also elevated in the duodenal mucosa of patients with *H. pylori*-related gastritis.[22] Finally, in response to duodenal acidification, duodenal ulcer patients release greater amounts of PGE_2 into the duodenal lumen than normal subjects.[23]

Two dopamine agonists, amantidine and bromocriptine, have been reported to be as effective as H_2-receptor antagonists in the prevention of duodenal ulcer relapse, but the mechanism is unclear.[24] Both systemic and central administration of selective dopamine agonists provide significant protection from experimental gastric ulcers, suggesting the existence of a functionally-significant, dopaminergic brain-gut axis.[25] The hypothesis that reactivation of a latent *Herpes simplex* virus may be a cause of recurrent duodenal ulceration appears unlikely, as maintenance treatment with acyclovir (400 mg bd) did not prevent ulcer recurrence,[26] but the dose was relatively low.

The incidence of *H. pylori* with duodenal ulceration is over 95%;

therefore any *H. pylori* negative ulceration should be evaluated carefully for other diagnoses. In one study, *H. pylori*-negative patients were more likely to be aspirin users, less likely to have a history of prior ulceration, more likely to be white, and more likely to present with bleeding rather than pain.[27] The diagnosis of Zollinger-Ellison syndrome should also be considered in *H. pylori*-negative duodenal ulcer patients.[28, 29]

CONTROL OF INTRAGASTRIC ACIDITY

Readers interested in the measurement of 24-h intragastric acidity may enjoy a supplement dedicated to this technique.[30] Wagner et al[31] measured 24-h acidity in 21 ulcer patients when in relapse with active ulceration and during remission after ulcer healing: they detected no difference, and concluded that the recurrent course of duodenal ulcer disease is not due to a fluctuation of intragastric acidity.

Merki et al[32] investigated the effect of eating snacks on 24-h intragastric acidity. It might be anticipated that eating a snack will have two effects on gastric function – it should neutralize intragastric acidity, but it may also stimulate gastric acid secretion. The results of these experiments suggest that the latter dominates, as intragastric acidity (particularly at night) was higher when the subjects ate snacks between meals. It may be sensible to recommend that ulcer patients should avoid eating between main meals or at bedtime. The timing of the evening meal can also cause a substantial change in intragastric acidity profile[33] – eating the evening meal at 5.30 pm resulted in higher intragastric acidity during the evening and early night, whereas eating a late evening meal at 9.30 pm resulted in a large increase of acidity in the late afternoon and early evening. Duodenal ulcer patients who eat in the early evening might benefit from splitting their dose of an H_2-blocker, taking half after the meal and half at bedtime. Similarly, patients who eat late in the evening may benefit from taking half their dose after lunch and the remainder at bedtime.

Another study suggested that nocturnal intragastric acidity is not quite as important as suggested by some experts. Bianchi-Porro et al[34] treated 130 duodenal ulcer patients with ranitidine 300 mg at either 8 am or 10 pm in a double-blind, placebo-controlled study. At 4 weeks the ulcers had healed in 67% of patients taking the morning dose, and 75% of those receiving the nocturnal dose – a non-significant difference. At 8 weeks the corresponding healing rates were 82% and 86%. Predictably, the morning dose of the drug decreased intragastric acidity during the daytime, whereas the bedtime dose decreased nocturnal acidity.

Kaufmann et al[35] reported the influence of cigarette smoking on 24-h intragastric acidity in duodenal ulcer patients, as compared with healthy volunteers. They analysed their records of 24-h profiles relating to 150 non-smokers and 174 smokers, while receiving placebo treatment. Daytime intragastric acidity was higher in smokers (median pH 1.56) as compared with non-smokers (median pH 1.70). However, there was no difference in 24-h or night-time median pH between the two groups. Although the increase of daytime acidity in the smoking subjects was statistically significant, the authors concluded that the difference is unlikely to account for the increased prevalence of peptic ulcer disease in cigarette smokers.

Burget et al[36] have developed their model relating the rate of duodenal ulcer healing to control of intragastric acidity achieved by a range of antisecretory regimens. They obtained the original results of acid suppression data from 21 studies performed by seven investigators, giving a total of 490 24-h profiles using 19 different treatment regimens. They performed a meta-analysis of published clinical trials of duodenal ulcer healing with these 19 treatment regimens, identifying 144 trials involving 14 208 patients. Using these two sets of data, the authors found a highly significant correlation between the rate of ulcer healing and the degree of acid suppression – the three main variables were the duration and degree of acid suppression throughout the 24 h, and the length of ulcer treatment. They identified pH 3 (1 mmol/L) as a particularly important threshold for ulcer healing.

Masoero et al[37] compared 24-h acidity in 15 'responder' and 10 'non-responder' duodenal ulcer patients. They found that median 24-h intragastric pH was significantly lower in patients with resistant duodenal ulcer, as compared with the responders (1.13 vs. 1.63, respectively). However, they could detect no difference in the response to either group after the administration of either ranitidine or famotidine. Hence, patients who do not heal their duodenal ulcers during H_2-blockade do not appear to have a resistance to the antisecretory effect of this class of drug.

Repeated dosing with an H_2-receptor antagonist results in a modest decrease of antisecretory potency; this decrease is termed 'tolerance'.[38] Tolerance has been shown with all the commonly used H_2-receptor antagonists after 14–28 days of dosing,[13] and this phenomenon probably affects even the second dose of an H_2-antagonist. The mechanism of tolerance is uncertain, but it may be partly due to a drug-induced release of gastrin that causes increased stimulation of gastric acid secretion.[39] Tolerance is not a progressive phenomenon; a placebo-controlled study using ranitidine 150 mg nocte demonstrated that the antisecretory effect of this regimen was unchanged between 1 and 5 months of dosing.[39]

Sudden withdrawal of dosing with H_2-receptor antagonists results in an increase of nocturnal intragastric acidity, which persists for up to 6 days.[39-41] The phenomenon does not appear to be gastrin-driven and it does not happen after dosing with sucralfate.[42]

Disordered gastro-duodenal motility may promote duodenal ulceration by allowing prolonged acid contact with the duodenal mucosa. Using a multilumen perfused-catheter incorporating three pH microelectrodes, Kerrigan et al[43] measured antral and duodenal pH and antro-pyloro-duodenal pressure activity in 36 subjects (10 with healed duodenal ulceration, 11 with active duodenal ulceration, and 15 healthy volunteers) during fasting and after a radiolabelled, solid test meal. The chief abnormalities in the ulcer groups consisted of an increase in postprandial duodenal retro-peristalsis, a reduction in pressure waves sweeping aborally through the duodenum after the meal, and an increased incidence of atypical, complex forms of coordinated duodenal motor activity throughout the study. Gastric emptying of the solid test meal was delayed in the group with healed duodenal ulceration, and the duodenal bulb pH was lower than 4 for a significantly greater time in the same group. The authors concluded that duodenal ulcer disease is associated with disturbed gastro-duodenal moti-lity and that a disturbance of motility in healed duodenal ulceration may promote ulcer relapse by impairing acid clearance from the bulb.

Omeprazole

The bioavailability of oral omeprazole increases with repeated oral dosing and this may be one of the reasons why the development of the drug's full antisecretory effect takes several days. The increased bioavailability is thought to be due to increased oral absorption, possibly related to less degradation of the acid-labile drug by gastric acid, and not to changes in systemic elimination,[44] and/or decreased first-pass elimination.[45] The return of intragastric acidity after dosing with omeprazole also takes 3–6 days in healthy volunteers (related to the time required to synthesize more H^+K^+-ATPase) – an effect which may contribute to the absence of rebound hyperacidity after abrupt withdrawal of dosing with omeprazole.[41] The effects of omeprazole and proximal gastric vagotomy on 24-h intra-gastric acidity and plasma gastrin concentration have been compared in eight duodenal ulcer patients before and after gastric surgery (Figs 7.1, 7.2). The decrease in intragastric acidity after 4 weeks' administration of omeprazole 20 mg daily was greater than that 4–6 months after the proxi-mal gastric vagotomy (-94% and -78%, respectively), whereas the increase in plasma gastrin concentration was greater after the vagotomy ($+285\%$) than during omeprazole treatment ($+186\%$).[46]

Omeprazole has been compared with placebo[47] and ranitidine in several recent clinical trials.[48, 49] A meta-analysis of 10 double-blind clinical studies in which 2225 patients were treated with either omeprazole 20 mg daily or ranitidine 300 mg daily provides a comparison of healing rates: there was a statistically significant advantage for omeprazole after 2 (69 vs. 53%; $P < 0.0001$) and 4 weeks (93 vs. 83; $P < 0.0001$).[50] A comparison of omeprazole 20 mg daily with famotidine 40 mg daily in 363 Japanese patients with duodenal ulcer demonstrated that omeprazole healed ulcers more quickly after 2 (56 vs. 33%; $P < 0.01$) and 4 weeks (88 vs. 72%; $P < 0.01$), but by 6 weeks the difference was not statistically significant (97 vs. 91%).[51] Symptom relief is quicker with omeprazole treatment; in one study 77% of the omeprazole-treated and 59% of the ranitidine-treated

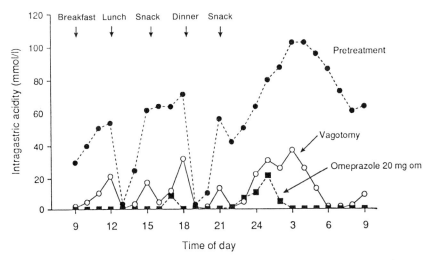

Fig. 7.1   Median 24-h intragastric acidity measured during treatment with omeprazole (20 mg daily) or after proximal gastric vagotomy, compared with pretreatment values in eight duodenal ulcer patients. (Reproduced with permission from Lind et al.[46])

patients were free of pain after 2 weeks of treatment.[52] A meta-analysis of the effect of treatment on symptom relief showed that 71% of patients had complete relief of symptoms within 2 weeks of omeprazole treatment, as compared to 58% with ranitidine ($P < 0.001$; $n = 2631$).[53] It is debatable whether these short-term advantages are clinically relevant, given the lifelong strategies of maintenance treatment that are required for most patients with duodenal ulcer disease.

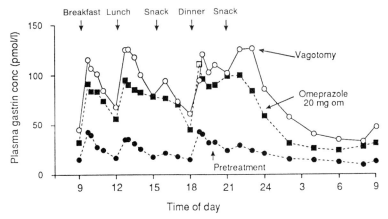

Fig. 7.2   Median 24-h plasma gastrin concentration measured during treatment with omeprazole (20 mg daily) or after proximal gastric vagotomy, compared with pretreatment values in eight duodenal ulcer patients. (Reproduced with permission from Lind et al.[46])

A multicentre trial assessed the early symptomatic relapse (within 10 weeks) after 2- and 4-week courses of either omeprazole 20 mg or ranitidine 300 mg daily. Follow-up 10 weeks after a 2-week course showed that symptoms had returned in 51% of the ranitidine-treated group and 31% of the omeprazole-treated group, but the return of symptoms was similar after a 4-week course of either omeprazole or ranitidine.[54] We still do not know whether rapid ulcer healing results in a robust duodenal ulcer scar. The proposal that the 'histological maturity' of the ulcer scar is associated with delayed ulcer relapse is most intriguing.[55]

The duodenal ulcer relapse rates 6 and 12 months after healing with omeprazole are 41–44% and 88%, respectively – these are very similar to the relapse rates after treatment with H_2-receptor antagonists.[56, 57] Two regimens of maintenance treatment with omeprazole (20 mg 3 days per week and 10 mg daily) were compared with placebo in 195 duodenal ulcer patients: the endoscopic relapse rates after 6 months were 23% and 27% for the omeprazole-treated groups, and 67% for the patients receiving placebo.[58] Low-dose omeprazole is probably a less effective strategy than long-term treatment with an H_2-receptor antagonist.[59, 60a,b]

The incidence and severity of adverse events of 19 000 patients in clinical trials with short-term omeprazole treatment (2–12 weeks) was similar to placebo,[61] although headache, rash, and diarrhoea have been reported often enough to make coincidence unlikely.[62] Omeprazole inhibits a specific subset of the cytochrome oxidase system in the liver responsible for the metabolism of certain drugs, but this seems clinically unimportant.[63]

The acceptability of omeprazole during long-term treatment is of considerable interest, because maintenance treatment will be necessary to prevent duodenal ulcer recurrence. Long-term toxicological experiments in rats showed hyperplasia of the enterochromaffin-like cells and carcinoid tumours which are probably related to sustained hypergastrinaemia.[64] In human beings, plasma gastrin rises 3–4 fold during acute treatment with omeprazole 20–40 mg daily, with occasionally a 10-fold rise. The plasma gastrin concentration did not continue to rise in one long-term study,[65] but Jansen et al[66] reported a gradual increase during the second year of dosing. Studies in man (up to 4 years) provide some reassurance that enterochromaffin-like cell hyperplasia is, at most, mild.[67–70]

There has been a debate concerning the potential genotoxicity of omeprazole following testing of this compound with a proposed assay of unscheduled DNA synthesis in the rat stomach.[71] There is general agreement that this assay also measures mucosal proliferation;[72, 73] the interpretation of this assay was also complicated by variation of results between different strains of rat.[74] The debate continues on whether omeprazole, or one of its metabolites, is genotoxic.[75, 76]

Omeprazole has a temporary suppressive effect on *H. pylori*, perhaps by a direct antimicrobial effect or related to bacterial overgrowth consequent to the profound acid suppression.[77] *H. pylori* density after 4 weeks of treatment with omeprazole decreases significantly, and this is associated with some improvement in the antral gastritis.[78, 79] This temporary effect on *H. pylori* has no direct advantage, although there is interest in combinations of omeprazole and antibiotics for eradication of *H. pylori*.[80] Omeprazole treatment for 3 days induces a significant increase in pepsinogen I and II concentrations, which falls again on withdrawal of treatment;[81] a similar elevation of both zymogens (approximately twofold) was also seen during 12–30 months of treatment with 20–40 mg of omeprazole,[66] but the significance of this finding is unknown.

Non-steroidal anti-inflammatory drugs

The occurrence of upper-gastrointestinal disease and the relevance of NSAID use were documented in 511 consecutive patients (63% female) over the age of 70 years old, referred for upper-gastrointestinal endoscopy in a District General Hospital.[82] Only 15% of these elderly patients were found to be normal – surprisingly, 43% had benign oesophageal disease, 12% gastric ulceration, and 11% duodenal ulceration. Gastric ulcers were more common in the patients taking NSAIDs. Haemorrhage was found to be as common in aspirin-takers (45%) as in standard-dose NSAID-takers (39%), even though 86% were taking only aspirin 300 mg per day or less.

A multi-centre study investigated the effect of ranitidine on the healing of NSAID-associated peptic ulcers – in a group of patients who stopped NSAID treatment and another group who continued with NSAID treatment; all patients received ranitidine 150 mg bd.[83] Endoscopy at 8 weeks showed that gastric ulcers had healed in 63% of those who continued to take an NSAID, as compared with 95% of those who had stopped NSAID treatment. For patients presenting with duodenal ulceration, the healing rates at 8 weeks were 84% in the group that continued NSAIDs, as compared with 100% in those who stopped NSAIDs. After 12 weeks of follow-up, 79% of gastric ulcers and 92% of duodenal ulcers were healed in the group that continued with NSAIDs, while all patients who had stopped taking NSAIDs were healed at 12 weeks. The authors concluded that healing is more successful when NSAID treatment is stopped, but, even if these drugs are continued, substantial healing rates are achievable by co-prescription with ranitidine 150 mg bd.

Edelson et al[84] used a model to coestimate the cost-effectiveness of misoprostol for prophylaxis against NSAID-induced gastrointestinal tract bleeding. They estimated that if misoprostol were to be prescribed for all non-steroidal users, the incremental cost to save a year of life would be $667 400. If the use were to be restricted to patients over the age of 60, or to patients with rheumatoid arthritis, the annual incremental costs would be $186 700 and $95 600, respectively. However, if the prophylactic use of misoprostol was restricted to those who need to continue to take NSAIDs, despite having had an episode of gastrointestinal bleeding in the previous year, the authors estimated that the incremental cost would be less than $40 000 per year of life saved.

New drugs

Ranitidine bismuth citrate is a new compound which not only has the acid antisecretory activity of ranitidine, but also the potential advantages of a bismuth compound – cytoprotective effects and anti-*H. pylori* activity.[41] The systemic absorption of bismuth is much less than that of tripotassium dicitrato bismuthate. Clinical trials are in progress but no results have been published. Bismuth appears to cause an improved histological maturity of the duodenal ulcer scar (as compared with cimetidine), which may explain the slower ulcer relapse rate in bismuth-treated ulcer patients.[55] There are several new compounds in clinical trial that are similar to established drugs: lansoprazole, a new proton pump inhibitor;[85, 86] arboprostil, a prosta-glandin analogue;[87] and roxatidine acetate, an H_2-receptor antagonist.[88]

Surgery

Johnston et al[89] have reported the outcome of 372 patients who had an elective proximal gastric vagotomy for duodenal ulceration between 1969 and 1979. The 10–20-year follow-up report of the group indicated that 15% had recurrent ulceration; 80% of these developed symptoms within 5 years and no patient had a recurrence after 13 years. Perhaps surprisingly, two-thirds of the relapsing patients went for further surgery rather than medical treatment – perhaps a disadvantage of follow-up in a surgical clinic. Penninckx et al[90] compared the recurrence rates after highly selective vagotomy when it was performed for either non-refractory duodenal ulceration (64 patients) or refractory ulceration (41 patients). The cumulative 5-year recurrence rate was 28.7% in refractory ulcers, as compared with 9.3% in non-refractory ulcers—a significant difference. The authors were unable to identify any variable to explain the early risk of recurrence in the refractory ulcer group, and they concluded that highly selective vagotomy cannot be considered a surgical procedure of choice for patients with refractory duodenal ulceration. Macintyre & Millar[91] reported the safety and efficacy of highly selective vagotomy in 500 patients, over a 15-year period. They reported no pre-operative or immediate postoperative mortality, although ulcers recurred in 18.5% of these patients. Bloating was the commonest long-term complication (8.8%) – yet highly selective vagotomy was found to have no effect on the gastric emptying of solids by Mistiaen et al.[92] ^{99m}Tc-HIDA scintigraphy was used to assess enterogastric reflux after gastric surgery; 16 patients selected by this test were helped by Roux-en-Y gastrectomy.[93]

Lundegardh et al[94] reported the long-term survival of 6459 patients who had undergone partial gastrectomy for benign ulcer disease, and who had survived the first year after operation. The cohort was followed for 27–35 years. There was a significant decrease in the relative survival rate of these patients, to 92% of expected survival, some 35 years after operation. This difference was not observed during the first 20 years after operation. Reasonably, the authors suggested that the effects of partial gastrectomy on survival are probably attributable to confounding factors linked with the peptic ulcer disease – for example, smoking – rather than to the surgical procedure itself. The risk of malignancy following gastric surgery was evaluated in several large studies. A Norwegian study suggested that the increased risk of cancer in digestive organs is mainly related to lifestyle factors, particularly tobacco-specific nitrosamines whose effect is enhanced by surgical sequelae.[95] In contrast, a Danish study showed a twofold increase in gastric carcinoma after 25 years of follow-up, but found that cancers related to smoking were close to expected numbers.[96] An Amsterdam study showed a 5-fold increased risk of gastric cancer for males and 3.5-fold increase for females 25 years after gastric surgery.[97] Interestingly, this increased risk of gastric cancer was not seen in Japanese patients after partial gastrectomy,[98] or 10 years after initial exposure to cimetidine.[99]

Finally, will laparoscopic vagotomy become the new fashion? Katkhouda & Mouiel[100] have described a 60-minute procedure which divides the right or posterior trunk of the vagus and denervates the anterior fundus by an anterior lesser curve seromyotomy. This operation decreased basal and insulin-stimulated secretion—and nine of ten ulcer patients were healed 60 days after the operation. This procedure could prove popular for the young, otherwise fit patient with an antibiotic-resistant *H. pylori* infection.

REFERENCES

1 Soll H. Pathogenesis of peptic ulcer and implications for therapy. N Engl J Med 1990; 322: 909–916
2. Peterson WL. *Helicobacter pylori* and peptic ulcer disease. N Engl J Med 1991; 324: 1043–1048
3 Feldman M, Burton ME. Histamine$_2$-receptor antagonists: standard therapy for acid-peptic diseases (in 2 parts). N Engl J Med 1991; 323: 1672–1678, 1749–1755
4 Maton PN. Omeprazole. N Engl J Med 1991; 324: 965–975
5 McCarthy DM. Sucralfate. N Engl J Med 1991; 325: 1017–1025
6 Ellard K, Beaurepaire J, Jones M, Piper D, Tennant C. Acute and chronic stress in duodenal ulcer disease. Gastroenterology 1990; 99: 1628–1632
7 McIntosh HH, Nasery RW, McNeil D, Coates C, Mitchell J, Piper DW. Perception of life event stress in patients with chronic duodenal ulcer: a comparison of the rating of life events by duodenal ulcer patients and community controls. Scand J Gastroenterol 1985; 20: 563–568
8 Hollander D, Tarnawski A. Dietary essential fatty acids and the decline of peptic ulcer disease – a hypothesis. Gut 1986; 27: 239–242
9 Grant HW, Palmer KR, Riermesma RR, Oliver MF. Duodenal ulcer is associated with low dietary linoleic acid intake. Gut 1990; 31: 997–998
10 Katschinski BD, Logan RF, Edmond M, Langman MJ. Duodenal ulcer and refined carbohydrate intake: a case-control study assessing dietary fibre and refined sugar intake. Gut 1990; 31: 993–996

11 Oderda G, Vaira D, Holton J et al. *Helicobacter pylori* in children with peptic ulcer and their families. Dig Dis Sci 1991; 36: 572–576
12 Prewett EJ, Bickley J, Owen RJ, Pounder RE. Deoxyribonucleic acid patterns in the body, antrum and duodenum. Gastroenterology 1992; 102: 829–833
13 Nwokolo CU, Bickley J, Attard AR, Owen JR, Fraser IA. DNA characterisation of *Helicobacter pylori* strains in three generations of a duodenal ulcer disease family. Gut 1991; 32(Abstract): 1207
14 Fraser AG, Prewett EJ, Pounder RE, Samloff M. Twenty-four hour hyperpepsinogenaemia in *Helicobacter pylori*-positive subjects is abolished by eradication of the infection. Aliment Pharmacol Ther 1992; 6: 389–394
15 Kang JY. Age of onset of symptoms in duodenal and gastric ulcer. Gut 1990; 31: 854–857
16 Lebovics E, Lee SS, Dworkia BM et al. Upper gastrointestinal bleeding following open-heart surgery. Predominant finding of aggressive duodenal ulcer disease. Dig Dis Sci 1991; 36: 757–768
17 Rabinovitz M, Schade RR, Dindzans V, Van-Thiel DH, Gavaler JS. Prevalence of duodenal ulcer in cirrhotic males referred for liver transplantation. Does the etiology of cirrhosis make a difference? Dig Dis Sci 1990; 35: 321–326
18 Singer AJ, Brandt LJ. Pathophysiology of the gastrointestinal tract during pregnancy. Am J Gastroenterol 1991; 86: 1695–1711
19 Ackerman Z, Karmeli F, Ligumsky M, Rachmilewitz D. Enhanced gastric and duodenal platelet-activating factor and leukotriene generation in duodenal ulcer patients. Scand J Gastroenterol 1990; 25: 925–934
20 Denizot Y, Sobhani J, Rambaud JC, Lewin M, Thomas Y, Benveniste J. PAF-acether synthesis by *H. pylori*. Gut 1990; 38: 1242–1246
21 Fukuda T, Kimura S, Arakawa T, Kobayashi K. Possible role of leukotriene in gastritis associated with *Campylobacter pylori*. J Clin Gastroenterol 1990; 12 (suppl 1): S131–S134
22 Gupta R, Moss S, Thomas DM, Abbot F, Rees A, Calam J. Abstract. *Helicobacter pylori* increases the release of interleukin 8, a potent attractant of neutrophils. Gut 1991; 32(Abstract): 1206
23 Bukhave K, Rask-Madesn J, Hogan DL, Koss MA, Isenberg JI. Proximal duodenal prostaglandin E_2 release and mucosal bicarbonate secretion are altered in patients with duodenal ulcer. Gastroenterology 1990; 99: 951–955
24 Sikiric P, Rotkvic I, Mise S et al. Dopamine agonists prevent duodenal ulcer relapse. A comparative study with famotidine and cimetidine. Dig Dis Sci 1991; 36: 905–910
25 Glavin GB. Dopamine and gastroprotection: the brain–gut axis. Dig Dis Sci 1991; 36: 1670–1672
26 Rune SJ, Linde J, Bonnevie O et al. Acyclovir in the prevention of duodenal ulcer recurrence. Gut 1990; 31: 151–152
27 Nensey YM, Schubert TT, Bologna SD, Ma CK. *Helicobacter pylori*-negative duodenal ulcer. Am J Med 1991; 91: 15–18
28 Saeed ZA, Evans DJJ, Evans DG et al. *Helicobacter pylori* and Zollinger-Ellison syndrome. Dig Dis Sci 1991; 36: 15–18
29 Fich A, Talley NJ, Shorter RG, Phillips SF. Zollinger-Ellison syndrome. Relation to *Helicobacter pylori*-associated chronic gastritis and gastric acid secretion. Dig Dis Sci 1991; 36: 10–14
30 Londong W, Pounder RE, Scarpignato C. Long-term intragastric pH measurement in man. Dig Dis 1990; 8 (suppl 1): 1–96
31 Wagner S, Gladziwa U, Gebel M, Schuler A, Freise J, Schmidt FW. Circadian pattern of intragastric acidity in duodenal ulcer patients: a study of variations in relation to ulcer activity. Gut 1991; 32: 1104–1109
32 Merki HS, Halter F, Wilder-Smith C et al. Effect of food on H_2-receptor blockade in normal subjects and duodenal ulcer patients. Gut 1990; 31: 148–150
33 Lanzon-Miller S, Pounder RE, McIsaac RL, Wood JR. The timing of the evening meal affects the pattern of 24-hour intragastric acidity. Aliment Pharmacol Ther 1990; 4: 547–553
34 Bianchi-Porro G, Parente F, Sangaletti O. Inhibition of nocturnal acidity is important but not essential for duodenal ulcer healing. Gut 1990; 31: 397–400

35   Kaufmann D, Wilder-Smith CH, Kempf M et al. Cigarette smoking, gastric acidity and peptic ulceration. What are the relationships? Dig Dis Sci 1990; 35: 1482–1487

36   Burget DW, Chiverton SG, Hunt RH. Is there an optimal degree of acid suppression for healing of duodenal ulcers? A model of the relationship between ulcer healing and acid suppression. Gastroenterology 1990; 99: 345–351

37   Masoero G, Roassanino A, Arossa W, De-La-Pierre M. Prolonged gastric pH monitoring in responder and nonresponder duodenal ulcer patients: response to placebo and to H_2-blockade administration. J Clin Gastroenterol 1991; 13: 291–295

38   Halter F, Mills JG, Wood JR. H_2-receptor antagonists: intragastric acidity after repeated doses. Aliment Pharmacol Therap 1990; 4 (suppl): 1–98

39   Nwokolo CU, Smith JTL, Sawyerr AM, Pounder RE. Rebound intragastric hyperacidity after abrupt withdrawal of histamine H_2-receptor blockade. Gut 1991; 32: 1455–1460

40   Fullarton GM, MacDonald AMI, McColl KEL. Rebound hypersecretion after H_2-antagonist withdrawal – a comparative study with nizatidine, ranitidine and famotidine. Aliment Pharmacol Ther 1991; 5: 391–398

41   Prewett EJ, Nwokolo CU, Hudson M, Sawyerr AM, Fraser A, Pounder RE. The effect of GR122311X, a bismuth compound with H_2-antagonist activity, on 24-hour intragastric acidity. Aliment Pharmacol Ther 1991; 5: 481–490

42   Kummer AF, Johnston DA, Marks IN, Young GO, Tigler-Wybrandi NA, Bridger SA. Changes in nocturnal and peak acid outputs after duodenal ulcer healing with sucralfate or ranitidine. Gut 1992; 33: 175–178

43   Kerrigan DD, Read NW, Houghton LA, Taylor ME, Johnson AG. Disturbed gastroduodenal motility in patients with active and healed duodenal ulceration. Gastroenterology 1990; 100: 892–900

44   Ching MS, Mihaly GW, Angus PW et al. Oral bioavailability of omeprazole before and after chronic therapy in patients with duodenal ulcer. Br J Clin Pharmacol 1991; 31: 166–170

45   Andersson T, Andren K, Cederberg C, Lagerstrom P-O, Lundborg P, Skanberg I. Pharmacokinetics and bioavailability of omeprazole after single and repeated oral administration in healthy subjects. Br J Clin Pharmacol 1990; 29: 557–563

46   Lind T, Cederberg C, Olausson M, Olbe L. 24-hour intragastric acidity and plasma gastrin after omeprazole treatment and after proximal gastric vagotomy in duodenal ulcer patients. Gastroenterology 1990; 99: 1593–1598

47   Graham DY, McCullough A, Sklar M et al. Omeprazole versus placebo in duodenal ulcer healing. The United States experience. Dig Dis Sci 1990; 35: 66–72

48   Valenzuela JE, Berlin RG, Snape WJ et al. U.S. experience with omeprazole in duodenal ulcer. Multicenter double-blind comparative study with ranitidine (The Omeprazole DU Comparative Study Group). Dig Dis Sci 1991; 36: 761–768

49   Cooperative Study Group. Double blind comparative study of omeprazole and ranitidine in patients with duodenal or gastric ulcer: a multicentre trial. Gut 1990; 31: 653–656

50   Mulder CJ, Schipper DL. Omeprazole and ranitidine in duodenal ulcer healing. Analysis of comparative clinical trials. Scand J Gastroenterol 1990; 178 (suppl): 62–66

51   Miyoshi A et al. The effect of omeprazole and famotidine on duodenal ulcer – a double-blind comparative study. Jpn Pharmacol Therap 1988; 16 (suppl 3): 563

52   McFarland RJ, Bateson MC, Green JR et al. Omeprazole provides quicker symptom relief and duodenal ulcer healing than ranitidine. Gastroenterology 1990; 98: 278–283

53   Blum AL. Treatment of acid-related disorders with gastric acid inhibitors: the state of the art. Digestion 1990; 47 (suppl 1): 3–10

54   Glise H, Martinson J, Solhaug JH et al. Two and four weeks' treatment for duodenal ulcer. Symptom relief and clinical remission comparing omeprazole and ranitidine (Scandinavian Clinics for United Research). Scand J Gastroenterol 1991; 26: 137–145

55   Pan S, Liao C-H, Lien G-S, Chen S-H. Histological maturity of healed duodenal ulcers and ulcer recurrence after treatment with colloidal bismuth subcitrate or cimetidine. Gastroenterology 1991; 101: 1187–1191

56   Farup PG, Rosseland AR, Halvorsen L, Anderson OK, Bernklev T. Duodenal ulcer treated with omeprazole: healing and relapse rates: does treatment duration influence subsequent remission? Scand J Gastroenterol 1989; 24: 1107–1112

57   Brook CW, Yeomans ND, McCarthy PG, Dudley FJ, Smallwood RA. Relapse of duodenal ulceration after healing with omeprazole. Med J Aust 1987; 147: 595–597

58   Lauristen K, Anderson BN, Laursen LS et al. Omeprazole 20 mg three days a week and 10 mg daily in prevention of duodenal ulcer relapse. Double-blind comparative trial. Gastroenterology 1991; 100: 663–669

59   Boyd EJ, Penston JG, Wormsley KG. Maintenance therapy of duodenal and gastric ulcer with H_2-receptor antagonists. Scand J Gastroenterol 1990 (suppl 178): 72–78

60a Penston JG, Wormsley KG. Efficacy and safety of long-term maintenance therapy of duodenal ulcers. Scand J Gastroenterol 1989; 24: 1145–1152

60b Penston JG, Wormsley KG. Review article: maintenance treatment with H_2-receptor antagonists for peptic ulcer disease. Aliment Pharmacol Ther 1992; 6: 3–29

61   Solvell L. The clinical safety of omeprazole. Digestion 1990; 47 (suppl 1): 59–63

62   Committee on Safety of Medicines. Diarrhoea, skin reactions, headaches following omeprazole therapy. Current Problems 1991; 31

63   Humphries TJ. Clinical implications of drug interactions with the cytochrome p450 enzyme system associated with omeprazole. Dig Dis Sci 1991; 36: 1665–1669

64   Karnes WE, Walsh JH. The gastrin hypothesis – implications for antisecretory drug selection. J Clin Gastroenterol 1990; 121 (suppl 2): S7–S12

65   Brunner G, Creutzfeldt W. Omeprazole in the long-term management of patients with acid-related diseases resistant to ranitidine. Scand J Gastroenterol 1989; 166 (suppl): 101–105

66   Jansen JB, Klinkenberg-Knol EC, Meuwissen GM et al. Effect of long-term treatment with omeprazole on serum gastrin and serum group A and C pepsinogens in patients with reflux oesophagitis. Gastroenterology 1990; 99: 621–628

67   D'Adda T, Pilato FP, Lazzaroni M, Robutti F, Bianchi-Porro G, Bordi C. Ultrastructural morphometry of gastric endocrine cells before and after omeprazole. A study in the oxyntic mucosa of duodenal ulcer patients. Gastroenterology 1991; 100: 1563–1570

68   Coupe M, Rees H, Springer CJ et al. Gastric enterochromaffin-like (ECL) cells in hypergastrinaemic duodenal ulcer disease. Gut 1990; 31: 144–147

69   Creutzfield W, Lamberts R, Stockmann F, Brunner G. Quantitative studies of gastric endocrine cells in patients receiving long-term omeprazole. Scand J Gastroenterol 1989; 24 (suppl 166): 122–128

70   Creutzfield W, Lamberts R. Is hypergastrinaemia dangerous to man? Scand J Gastroenterol 1991; 26 (suppl 180): 179–191

71   Burlinson B, Morris S, Gatehouse DG, Tweats DJ, Jackson MR. Uptake of tritiated thymidine by cells of the rat gastric mucosa after exposure to loxtidine or omeprazole. Mutagenesis 1991; 6: 11–18

72   Larsson H, Fryklund J, Helander HF, Wallmark B. Partial pronase digestion of the rat gastric mucosa isolates cells undergoing replicative DNA synthesis. Mutagenesis 1991; 6: 3–9

73   Holt S, Zhao-Hua Z, Powers R. Observations on a proposed measure of genotoxicity in rat gastric mucosa. Gastroenterology 1991; 101: 650–656

74   Pounder RE, Fraser AG. Safety concerns related to treatment of peptic ulceration. Curr Opin Gastroenterol 1991; 7: 894–899

75   Furihata C, Hirose K, Matsushima T. Genotoxicity and cell proliferative activity of omeprazole in rat stomach mucosa. Mutat Res 1991; 262: 73–76

76   Rosenkranz HS, Klopman G. Omeprazole: an exploration of its reported genotoxicity. Mutagenesis 1991; 6: 381–384

77   Weil J, Bell GD, Powell K et al. Omeprazole and *Helicobacter pylori*: temporary suppression rather than true eradication. Aliment Pharmacol Ther 1991; 5: 309–313

78   Hui WM, Lam SK, Ho J et al. Effect of omeprazole on duodenal ulcer-associated antral gastritis and *Helicobacter pylori*. Dig Dis Sci 1991; 36: 577–582

79   Rauws EA, Langenberg W, Bosma A, Dankert J, Tytgat GN. Letter. Lack of eradication of *Helicobacter pylori* after omeprazole. Lancet 1991; 337: 1093

80   Lamouliatte H, Bernard PH, Boulerd A, Megraud F, De Mascoel A, Quinton A. Controlled study of omeprazole-amoxycillin-tinidazole vs ranitidine-amoxycillin-tinidazole in *Helicobacter pylori*-associated duodenal ulcers. Gastroenterology 1991; 100(Abstract): A104

81   Biemond I, Crobach LF, Jansen JB, Lamers CB. Effect of intermittent administration of omeprazole on serum pepsinogens in duodenal ulcer patients and healthy volunteers. Br J Clin Pharmacol 1990; 29: 465–472

82   Bellary SV, Isaacs PE, Lee FI. Upper gastrointestinal lesions in elderly patients for presenting for endoscopy: relevance of NSAID usage. Am J Gastroenterol 1991; 86: 961–964

83   Lancaster-Smith MJ, Jaderberg ME, Jackson DA. Ranitidine in the treatment of non-steroidal anti-inflammatory drug associated gastric and duodenal ulcers. Gut 1991; 32: 252–255

84   Edelson JT, Tosteson AN, Sax P. Cost-effectiveness of misoprostol for prophylaxis against nonsteroidal anti-inflammatory drug-induced gastrointestinal tract bleeding. JAMA 1990; 264: 41–47

85   Londong W, Barth H, Dammann HG et al. Dose-related healing of duodenal ulcer with the proton pump inhibitor lansoprazole. Aliment Pharmacol Ther 1991; 5: 245–254

86   Hotz J, Kleinert R, Gyrmbowski T, Henning U, Schwarz JA. Lansoprazole versus famotidine: efficacy and tolerance in the acute management of duodenal ulceration. Aliment Pharmacol Ther 1992; 6: 87–95

87   Euler AR, Krawiec J, Odes H et al. An evaluation of arbaprostil at multiple doses for the treatment of acute duodenal ulcer: a randomized double-blind placebo-controlled international trial. Am J Gastroenterol 1990; 85: 145–149

88   European Cooperative Roxatidine Study Group. Roxatidine acetate as maintenance treatment for patients with peptic ulcer disease. Clin Ther 199; 13: 47–57

89   Johnston GW, Spencer EF, Wilkinson AJ, Kennedy TL. Proximal gastric vagotomy: follow-up at 10–20 years. Br J Surg 1991; 78: 20–23

90   Pennickx F, Vuylsteke P, Kerremans R. Recurrences after highly selective vagotomy in refractory and non-refractory duodenal ulcer disease. Acta Chir Belg 1990; 90: 41–45

91   Macintyre IM, Millar A. Highly selective vagotomy – a safe operation for duodenal ulcer. Immediate and long-term complications and sequelae in 500 patients. Eur J Surg 1990; 157: 261–265

92   Mistiaen W, Van-Hee R, Blockx P, Hubens A. Gastric emptying for solids in patients with duodenal ulcer before and after highly selective vagotomy. Dig Dis Sci 1990; 35: 310–316

93   Xynos E, Vassilakis JS, Fountos A, Pechlivanides G, Karkavitsas N. Enterogastric reflux after various types of antiulcer gastric surgery: quantitation by ^{99m}Tc-HIDA scintigraphy. Gastroenterology 1991; 101: 991–998

94   Lundegardh G, Holmberg L, Krusemo UB. Long-term survival in patients operated on for benign peptic ulcer disease. Br J Surg 1991; 78: 234–236

95   Eide TJ, Viste A, Andersen A, Sooreide O. The risk of cancer at all sites following gastric operation for benign disease. A cohort study of 4224 patients. Int J Cancer 1991; 48: 333–339

96   Moller H, Toftgaard C. Cancer occurrence in a cohort of patients surgically treated for peptic ulcer. Gut 1991; 32: 740–744

97   Tersmette AC, Goodman SN, Offerhaus GJ et al. Multivariate analysis of the risk of stomach cancer after ulcer surgery in an Amsterdam cohort of postgastrectomy patients. Am J Epidemiol 1991; 134: 14–21

98   Tersmette AC, Giardiello FM, Offerhaus GJ et al. Geographical variance in the risk of gastric stump cancer: no increased risk in Japan? Jpn J Cancer Res 1991; 82: 266–272

99   Colin-Jones DG, Langman MJS, Lawson DH, Logan RFA, Paterson KR, Vessey MP. Post-cimetidine surveillance for up to ten years: incidence of carcinoma of the stomach and oesophagus. Q J Med 1991; 285: 13–19

100 Katkhouda N, Mouiel J. Laparoscopic treatment of duodenal ulcer: a plea for clinical trials. Am J Surg 1991; 161: 361–364

8

Paediatric gastroenterology

R. Nelson

Since the previous review of paediatric gastroenterology in 1988, the most important advances have been related to diagnostic problems in coeliac disease and the research progress on the basic defect of cystic fibrosis and its treatment. This report will therefore concentrate on these two common causes of chronic malabsorption in children.

COELIAC DISEASE

Coeliac disease may present at any age but is most commonly diagnosed under the age of 5. Significant changes in the epidemiology of coeliac disease have occurred.[1] In most parts of Europe the annual rate of diagnosis has fallen from the peak years of the mid-1970s. The mode of presentation has not changed significantly, but there has been an increase in the age of presentation and diagnosis.[2] This is probably related to increased prevalence of breast-feeding and to delay in the age of weaning onto gluten-containing foods in infancy.

Diagnosis of coeliac disease

Despite extensive research the basic aetiology remains unknown. Knowledge is incomplete about the genetic components and environmental factors, including the reaction to gluten. The various theories on the pathogenesis of coeliac disease have been well summarized by Walker-Smith.[3] Since 1970 the diagnosis in childhood, based upon the recommendations of the European Society of Paediatric Gastroenterology and Nutrition (ESPGAN), has required three jejunal biopsies.[4] The main diagnostic criteria are the following:

1. Demonstration of abnormal jejunal mucosa at presentation on a gluten-containing diet
2. A clear clinical and histological improvement on a gluten-free diet
3. Deterioration of the jejunal mucosa after oral challenge with gluten.

Reviews at an international symposium[5] and by ESPGAN[6] repeated the advice. The Italian Working Group for Paediatric Gastroenterology[7] advocated changes. ESPGAN revised the diagnostic criteria at its annual meeting in Budapest in 1989.[8] The new criteria are summarized as follows:

1. The initial diagnosis of coeliac disease must still depend upon demonstration of the characteristic small intestinal histology.
2. There must be a clear-cut clinical remission on a strict gluten-free diet with relief of all symptoms of the disease.
3. Gluten challenge is not mandatory in all patients.
4. A control jejunal biopsy on a gluten-free diet is recommended if:
    (a) The patient was asymptomatic at the time of diagnosis, for example, asymptomatic relatives diagnosed in a family study.
    (b) The clinical response to a gluten-free diet is equivocal.
5. The jejunal biopsy should be obtained via a biopsy capsule. This allows examination and correct orientation of the biopsy specimen under dissecting microscope control.
6. The working party acknowledges recent developments in the use of circulating antibodies to aid the diagnosis (see p. 124).
7. Gluten challenge followed by jejunal biopsy is recommended in the following circumstances:
    (a) If there is doubt about the initial diagnosis.
    (b) In communities with high incidence of other causes of enteropathy – for example, cow's milk intolerance, post-gastroenteritis syndrome, and *Giardia lamblia* infestation.
    (c) If the initial diagnosis is made under the age of 2 years.
    (d) In adolescents intending to abandon the previous gluten-free diet.

It was recommended that the challenge should not be undertaken for at least 2 years after initial diagnosis and treatment with a gluten-free diet. Gluten challenges should be carried out beyond the age of 6 years to reduce the risk of damage to dentition.[9] Although these criteria enable a confident diagnosis of coeliac disease in most patients, several reported situations demonstrate that short-term diagnosis is impossible in a significant minority.

Emerging diagnostic problems

The definition of coeliac disease involves permanent intolerance of gluten. On gluten challenge, most patients earlier diagnosed on satisfactory criteria show a deterioration in morphological damage to the jejunal mucosa within 3–6 months of an oral intake of either at least 2 slices of bread or 10 g of gluten powder daily. Several reports, however, have confirmed that a sizable minority (5–16%) failed to show a histological or clinical relapse after prolonged gluten challenge. In most patients evidence of sensitization to gluten is delayed because histological changes and clinical symptoms develop within 2 years of normal gluten intake. Several reports describe failures to relapse after 5–7 years of gluten provocation.[10] Some of these cases may warrant a diagnosis of transient gluten intolerance[11] rather than coeliac disease. Prolonged follow-up of these patients is recommended strongly, particularly after the recent report supporting the role of a gluten-free diet in the protection against long-term malignancy.[12]

Gluten challenge to confirm the persistence of gluten intolerance will often occur during adolescence. This period of life may be associated with a reduced clinical and mucosal sensitivity to gluten.[13] At this age, reduced compliance to a strict gluten-free diet is common.[14] Many of these adolescent patients remain well, showing satisfactory height velocities on gluten despite evidence of jejunal mucosal relapse.[15] Ten patients have been described whose abnormal jejunal mucosa on a normal gluten-containing diet has recovered spontaneously despite continuing to take gluten.[16]

In coeliac disease, symptoms leading to diagnosis may develop at any period of life. Until recently, it was assumed that patients who developed symptoms after many years' gluten ingestion had prolonged subclinical small-intestinal villous atrophy before final diagnosis. Several reports of late concordancy for coeliac disease in monozygotic twins indicate that coeliac disease may remain latent, with normal jejunal mucosa on prolonged gluten intake.[17] Four patients, (two children, one adolescent and one adult) had a normal jejunal biopsy after several years of a normal diet. A gluten-containing diet was contined from 2.6–9 years after the initial biopsy before a second small-intestinal biopsy showed villous atrophy with crypt hyperplasia compatible with a diagnosis of coeliac disease.[18] On a gluten-free diet all patients showed a reduction of IgA antibodies to gliadin, reticulin, and endomesium (see p. 124), and two patients showed improvement in jejunal mucosal histology on repeat biopsy.

A normal jejunal mucosal biopsy taken when a patient is on a normal, gluten-containing diet does not rule out the possibility that clinical and histological features of coeliac disease may later develop. The reason why some patients develop coeliac disease within a few months of dietary introduction of gluten, whereas others do not acquire gluten sensitivity for many years, is difficult to explain. It is unlikely that these differences are related to low gluten-containing diets in patients who relapse late in life.[19, 20] Trigger factors other than genetic susceptibility and gluten ingestion may be needed to induce mucosal damage and the development of symptoms. Gastrointestinal infection may trigger histological and clinical relapse in latent cases. Adenovirus infection has been investigated as a potential candidate, as there is a remarkable sequence homology between alpha-gliadin and an early protein component of adenovirus 12.[21, 22]

Method of small-intestinal biopsy

The ESPGAN working party continues to recommend that jejunal biopsies should be obtained by intestinal biopsy capsule. This is surprising, considering the widespread use of endoscopic small-bowel biopsies for the diagnosis of coeliac disease among adult patients. Jejunal mucosal material for histological examination can be obtained by three methods – by Watson–Crosby or other biopsy capsule, by endoscopic forceps biopsy, or by a biopsy capsule muzzle loaded onto an endoscope. In experienced hands there is probably little difference, in time taken and discomfort to the patient, between capsule and endoscopic biopsy. The current differences in practice between adult gastroenterologists and paediatricians probably reflects the differing levels of expertise in each method between specialities. In adult patients there are several reports showing that diagnostic accuracy is similar in both methods of biopsy.[23, 24] At least one report confirms these findings in infants and children.[25]

Additional relevant investigations

Diagnosis of coeliac disease depends upon the histological demonstration of villous atrophy and crypt hyperplasia in jejunal mucosa. Whatever method is used, small-bowel biopsy is an invasive and unpleasant investigation which may need to be repeated many times before a confident diagnosis of coeliac disease is made. Considerable effort to discover less invasive ways of predicting the diagnosis of coeliac disease and the presence of villous atrophy has been made. The major supportive investigations are listed in

Table 8.1 Investigations in addition to jejunal biopsy to aid the diagnosis and management of coeliac disease

Folate status	Red cell folate
	Whole blood folate
HLA groups (associated with a high incidence of coeliac disease)	HLA-B8
	HLA-DR3
	HLA-DR7
	HLA-DQw2
	HLA-DR2G
Xylose absorption	Timed urinary xylose excretion
	1-hour blood xylose level
Passive intestinal permeability	Sugar markers – mannitol/rhamnose
	lactulose/cellibiose
	^{51}C-EDTA
	Polyethylene glycols
Rectal gluten challenge	
Antibodies to	Gliadin
	Reticulin
	Endomysium
	Jejunum

Table 8.1. None of them are 100% reliable. Some (e.g. folate status) are useful only as screening tests at initial presentation.[26] Some may be used during oral gluten challenge to predict the timing of subsequent jejunal biopsies. The ESPGAN working party has recently suggested that circulating antibody levels and intestinal permeability tests may, in certain situations, be used in place of jejunal biopsy to indicate the presence of jejunal mucosal damage.

HLA genes on chromosome 6 encode for antigens expressed on the cell surface of lymphocytes and other tissues. Three series of class 1 (HLA-A, HLA-B, and HLA-C) and three series of class 2 (HLA-DR, HLA-DQ, and HLA-DP) antigens are now clearly defined. Several HLA antigenic types have been shown in population studies to be associated with a high incidence of coeliac disease. They are probably markers of closely linked genes which confer susceptibility to coeliac disease, because not all patients with coeliac disease have the commonly associated HLA groups, and family members and normal individuals in the community may share the same HLA groups without developing coeliac disease. This topic is well-reviewed by Walker-Smith.[3]

One of the earliest tests of intestinal absorption used to screen for coeliac disease has been xylose absorption. During the 1970s the 1-hour blood xylose test was introduced to deal mainly with the problem of obtaining accurately timed urine specimens in young children. Recent investigations confirm previous reports that the d-xylose absorption test is limited by poor specificity as a screening test for coeliac disease.[27, 28]

Several methods have been developed to measure passive permeability of the upper intestinal mucosa. Several probe markers have been used, including ^{51}Cr-EDTA, polyethylene glycols, and various sugar molecules, for example, rhamnose or mannitol, which are probably absorbed by the transcellular pathway, and lactulose or cellobiose, which are probably absorbed by the paracellular route.[29] These investigations have been shown to be sensitive markers of small-intestinal damage in a variety of disease states including coeliac disease.[30] The high sensitivity has recently been demonstrated by the rapid change in intestinal permeability occurring in coeliac disease within 6 hours of a single challenge with 50 g of gluten.[31]

It is over 30 years since research demonstrated that the small-intestinal mucosa throughout the jejunum and ileum is sensitive to gluten in coeliac disease. Recent research has indicated that the colonic mucosa also reacts to luminal challenge with gluten. Patients with coeliac disease show a significant increase in total intraepithelial lymphocytes within rectal biopsies following challenge with gluten, as compared with beta-lactoglobulin and with non-coeliac controls.[32] Authors recommend this test as an alternative to jejunal biopsy when this is difficult, hazardous, or contraindicated.

Jejunal mucosal damage resulting from exposure to gluten in coeliac disease probably involves immunological reactions, although final proof is absent. Many cellular and humoral immunological phenomena have been demonstrated in the serum and the gut in coeliac disease, and several of these have now been shown to be useful in final diagnosis. The formation of small quantities of antibody to ingested protein including gluten is a normal physiological occurrence. Several methods have been developed for the measurement of antibodies of various immunoglobulin classes to gliadin. The most frequently used method of detection of IgG and IgA antigliadin antibodies is the enzyme-linked immunosorbent assay (ELISA). Other methods include fluorescent immunosorbent test, immunobinding assay, and enzyme immunoassay.[33, 34]

Over 30 papers have been published on antigliadin antibody measurement in childhood coeliac disease. Comparison of their findings, even of those papers using the ELISA technique, is difficult because of different methodologies.[34] Most papers have assessed the diagnostic sensitivity (percentage of positive results in patients with coeliac disease) and specificity (the percentage of negative results in subjects not suffering from coeliac disease) of each antibody measurement. Most agreed that IgG antigliadin antibodies had a greater sensitivity and a lower specificity than IgA antibodies.[27, 35] Studies analysing results according to age show a higher sensitivity below the age of 2 years and a lower sensitivity in adults.

Other circulating antibodies which correlate with coeliac disease include IgA antibodies to reticulin, endomysium, and jejunum.[36] Global evidence shows these antibodies to be less sensitive but more specific than antigliadin. Several papers recommend measurement of a combination of antibodies for the assessment of potential coeliac disease.[37] The most widely used are IgG and IgA antibodies to gliadin and IgA antibodies to endomysium.[35] Circulating antibodies cannot be the sole basis for the diagnosis because occasional false positive and false negative results do occur. Coeliac disease has been diagnosed in patients with hypogammaglobulinaemia and is more common in individuals with IgA deficiency than in the normal population.

Measurement of these antibody levels has three major functions in the diagnosis and management of coeliac disease. They are as follows:

1. Preliminary screening tests before the final decision to perform an initial jejunal biopsy. They are particularly useful where clinical suspicion of coeliac disease is relatively low – for example, healthy patients with unexplained short stature, healthy relatives, etc.
2. Follow-up of patients on a gluten-free diet. Their disappearance on a gluten-free diet is further evidence in favour of coeliac disease. Their persistence or reappearance may indicate that patients are not following a strict gluten-free diet.
3. Useful measurements at intervals during a diagnostic gluten challenge.[38, 39] Their reappearance may be used to indicate the timing of post-gluten challenge jejunal biopsies.

Summary

ESPGAN has recently simplified the diagnostic criteria for selected patients who do not require a gluten challenge. Diagnosis still depends upon an initial demonstration of small-intestinal pathology and its relationship to gluten ingestion. Patients with a previously abnormal jejunal biopsy who fail to relapse on gluten challenge require long-term follow-up on their normal diet.

The basic aetiology (that is the genetics, the nature of the reaction to gluten, and possible trigger factors) remains unknown. Further long-term studies, involving repeated biopsies and supportive studies of intestinal permeability and circulating antibodies on and off gluten ingestion, are needed to clarify the diagnostic principles applicable to all cases.

CYSTIC FIBROSIS (CF)

Since the last review of Paediatric Gastroenterology in 1988, there have been major advances towards eventual discovery of the basic defect. Since the early 1980s increasing evidence has confirmed that active transport of chloride through specialized channels on the apical membranes of the surface epithelium of various organs is defective in CF. This defect in chloride transport has been demonstrated within the collecting ducts of sweat glands,[40] in the respiratory epithelium of the nasopharynx and bronchial airways,[41] within the epididymis, in the small-intestinal[42] and colonic mucosa, within pancreatic ductules,[43] and within the intrahepatic biliary cannaliculi.[44]

In late 1989 the enormous research effort to localize the mutation on chromosome 7 responsible for the inheritance of CF was finally successful.[45] The mutation occurs in a large gene encoding for a large membrane-associated protein of 1480 amino acids, which has been named the cystic fibrosis transmembrane regulator (CFTR[46, 47]). This protein is one of a large family of membrane-associated proteins. At the discovery of CFTR, the only other family member known to exist in human beings was the p-glycoprotein responsible for multiple resistance to chemotherapeutic drugs among some oncology patients. The DNA sequence of the gene and the amino-acid structure of the protein were established. The mutation delta-F508, deletion of a 3-base pair encoding for phenylalanine at amino-acid position 508 of CFTR, was found to be responsible for the inheritance of CF in the majority of patients. CF is a multiple gene disease, and to date over 100 mutations involving different changes to the structure of CFTR have been found to be associated with its inheritance. In most populations, delta-F508 is the commonest mutation, accounting for approximately 70% of mutant genes responsible for CF. There are geographical differences in the distribution of delta-F508, which is much commoner in north-western

Europe than in southern Europe, the Middle East, eastern Russia, and among certain racial groups such as Afro-Americans.[48]

The discovery that CF can be inherited by many variant genes has confirmed previous suspicions that some patients have genetically determined milder disease than others. Patients who are homozygous for delta-F508 tend to have more severe disease than those who are either heterozygous for delta-F508[49] and another mutation, or homozygous for mutations other than delta-F508. Patients who are delta-F508 homozygous tend to have more severe pancreatic disease[50] and more rapid deterioration in pulmonary function than other patients,[51] although most clinical studies have suggested that there is a close link between mild pancreatic disease and mild respiratory disease, whatever the genetic component.[52]

To date, despite advances in our understanding of the genetics and the cellular biology involved with CF, the basic defect is still incompletely understood. Recent research, however, is providing increasing evidence to support the concept that the defective protein CFTR is the abnormal chloride channel, which is responsible for defective chloride transport across the apical membrane of epithelial cells. Further advances in our understanding of the basic defect may lead to major improvements in treatment. It is already technically possible to transfer the cloned normal gene for CFTR into CF cells, restoring normal chloride transport.[53,54] It may be several years before gene therapy becomes a realistic possibility for CF.[55]

There have also been recent advances in understanding of the mechanisms of lung damage caused by chronic *Pseudomonas* infection. These advances, in addition to gene therapy and further developments in heart-lung transplantation, are likely to produce further improvements in the prognosis in future decades. This treatment is likely to be centred upon the respiratory tract, the site of the most serious complications. As patients live longer, they are likely to develop more and more complications involving other organs (such as the gastrointestinal tract) which are less amenable to primary therapy.

CF is characterized by the very large number of complications which can affect individual patients with the disease. These complications affect many organ systems, but none can compare with the gastrointestinal tract for the number and diversity of potential problems and complications.[56] All regions from the oesophagus to the rectum, including the liver and biliary system, may be involved (Table 8.2). To date, over 40 complications have been described. These include several disorders which are otherwise rare in children and young adults, such as duodenal ulcer, non-pigment gallstones with cholecystitis, biliary cirrhosis, and acute pancreatitis. There are also several seemingly unconnected diseases which appear to occur more commonly than expected in CF. These include coeliac disease, cow's-milk-protein intolerance with enteropathy, Crohn's disease, giardiasis, and several rare carcinomas of the gastrointestinal tract.

Table 8.2 Major gastrointestinal
complications of cystic fibrosis

Gastro-oesophageal reflux[81]
Gastro-oesophageal varices*
Pancreatic exocrine hyposecretion
Neonatal cholestasis
Gallstone* ⎫ Cholecystitis[82]
Non-gallstone* ⎭
Bile-duct stenosis*[83, 84]
Multifocal biliary cirrhosis*
Duodenal ulcer*
Meconium ileus
Distal intestinal obstruction*[85, 86]
Chronic intussusception[87]
Encopresis
Rectal prolapse

* Complications which are more common in
older children and adults.

GASTROINTESTINAL DISEASES WHICH ARE POSSIBLY ASSOCIATED WITH CYSTIC FIBROSIS

Coeliac disease

Several anecdotal cases of coexistence of CF and coeliac disease have been reported. In a population of 11 000 CF patients, the incidence of coeliac disease was 1 in 220. This is greater than the highest reported incidence in a normal population.

Cow's-milk-protein intolerance with enteropathy

Eight CF children under the age of 3 years with abnormal small-bowel histology have been reported.[57] They presented with diarrhoea and failure to thrive despite adequate treatment of the pancreatic steatorrhoea. Seven showed an improvement in diarrhoea and weight gain on a diet not containing cow's milk protein.

Giardiasis

CF patients were found to have a significantly higher rate of infestation with *Giardia lamblia* (28.0%), as compared with a control group of normal members of the same household (6.3%).[58] CF appeared to be the only risk factor likely to account for the difference in infestation discovered by counterimmune electrophoresis of stool samples.

Crohn's disease

Coexistence of CF and inflammatory bowel disease has been reported occasionally. Three cases of Crohn's disease were diagnosed over a 5-year period in a CF clinic of 120 patients.[59] The author suggested that the coexistence of the two conditions was not coincidental, since the frequency was much higher than what could have occurred by chance. Fistula formation seemed to be more common in CF patients.

Intestinal carcinomas

Since 1982, nine adenocarcinomas of the gastrointestinal tract have been described in young adults with CF,[60] including one adenoma of the extrahepatic biliary duct system, four adenocarcinomas of the ileum, and four adenocarcinomas of the pancreas. Clearly, these carcinomas may be associated with CF by chance, but the rarity of these tumours in the normal population and the young age of the patients affected (23–42 years; mean 30 years), suggest that young adults with CF may have an increased risk of certain gastrointestinal malignancies.

Causes of malabsorption in cystic fibrosis

There has been a significant improvement in the prognosis and life expectancy of patients with CF during the past 30 years. Today increasing numbers of patients are surviving well into adult life. In many regions of the UK adults over the age of 16 account for about one-third of all patients. This improvement in life expectancy has not resulted from any major breakthrough in treatment but has been due to many minor advances. Reasons for the improved prognosis are difficult to define, but there is increasing evidence that the greater emphasis on aggressive nutritional rehabilitation and maintenance[61] has made a major contribution to the reduced rate of deterioration in pulmonary function that patients experience today, as compared with previous generations.

The maintenance of satisfactory nutrition depends upon increased calorie and nitrogen intake; aggressive management of pancreatic steatorrhoea with pancreatic enzyme supplements; and identification and supplementation of potential deficiencies in vitamins, minerals and trace elements, essential fatty acids, etc. As pulmonary infection and disease progress, there is often a reduction in spontaneous food intake and an increase in nutritional requirements. This frequently requires more aggressive calorie and nitrogen supplementation – for example, by overnight supplementation via nasogastric tube or feeding gastrostomy. Patients with advanced pulmonary disease, who are potential candidates for heart-lung transplantation, particularly require aggressive supplementation to maintain adequate nutrition to support major surgery.

In many patients the malabsorption of CF is not simply related to the pancreatic exocrine damage. Other gastrointestinal problems, such as gastric acid hypersecretion,[62] decreased duodenal bicarbonate concentration and pH,[63] disorders of bile acid metabolism,[64] and altered intestinal motility and permeability,[65] may all contribute to the malabsorption or affect its response to treatment.

The basis for treatment of pancreatic exocrine failure is the administration of enzyme supplements with each meal. In modern preparations the active enzymes are packaged in microspheres surrounded by a pH-sensitive hydrocarbon membrane, which protects them from destruction by gastric acidity when they have been swallowed into the stomach. At a pH of 5.5–6.0 the microspheres dissolve, releasing the active enzymes into the duodenal lumen.[66] Currently there are three preparations in use in the UK: Pancrease, Creon, and Nutrizym GR. There are differences in enzyme content and in the release of enzymes at different duodenal pH levels. Clinically there is little difference in their ability to control pancreatic steatorrhoea.[67]

In most patients pancreatic enzyme supplements correct the malabsorption enough to support satisfactory growth and weight gain. A few patients continue to have severe steatorrhoea despite taking large doses of enzyme with each meal. A further increase in enzyme supplements is unlikely to improve the malabsorption, as this is probably related to gastrointestinal factors in addition to pancreatic exocrine hyposecretion. In one study, patients' large doses of enzymes were reduced by 50% without significantly affecting fat excretion.[68]

The most important factor affecting the treatment of malabsorption in CF is probably the decreased duodenal pH. Not only will a duodenal pH below 5 prevent efficient release of enzymes from the microspheres, but also the pancreatic enzymes will be inactivated if released from the microspheres. Studies of fasting ambulatory recordings of pH throughout the upper small intestine show prolonged periods below 5.[69]

Patients with persistent severe malabsorption despite aggressive pancreatic enzyme supplementation should be investigated for other factors in addition to severe pancreatic involvement. Particularly in young patients, a jejunal biopsy should be considered to investigate the possibility of associated coeliac disease or other cause of enteropathy. The most effective additional treatment is likely to be therapy to increase duodenal pH and to correct the effects of acid duodenal lumen on the efficiency of pancreatic supplementation, bile acid metabolism, etc.[70] This means long-term treatment to decrease gastric acid secretion with drugs such as cimetidine, ranitidine,[71] misoprostol,[72] or omeprazole.[73] Misoprostol may be particularly indicated, as it increases gastric, duodenal, and pancreatic secretion of bicarbonate as well as decreasing gastric acid secretion in normal control subjects, but, unfortunately, there is no published study confirming this effect in CF. Omeprazole produces more profound suppression of gastric acidity than the commonly used H_2-antagonists. In some CF patients in whom H_2-antagonists have failed to improve fat absorption, omeprazole has been associated with a significant improvement in fat excretion.

There remains considerable doubt about the safety of prolonged suppression of gastric acid secretion,[74] but there is no evidence that prolonged use of these drugs does produce an increased risk of gastric tumours. Suppression of gastric acidity to correct severe steatorrhoea in CF should be considered only if other means of correcting malnutrition have failed. Patients with CF may already have an increased risk of gastrointestinal tumours.

Ursodeoxycholic acid has been used in patients with CF with abnormal liver function tests. Its use has been associated with an improvement in liver function[75] and this treatment may protect susceptible patients from long-term liver damage and development of biliary cirrhosis.

Although ursodeoxycholic acid has less fat detergent property than do naturally occurring bile acids, its use has been associated with an improvement in steatorrhoea[75] and in weight gain.[76] Patients with CF tend to have high glycine/taurine ratios of duodenal bile acids, the result of the increased faecal excretion of bile acids. Supplementation with taurine reduces the glycine/taurine ratio[77] and improves fat absorption.[78, 79] Duodenal bile acids are inactivated by precipitation at a duodenal pH below 5. Glycine-conjugated bile acids are more susceptible to this defect than are taurine conjugates. Ursodeoxycholic acid administration further increases the glycine/taurine ratio,[80] and taurine supplements should also be administered.

SUMMARY

Research in CF is getting closer to the discovery of the basic defect. Future advances in therapy are likely to be aimed at the lung disease, the overwhelming cause of premature death.

CF is characterized by the wide range and variety of clinical complications affecting particularly the gastrointestinal tract. Several occur more frequently in adults. Aggressive nutritional and enzyme supplementation has significantly contributed to the improved prognosis of CF. Malabsorption may be due to other gastrointestinal problems, in addition to pancreatic exocrine hyposecretion. Some of these problems may be improved by controlling gastric acid secretion.

Many children and most adults with CF are managed by respiratory physicians. Regular expert review of nutrition and gastrointestinal status should be part of their long-term care.

REFERENCES

1 Kelly DA, Phillips AD, Elliot EJ, Dias JA, Walker-Smith JA. Rise and fall of coeliac disease 1960–85. Arch Dis Child 1989; 64: 1157–1160
2 Ascher H, Krantz I, Kristiansson B. Increasing incidence of coeliac disease in Sweden. Arch Dis Child 1991; 66: 608–611

3 Walker-Smith JA (ed). Coeliac disease. In: Diseases of the small intestine in childhood. 3rd edn. London: Butterworth, 1988: pp 88–143
4 Meuwisse GW. Diagnostic criteria in coeliac disease. Acta Paediatr Scand 1970; 59: 461–463
5 Visakorpi JK. Definition of coeliac disease in children. In: Hekkens WTh JM, Pena AS, eds. Coeliac disease (Proceedings of the second international coeliac symposium, Noordwijkerhout, Netherlands). Leyden: Stenfert Kroese, 1974: pp 10–16
6 McNeish AS, Harms K, Rey J, Shmerling DH, Walker-Smith JA. Re-evaluation of diagnostic criteria for coeliac disease. Arch Dis Child 1979; 54: 783–786
7 Guandalini S, Ventura A, Ansaldi N et al. Diagnosis of coeliac disease: time for a change? Arch Dis Child 1989; 64: 1320–1325
8 Walker-Smith JA, Guandalini S, Schmitz J, Shmerling DH, Visakorpi JK. Revised criteria for the diagnosis of coeliac disease. Report of working group of ESPGAN. Arch Dis Child 1990; 65: 909–911
9 Aine L. Dental enamel defects and dental maturity in children and adolescents with coeliac disease. Proc Finn Dent Soc 1986; 82 (suppl 3): 1–71
10 Shmerling DH, Francx J. Childhood coeliac disease: a long-term analysis of relapses in 91 patients. J Pediatr Gastroenterol Nutr 1986; 5: 565–569
11 Walker-Smith JA. Transient gluten intolerance: does it exist? Neth J Med 1987; 31: 269–278
12 Holmes GKT, Prior P, Lane MR, Pope D, Allan RN. Malignancy in coeliac disease – effect of a gluten-free diet. Gut 1989; 30: 33–39
13 Maki M, Ladheaho M-L, Hallstrom O, Viande M, Visakorpi JK. Postpubertal gluten challenge in coeliac disease. Arch Dis Child 1989; 64: 1604–1607
14 Mayer M, Greco L, Troncome R, Auricchio S, Marsh MN. Compliance of adolescents with coeliac disease with a gluten-free diet. Gut 1991; 32: 881–885
15 Kumar PJ, Walker-Smith J, Milla P, Harris G, Colyer J, Halliday R. The teenage coeliac: follow-up study of 102 patients. Arch Dis Child 1988; 63: 916–920
16 Schmitz J, Arnand-Battandier F, Jos J, Rey J. Long-term follow-up of childhood coeliac disease (CD). Is there a 'natural recovery'? Pediatr Res 1984; 18: 1052
17 de Sonya JS, de Almeida JMR, Monteiro MV, Ramalto-Magalhaes P. Late onset coeliac disease in the monozygotic twin of a coeliac child. Acta Paediatr Scand 1987; 76: 172–174
18 Maki M, Holm K, Koskinnes S, Hallstrom O, Visakorpi JK. Normal small bowel biopsy followed by coeliac disease. Arch Dis Child 1990; 65: 1137–1141
19 Polanco I, Mearin ML, Larrauri I, Bremond I et al. Effects of gluten supplementation in healthy siblings of children with celiac disease. Gastroenterology 1987; 92: 678–681
20 Montgomery AMP, Goka AKJ, Kumar PJ, Farthing MJG, Clark ML. Low-gluten diet in the treatment of adult coeliac disease: effect on jejunal morphology and serum anti-gluten antibodies. Gut 1988; 29: 1564–1568
21 Kagnoff MF, Peterson YJ, Kumar PJ et al. Evidence for the role of a human intestinal adenovirus in the pathogenesis of coeliac disease. Gut 1987; 28: 995–1001
22 Maho J, Blair GE, Wood GM, Scott BB, Losowsky M, Howde PD. Is persistent adenovirus 12 infection involved in coeliac disease? A search for viral DNA using the polymerase chain reaction. Gut 1991; 32: 1114–1116
23 Mee AS, Burke M, Vallon AG, Newman J, Cotton PB. Small bowel biopsy for malabsorption: comparison of the diagnostic accuracy of endoscopic forceps and capsule biopsy specimens. BMJ 1985; 291: 769–772
24 Achtar E, Carey WD, Petras R, Sivak MV, Revta R. Comparison of suction capsule and endoscopic biopsy of small bowel mucosa. Gastrointest Endosc 1986; 32: 278–281
25 Kirberg A, Latorre JJ, Hartard EJ. Endoscopic small intestinal biopsy in infants and children: its usefulness in the diagnosis of coeliac disease and other enteropathies. J Pediatr Gastroenterol Nutr 1989; 9: 178–181
26 Halsted CH, Reisenauer AM, Romero JJ. Jejunal perfusion of simple and conjugated folate in coeliac sprue. J Clin Invest 1977; 59: 933–940
27 Rich EJ, Christie DL. Anti-gliadin antibody panel and xylose absorption test screening for celiac disease. J Pediatr Gastroenterol Nutr 1990; 10: 174–178
28 Lifschitz CH, Shulman RJ, Langston C, Gopalakrishna GS. Comparison of the d-xylose and polyethylene glycol absorption tests as indicators of mucosal damage in infants with chronic diarrhoea. J Pediatr Gastroenterol Nutr 1989; 8: 47–50

29 Lifschitz CL. Intestinal permeability. J Pediatr Gastroenterol Nutr 1985; 4: 520–523
30 Stenhammer L, Falth-Magnusson K, Jansson G, Magnusson KE, Sandquist T. Intestinal permeability to inert sugars and different sized polyethyleneglycols in children with celiac disease. J Pediatr Gastroenterol Nutr 1989; 9: 281–289
31 Greco L, D'Adamo G, Truscelli A, Parrilli G, Mayer M, Budillon G. Intestinal permeability after single dose gluten challenge in coeliac disease. Arch Dis Child 1991; 68: 870–872
32 Loft DE, Marsh NM, Crowe PT. Rectal gluten challenge and diagnosis of coeliac disease. Lancet 1990; 335: 1293–1295
33 Lerner A, Lebenthal E. The controversy of the use of anti-gluten antibody (AGA) as a diagnostic tool in celiac disease. J Pediatr Gastroenterol Nutr 1991; 12: 407–409
34 Troncone R, Ferguson A. Antigliadin antibodies. J Pediatr Gastroenterol Nutr 1991; 12: 150–158
35 Burgin-Wolff A, Gaze H, Hadzibelimovic F et al. Antigliadin and antiendomysial antibody determination for coeliac disease. Arch Dis Child 1991; 66: 941–947
36 McMillan SA, Haughton DJ, Biggard JD, Edgar JD, Porter KJ, McNeill TA. Predictive value for coeliac disease of antibodies to gliadin, endomysium and jejunum in patients attending for jejunal biopsy. BMJ 1991; 303: 1163–1165
37 Calabuig M, Torregosa R, Polo P et al. Serological markers and celiac disease: a new diagnostic approach? J Pediatr Gastroenterol Nutr 1990; 10: 435–442
38 Ascher H, Launer A, Kristiansson B. A new laboratory kit for antigliadin IgA at diagnosis and follow-up of childhood celiac disease. J Pediatr Gastroenterol Nutr 1990; 10: 43–45
39 Valletta EA, Trevisiol D, Mastella G. IgA anti-gliadin antibodies in the monitoring of gluten challenge in celiac disease. J Pediatr Gastroenterol Nutr 1990; 10: 169–173
40 Quinton P. Chloride impermeability in cystic fibrosis. Nature 1983; 301: 431–432
41 Frizzell RA, Reihkemmer G, Shoemaker RL. Altered regulation of airway epithelial cell chloride channels in cystic fibrosis. Science 1986; 233: 558–569
42 Baxter PS, Read NW, Hardcastle PT, Wilson AJ, Hardcastle J, Taylor CJ. Abnormal jejunal potential difference in cystic fibrosis. Lancet 1989; 1: 464–466
43 Kopelman HR, Corey M, Gaskin KJ, Durie P, Forstner GG. Impaired chloride secretion as well as bicarbonate secretion underlies fluid secretory defect in the cystic fibrosis pancreas. Gastroenterology 1988; 95: 349–355
44 Sinaasappel M. Hepatobiliary pathology in patients with cystic fibrosis. Acta Paed Scand (suppl) 1989; 363: 45–51
45 Rommens JM, Iannuzzi MC, Kerena B-S et al. Identification of the cystic fibrosis gene: chromosome walking and jumping. Science 1989; 245: 1059–1065
46 Kerena B-S, Rommens JM, Buchanan JA et al. Identification of the cystic fibrosis gene: genetic analysis. Science 1989; 245: 1073–1079
47 Riordan JR, Rommens JM, Kerena B-S et al. Identification of the cystic fibrosis gene: cloning and characterisation of complementary DNA. Science 1989; 245: 1066–1073
48 The Cystic Fibrosis Genetic Analysis Consortium. Worldwide survey of the delta F508 mutation – report from the cystic fibrosis genetic analysis consortium. Am J Hum Genet 1990; 47: 354–359
49 Johansen HK, Nir M, Hoiby N, Koch C, Schartz M. Severity of cystic fibrosis in patients homozygous and heterozygous for ΔF508 mutation. Lancet 1991; 337: 631–636
50 Borgo G, Mastella G, Gasparini G, Zorzanello A, Doro R, Pignatti PF. Pancreatic function and gene deletion F508 in cystic fibrosis. J Med Genet 1990; 27: 665–669
51 Campbell PW, Phillips JA, Krishnainain MRS, Maness KJ, Hazinski TA. Cystic fibrosis: relationship between clinical status and F508 deletion. J Pediatr 1991; 118: 239–241
52 Santis G, Osborne L, Knight RA, Hodson ME. Independent genetic determinants of pancreatic and pulmonary status in cystic fibrosis. Lancet 1990; 336: 1081–1084
53 Drumm ML, Pope HA, Cliff WK et al. Correction of the cystic fibrosis defect in vitro by retrovirus-mediated gene transfer. Cell 1990; 62: 1227–1233
54 Rich DP, Anderson MP, Gregory RJ et al. Expression of cystic fibrosis transmembrane conductance regulator corrects defective chloride channel regulation in cystic fibrosis airway epithelial cells. Nature 1990; 347: 358–363
55 Editorial. Cystic fibrosis: towards the ultimate therapy slowly. Lancet 1990; 336: 1224–1225

56 Zentler-Munro PL. Cystic fibrosis: a gastrointestinal cornucopia. Gut 1987; 28: 1531–1547
57 Hill SM, Phillips AD, Mearns M, Walker-Smith JA. Cow's milk sensitive enteropathy in cystic fibrosis. Arch Dis Child 1989; 64: 1251–1255
58 Roberts DM, Craft JC, Mather FJ, Davis SH, Wright JA. Prevalence of giardiasis in patients with cystic fibrosis. J Pediatr 1988; 112: 555–559
59 Behrens R, Segerer H, Bowing B, Bender SW. Crohn's disease in cystic fibrosis. J Pediatr Gastroenterol Nutr 1989; 9: 528–553
60 Lloyd-Still JD. Cystic fibrosis, Crohn's disease, Biliary abnormalities and Cancer. J Pediatr Gastroenterol Nutr 1990; 11: 434–437
61 Shepherd RW, Holt TL, Thomas BJ et al. Nutritional rehabilitation in cystic fibrosis: controlled studies on effects on nutritional growth retardation, body protein turnover and course of pulmonary disease. J Pediatr 1986; 109: 788–794
62 Cox KL, Isenberg JN, Ament ME. Gastric acid hypersecretion in cystic fibrosis. J Pediatr Gastroenterol Nutr 1982; 1: 559–565
63 Zentler-Munro PL, Fitzpatrick WJF, Batten JC, Northfield TC. Effect of intraluminal acidity on aqueous phase bile acid and lipid concentration in pancreatic steatorrhoea due to cystic fibrosis. Gut 1984; 23: 500–507
64 Weizman Z, Durie PR, Kopelman HR, Vesely SM, Forstner GG. Bile acid secretion in cystic fibrosis: evidence for a defect unrelated to fat malabsorption. Gut 1986; 27: 1043–1048
65 Le Clercq-Foucart J, Forget P, Sodoyez-Goffaux F, Zapitelli A. Intestinal permeability to [^{51}Cr] EDTA. in children with cystic fibrosis. J Pediatr Gastroenterol Nutr 1986; 5: 384–387
66 Littlewood JM, Kelleher J, Walters MP, Johnson AW. In vivo and in vitro studies of microsphere pancreatic supplements. J Pediatr Gastroenterol Nutr 1988; 7 (suppl 1): 522–529
67 Beverley DW, Kelleher J, McDonald A, Littlewood JM, Robinson T, Walters MP. Comparison of four pancreatic extracts in cystic fibrosis. Arch Dis Child 1987; 62: 564–568
68 Robinson PJ, Sly PD, High dose pancreatic enzymes in cystic fibrosis. Arch Dis Child 1990; 65: 311–312
69 Robinson PJ, Smith AL, Sly PD. Duodenal pH in cystic fibrosis and its relationship to fat malabsorption. Dig Dis Sci 1990; 35: 1299–1304
70 Zentler-Munro PL, Fine DR, Batten JC, Northfield TC. Effect of cimetidine on enzyme inactivation, bile acid precipitation and lipid solubilisation in pancreatic steatorrhoea due to cystic fibrosis. Gut 1985; 26: 892–901
71 Heijerman HG, Lamers CB, Dijkman JH, Bakker W. Ranitidine compared with the dimethyl prostaglandin E2 analogue enprostil as adjunct to pancreatic replacement in adult cystic fibrosis. Scand J Gastroenterol 1990; 25 (suppl 178): 26–31
72 Robinson P, Sly PD. Placebo-controlled trial of misoprostol in cystic fibrosis. J Pediatr Gastroenterol Nutr 1990; 11: 37–40
73 Heijerman HG, Lamers CB, Bakker W. Omeprazole enhances the efficacy of pancreatin (pancrease) in cystic fibrosis. Ann Int Med 1991; 114: 200–201
74 Selway SAM. Potential hazards of long-term acid suppression. Scand J Gastroenterol 1990; 25 (suppl 178): 85–92
75 Colombo C, Setchell KDR, Podda M et al. Effects of ursodeoxycholic acid therapy for liver disease associated with cystic fibrosis. J Pediatr 1990; 117: 482–489
76 Cotting J, Lentze MJ, Reichen J. Effects of ursodeoxycholic acid treatment on nutrition and liver function in patients with cystic fibrosis and long-standing cholestasis. Gut 1990; 31: 918–921
77 Darling PB, Lepage G, Leroy C, Masson P, Roy CC. Effect of taurine supplements on fat absorption in cystic fibrosis. Pediatr Res 1985; 19: 578–582
78 Belli DC, Levy E, Darling P, Leroy C, Lepage G, Giguere R, Roy CC. Taurine improves the absorption of a fat meal in patients with cystic fibrosis. Pediatrics 1987; 80: 517–523
79 Thompson GN, Robb TA, Davidson GP. Taurine supplementation, fat absorption and growth in cystic fibrosis. J Pediatr 1987; 111: 501–506
80 Marteau P, Chazouilles O, Mejara A, Jian R, Rambaud J-C, Poupon R. Effect of chronic administration of ursodeoxycholic acid on ileal absorption of endogenous bile acids in

man. Hepatology 1990; 12: 1206–1208

81 Cucchiara S, Santamaria F, Andreotti MR et al. Mechanisms of gastro-intestinal reflux in cystic fibrosis. Arch Dis Child 1991; 66: 617–622

82 Snyder CL, Ferrel KL, Salzman DA, Warwick WJ, Leonard AS. Operative therapy of gallbladder disease in patients with cystic fibrosis. Am J Surg 1989; 157: 557–561

83 Gaskin KJ, Walters DLM, Howman-Giles R et al. Liver disease and common bile-duct stenosis in cystic fibrosis. N Engl J Med 1988; 318: 340–346

84 Nagel RA, Westaby D, Javaid A et al. Liver disease and bile-duct abnormalities in adults with cystic fibrosis. Lancet 1989; 2: 1422–1425

85 Koletyko S, Stringer DA, Cleghorn GJ, Durie PR. Lavage treatment of distal intestinal obstruction syndrome in children with cystic fibrosis. Pediatrics 1989; 83: 727–733

86 Koletyko S, Corey M, Ellis L, Spino M, Stringer DA, Durie PR. Effects of cisapride in patients with cystic fibrosis and distal intestinal obstruction syndrome. J Pediatr 1990; 117: 815–822

87 Holmes M, Murphy V, Taylor M, Denham B. Intussusception in cystic fibrosis. Arch Dis Child 1991; 66: 726–727

9

Upper-gastrointestinal haemorrhage

C. P. Swain

It used to be the case that most articles on the management of gastro-intestinal (GI) bleeding would start from the thesis that the mortality from GI bleeding in the last 30 years had not altered despite apparent improvements.

Management was formerly organized on authoritarian lines. Patients were fed, transfused whole blood to maintain their CVP, put on the most potent drug regimens to suppress acid secretion and automatically operated on (preferably early) if they re-bled in hospital.

The subject is humming with controversy at present. The value of traditional management has been seriously questioned. Controlled studies have particularly denied the expected advantages of treatment with potent acid-suppressing drugs. Epidemiologists and some units suggest that there has been no overall alteration in mortality rates, but suggest that there is a trend towards increased mortality, especially in elderly females, perhaps related to the increasing consumption of non-steroidal anti-inflammatory drugs (NSAIDs). Others suggest that the use of defined protocols and combined surgical and medical management have reduced mortality rates in their units. There is perhaps reasonably convincing evidence from controlled trials that certain endoscopic therapeutic techniques can sometimes improve outcome, but there is controversy, especially between proponents of thermal and injection methods. The role of surgery, in particular, has become uncertain, with some surgeons advocating early surgery for elderly patients, while some therapeutic endoscopists treat rebleeding episodes on several occasions before referring patients for surgery. Statisticians indicate that controlled clinical trials in GI bleeding probably have rarely randomized sufficient patients to answer any questions on the management of GI bleeding. The technique of meta-analysis, applied to drug trials in peptic-ulcer bleeding with inadequate numbers, has suggested a possible benefit which has not been confirmed by larger trials – but meta-analysis appears to confirm the efficacy of endoscopic therapeutic methods.

An authoritarian approach to the management of GI bleeding is difficult to justify in view of the paucity of evidence that conventional treatment is effective. Despite this uncertainty, there is no excuse for failing to make an early, accurate diagnosis of the source of bleeding, or for delay in recognition of rebleeding and arranging necessary surgery.

EPIDEMIOLOGY

A study of the epidemiology of peptic-ulcer disease in Britain from 1970 to 1985 by Bloom et al[1] suggests the overall mortality for gastric-ulcer and peptic-ulcer disease has changed little over this period, but there had been an important shift in the age and sex of patients dying of ulcer-related complications. While there has been a steady trend in reducing the mortality in men, there has been an increase in mortality for women over 65. By 1985, 95% of the mortality was in the over-65 age group, especially for women (46% increase for gastric ulcer; 100% for duodenal ulcer). An Australian study by Turner et al[2] of 272 patients with bleeding peptic ulcer over a 2-year period from 1986 to 1987 showed a mortality rate of 9.6% with a higher mortality rate for duodenal (11.4%) than gastric ulcers (6.7%). This study suggests that the commonly quoted mortality rate of 10%, reported in series over the previous 20 years, has changed little. In a US study of the evolving epidemiology of GI bleeding, Gilbert[3] points out that over the same period in the US the admission rate for bleeding gastric ulcer doubled while the admission rate for bleeding duodenal ulcer remained much the same. This large study by Gilbert for the American Society of Gastrointestinal Endoscopy found a mortality rate of 11% in a series of 2225 patients with upper-gastrointestinal (UGI) bleeding admitted between 1978 and 1979. Kafetz & Wijesuriya[4] compared mortality in 155 patients aged over 75 years with 243 patients aged less than 75. The mortality rates in patients with gastric ulcer were similar (14% for those above 75; 18% for those below), but duodenal ulceration was both significantly less common and significantly more lethal (26% for those above 75; 5.2% for those below).

In contrast, some individual units have published a traditional type of paper, now fashionably called an 'audit', in which admissions over a certain period are presented with a relatively low mortality rate for bleeding peptic ulcer; for example, 4.2%, 4.3%, 5.3%, and 5.6%, respectively, in studies by Holman et al,[5] Sanderson et al,[6] Jeans et al,[7] and Branicki et al.[8] These good results are ascribed to close co-operation between physicians and surgeons; none of these units used endoscopic therapy. The absence of controlled trial evidence to support the contention that any conventional aspect of management (such as drug manipulation, transfusion, or surgery) influences the outcome following admission with peptic-ulcer bleeding makes it more likely that chance, or some factor such as a low mean age of the patients, rather than joint management has influenced outcome.

NON-STEROIDAL ANTI-INFLAMMATORY DRUGS AND PEPTIC-ULCER BLEEDING

This increased mortality rate in females over 65 might be due, at least in part, to the increased use of NSAIDs. Two recent case-control studies have suggested that NSAIDs were used more commonly by patients with UGI bleeding, whereas paracetamol was equally used in the two populations. The odds ratio of aspirin and NSAID use was about seven times higher in 875 patients with haemorrhage when compared with 2682 hospitalized controls in Laporte et al's study[9] from Spain and was similar in a Belgian study[10] by Holvoet et al. Although some drugs such as misoprostol or ranitidine have been shown to reduce the frequency of endoscopically observed erosions in the stomach or duodenum, it remains to be proven that prophylaxis with such medication can reduce the incidence of bleeding in patients on these drugs. A study[11] by Edelson et al of the costs involved and the potential years of life saved suggests that primary prevention with misoprostol for all NSAID takers is too costly ($667 400 per year of life saved), but that secondary prevention in patients with a proven history of GI haemorrhage may be more cost-effective ($40 000 per year of life saved).

CLINICAL INVESTIGATIONS

Nasogastric aspirate

Nasogastric tube aspirate was shown by Cuellar et al[12] to be of little value in the prediction of active bleeding (sensitivity of 79% and specificity of 55%) in a prospective study in which a nasogastric tube was passed just before endoscopy and the two evaluations compared.

Urea:creatinine ratio

In Olsen & Andreassen's prospective study[13] in 76 patients who presented with altered blood in their stool within the previous 24 hours, but without haematemesis, the urea:creatinine ratio was compared with ultimate diagnosis for the bleeding source. A ratio of 90 or higher was found in 30 of 42 patients (70%) of those with an upper gastrointestinal source, and a ratio of lower than 90 was found in 32 of 34 (94%) of those with a lesion in the lower part of the intestine.

Endoscopic stigmata, the visible vessel, and the prediction of further bleeding and mortality

A review of the significance and predictive value of endoscopic risk factors for bleeding peptic ulcer by Johnston[14] has suggested an evolutionary scheme for the natural history of stigmata of haemorrhage for peptic ulcer.

Major bleeding from a peptic ulcer is arterial in origin. The bleeding point becomes plugged with a large red clot which reduces in size, to appear as a raised 'visible vessel'. The haemoglobin changes in colour from red to a darker colour. Later the red cells are lysed, leaving a white plug of fibrin and platelets. The raised plug disappears as the healing process is completed.

Is it possible to predict the endoscopic findings in patients with GI bleeding from history and physical examination? Stolzing et al's[15] prospective study which used computer-aided diagnosis, based on 28 variables from the history and eight from the physical examination, indicated that neither a bleeding ulcer nor stigmata of bleeding could be reliably predicted from the patient's history and clinical examination. The authors conclude that all patients with GI bleeding should have an emergency endoscopy if possible. Another study by Coleman et al[16] of risk models for rebleeding and postoperative mortality, based on a prospectively collected database on 387 patients with a benign bleeding ulcer, found that multivariate models for the prediction of rebleeding were rather unsatisfactory (accuracy of 86% but sensitivity of only 54%). However models predicting postoperative mortality were more reliable, with an accuracy of 93% and a sensitivity of 80%.

A study evaluating risk factors for rebleeding and death in 433 patients with bleeding duodenal ulcer, by Branicki et al[17] from Hong Kong, identified large ulcer size and presence of endoscopic stigmata of recent haemorrhage as being the two factors most significantly associated with further bleeding. Ulcer size greater than 1 cm was the factor most strongly predictive of mortality (0.4% vs. 12.5%) in this series, with a low overall mortality of 2.8% and a mean age of 55 years.

THE INCIDENCE AND NATURE OF BLEEDING PEPTIC ULCER IN PATIENTS WITH OTHER MEDICAL AND SURGICAL CONDITIONS

Bleeding peptic ulcer occurs with increased frequency in some medical and surgical conditions and may be associated with a particularly poor prognosis. In a retrospective survey of 112 patients with an abdominal aortic aneurysm, Konno et al[18] reported that 16.7% had a history of peptic ulcer and 6.3% had ulcer bleeding after surgical repair of the aneurysm. A prospective endoscopic study found that 52% (that is, 25 of 48 patients with an abdominal aortic aneurysm) had ulcers or erosions prior to surgery, but none had ulcer bleeding with active medical treatment and reversal of coagulopathy prior to aneurysm surgery.

A lower incidence of 0.4% (18 of 4892) of major bleeding from peptic ulcer was reported by Lebovics et al[19] in patients having open-heart surgery. Most (89%) were found to have a duodenal ulcer at urgent endoscopy.

A study[20] by Allum et al of 30 patients with GI bleeding from gastric malignancies indicated that these patients had a poor prognosis. Twenty-three per cent died during the presenting hospital admission. Twelve of 20 in whom an operation was undertaken had a resection: the median survival of patients with unresectable tumours was 2.5 months, but it was 17 months in those with resectable tumours.

In Parente et al's study[21] of GI bleeding in 15 patients with AIDS, nine had AIDS-related causes (three had UGI lymphoma, one had duodenal Kaposi, two had candidal oesophagitis, two had CMV oesophagitis, one had HSV oesophagitis, and one had *Mycobacterium avium intracellulare*), while six had non-AIDS-related causes (three had peptic ulcer, two had oesophageal varices, and one had erosive gastritis). The authors argue for active investigation with endoscopy except in terminally ill patients, since many causes were treatable. Their patients had a poor overall prognosis with 8% surviving at 1 year, as compared with 64% of 438 patients who had not bled.

The major complications of peptic ulcers are bleeding and perforation. Occasionally patients present with both bleeding and perforation in the course of the same admission. In Hunt & Clarke's[22] series of 840 patients with peptic-ulcer bleeding, 12 (1.4%) were subsequently found to have perforation.

PATHOPHYSIOLOGY

A review of the pathophysiology of bleeding peptic ulcer by Swain[23] outlines three theories which seek to explain why some ulcers bleed recurrently and massively, while others do not, and why peptic-ulcer bleeding is perhaps more prone to recurrent bleeding than ulcers at other sites. He called these theories, respectively, the big-artery, big-bleed theory; the rotten-artery, recurrent-bleed theory; and the pepsin, pH, and adverse-environment theory.

A study[24] by Allison et al of gastric-mucosal bleeding time in 61 control patients and 47 patients with bleeding peptic ulcers or erosions found that bleeding times were significantly shorter (0–5 min) in patients with bleeding than in those without (2–8 min). The authors suggest that enhanced gastric haemostasis may reflect a local protective response to minimize blood loss from the bleeding lesion.

Fullarton et al[25] studied the effect of simulated intragastric haemorrhage on gastric-acid secretion and gastric motility. They infused 160 ml autologous blood or 160 ml egg-white in random order on separate days into the stomach in six volunteers. When compared with the equivalent protein meal, intragastric blood stimulated less acid secretion and delayed gastric emptying. The authors argue that this effect may facilitate haemostasis after gastric bleeding.

DRUG TREATMENT

The results of drug treatment in peptic-ulcer bleeding have been disappointing. The main problem in assessing the effect of drugs has been that no studies have recruited a sufficient number of patients to ensure that a treatment effect has not been missed. Langman's review[26] of the pharmacological treatment of GI bleeding indicates that the technique of meta-analysis when applied to the numerous drug trials appears to suggest that treatment with H_2-receptor antagonists and tranexamic acid is associated with a modest but significant reduction in the rebleeding rate when compared with control treatment, especially in patients with bleeding gastric ulcers. Two large randomized studies, one of famotidine in 1005 patients by Walt et al,[27] and another of omeprazole in 1154 patients by Daneshmend et al,[28] have been published in abstract form with negative results – suggesting that positive conclusions based on meta-analyses of trials with small numbers may have to be viewed with caution.

pH, drugs and recurrent bleeding from peptic ulcer

In a controlled study by Fullarton et al[29] of intravenous famotidine in 20 patients with recent bleeding from peptic ulcer, the treatment group maintained intragastric pH above 6 for a median of 22 hours of treatment, as compared with 13% of the control group. Rebleeding occurred in four of the control group but none of the treatment group (NS). A report in abstract form by Walt et al[27] presented data on the use of intravenous famotidine at the same dose regimen for 72 hours in a placebo-controlled study of 1005 patients with acute peptic-ulcer haemorrhage recruited from 67 different centres. The incidence of further bleeding, the need for urgent surgery, and mortality were the same for the two groups.

Although these studies are depressing news for all of us who hoped that antisecretory treatment might be an easy option to improve the outcome for patients with peptic-ulcer bleeding, the studies by no means indicate that gastric acidity is unimportant in the pathogenesis of further bleeding in patients with bleeding peptic ulcer. Antisecretory drugs might be effective if used in doses sufficient to neutralize gastric and duodenal acidity. The relative merits of continuous and bolus intravenous infusion of H_2 blocker with or without nasogastric antacids to maintain a high intragastric pH for the control of peptic-ulcer bleeding are discussed by Arora et al.[30] It may seem quite an achievement to maintain an intragastric pH of 6.0, but even that may not be good enough. At pH 6.8, platelet aggregation is only 23% of normal, while conventional measurements of extrinsic and intrinsic clotting function (prothrombin time and kaolin partial thromboplastin time) are prolonged by a factor of 4. No gastroenterologist would undertake a liver biopsy with clotting function as deranged as this. Clamping the pH in the stomach and duodenum at 7.4 will require some pharmacological ingenuity.

It is commendable that gastroenterologists have at last begun to mount trials randomizing more than 1000 patients with GI bleeding, but is this enough? The numbers are designed so as not to miss a halving of an expected mortality rate of 10% associated with drug treatment. This seems a lot to ask of a drug; with the possible exception of meningococcal meningitis, it is hard to think of any medical conditions in which any drug halves the mortality rate. Our cardiological colleagues randomize far larger numbers of patients to show small benefits from treatments for hypertension or myocardial infarction, and it is time that gastroenterologists organized themselves to follow in their footsteps. Langman[31] argues that the possible degree of benefit, a 30–40% reduction in rebleeding, with attendant reduced operation and mortality rates, makes it worthwhile to confirm the existence of a 'Holy Grail' of pharmacological benefit by larger studies.

ENDOSCOPIC TREATMENT OF BLEEDING PEPTIC ULCER

Randomized controlled trials

Only randomized trials that include a control (that is, a non-endoscopic treatment group) can hope to provide evidence that a method of endoscopic treatment of peptic ulcer is superior to no treatment. The continued conduct of controlled trials, assessing endoscopic methods for the control of GI bleeding, is an important freedom that must be stressed to ethics committees.

Rajgopal & Palmer[32] have reported a randomized controlled trial of injection of adrenaline and ethanolamine for bleeding peptic ulcer: 25 of 53 (47%) controls re-bled as compared to seven of 56 (7%) patients treated with injection of adrenaline 1:100 000 and 5% ethanolamine ($P < 0.05$). This controlled trial suggests a significant reduction in rebleeding rate but no other end-points for treatment with injection scleropathy. The rebleeding rate in the control group (47%) seems rather high, and the decision to allow some control patients who re-bled to have endoscopic treatment may have reduced the chance of showing that injection altered the need for urgent surgery or the mortality rate.

Lin et al[32] compared a heater probe, alcohol injection, and control treatment. The heater probe was significantly superior to no endoscopic therapy with a lower rebleeding rate (3/45 vs. 22/46), lower requirement for urgent surgery (3/45 vs. 12/46), and lower mortality (1/45 vs. 7/46), (all $P < 0.05$) and it reduced the mean number of days in hospital from 13.8 to 6.2. The heater probe was also significantly superior to injection with absolute alcohol with a lower rebleeding rate (3/45 vs. 15/46) and was better at achieving an initial haemostatic effect (44/45 vs. 31/46). The data on the effect of alcohol injection on surgery or mortality are difficult to interpret, since one-third of patients receiving alcohol re-bled and were treated by the heater probe. Matthewson et al[34] reported a randomized controlled trial comparing Nd:YAG laser, heater probe, and no endoscopic therapy. A total of 143 consecutive patients with stigmata of recent haemorrhage accessible to endoscopic therapy were included in the trial. Rebleeding was significantly reduced in the laser-treated group, as compared with the control group. Although there was a trend suggesting that the heater probe had a lower incidence of rebleeding when compared with control, this was not statistically significant. These results suggested that heater probe and control treatment were inferior to laser treatment. Of 44 laser-treated patients, nine (20%) had further bleeding, including one (2%) death. Of 57 heater probe-treated patients, 16 (28%) had further bleeding and six (10%) died. Of 42 control (no endoscopic treatment) patients, 18 (42%) had further bleeding, and four (9%) died.

A randomized controlled trial comparing heater probe, bipolar probe, and control (that is, no endoscopic therapy) treatment was reported by Jensen.[35] Of 32 heater probe-treated patients, seven (22%) had further bleeding, one (3%) required urgent surgery, and one (3%) died. Of 32 control (no endoscopic treatment) patients, 23 (72%) had further bleeding, 13 (41%) required urgent surgery, and three (9%) died. The heater probe-treated patients had significantly less further bleeding and required significantly fewer urgent operations. Of 30 bipolar electrocoagulation treated-patients, 13 (44%) had further bleeding, 10 (33) required urgent surgery, and one (3%) died. Although the bipolar electrocoagulation results seem better than control and worse than heater probe results, the differences were not statistically significant.

Laine[36] has presented data on the efficacy of bipolar electrocoagulation in two randomized controlled trials. The first compared the efficacy of bipolar electrocoagulation in the treatment of patients with active bleeding from peptic ulcers (with a few Mallory-Weiss tears): 21 were treated with a large, 3.2 mm bipolar probe with a mean 40 s of coagulation. Two of 21 (10%) bipolar-treated patients had further bleeding, and three of 21 (14%) required urgent surgery, as compared with non-endoscopically-treated control patients of whom 19 of 23 (87%) and 13 of 23 (57%) had further bleeding. Bipolar electrocoagulation-treated patients had significantly less further bleeding; fewer urgent operations, transfusions, and days in hospital; and lower hospital costs. In a randomized controlled study of bipolar electrocoagulation in ulcers with non-bleeding visible vessels, bipolar-treated patients had a significantly lower incidence of further bleeding and urgent operations, shorter hospital stays and lower hospital costs. Seven of 38 (18%) bipolar-treated patients had further bleeding, and three of 38 required urgent operation, as compared with non-endoscopically treated patients of whom 15 of 37 (41%) had further bleeding, and 11 of 37 (30%) had further bleeding.

Randomized uncontrolled trials

Trialists, who have already completed one randomized controlled trial which showed significant benefit for one therapeutic modality, have problems if they want to compare one previously successful method with another. These problems include, firstly, the difficulty of convincing an ethics committee that it is ethical to randomize patients to a non-treatment group. Secondly, there is the numbers problem which is due to the amplification of the type-2 or type-B error (that bedevils GI-bleeding trials, since, if both treatments are more effective than no treatment, very much larger numbers of patients are needed to show a significant difference between two treatments than the numbers needed to show a difference between control and treatment group). Trialists are also likely to start with more clinical experience with their first than with their second therapeutic modality.

Chung et al[37a] compared injection of adrenaline with the heater probe, having completed a controlled trial showing that adrenaline alone was superior to no endoscopic therapy in reducing rebleeding rate and requirement for urgent surgery.[37b] They randomized 132 patients with active ulcer bleeding to receive either endoscopic adrenaline injection or heater probe treatment. There were no significant differences in outcome as measured by transfusion requirement (4.5 units vs. 3.8 units), emergency surgery (20% vs. 22%), hospital stay (8 d vs. 7 d), and mortality (two vs. four deaths) between the injection group and the heat probe group.

Laine[38] has carried out a controlled trial showing that bipolar electrocoagulation is superior to no endoscopic treatment in reducing rebleeding rate, requirement for surgery, transfusion requirement, hospital stay, and cost. He has now reported a randomized study[39] without a control group comparing bipolar electrocoagulation with injection of absolute alcohol in 60 high-risk patients with bleeding peptic ulcers. No significant differences were observed in outcome: comparing bipolar electrocoagulation vs. absolute alcohol rebleeding rates, 6% vs. 10%; units of blood transfused, 1.8 vs. 1.3; surgery for bleeding, 6% vs. 7%; and mortality rates, 3% vs. 3%, respectively.

Balanzo et al[40] have reported a controlled trial, comparing adrenaline and polidocanol with no endoscopic treatment, which showed a significant reduction in bleeding for patients treated with injection. The new randomized but not controlled trial[41] compared adrenaline alone with adrenaline and thrombin. Sixty-four bleeding-ulcer patients (visible vessel or active bleeding) were treated randomly with injections of adrenaline $1:10\,000$ ($4-7 \times 1-2\,ml$) alone or adrenaline and thrombin ($5-10\,ml$ of 30 U.l/ml dilution). The rebleeding rate was 6/32 (19%) with adrenaline alone; 5/32 (16%) with adrenaline and thrombin.

The results of these three trials comparing two methods of endoscopic haemostasis without a control group all fail to show significant differences. Should we conclude, with Cole Porter, that anything goes – it doesn't matter what we use? Or should we rather think that GI bleeding is a difficult subject in which it is hard to show anything convincingly? The latter view seems more probable. None of these operators have yet shown a significant reduction in mortality rate, and these studies would have been strengthened, but made more difficult, by the inclusion of a control group. How do we reconcile the results of Laine[39] and Chung et al,[37a] which appear to show that the heater probe and bipolar electrocoagulation are no different from injection, with the results of Lin et al,[33] which seem to show a clear superiority of the heater probe over injection? The answer is by larger studies, preferably with a control group.

If an investigator has carried out a controlled trial which shows that a treatment is superior to no treatment, it may be reasonable to assume, if a subsequent trial compares two treatments and they are not different, that both treatments might be similarly superior to no treatment. There still remains the fear that this may not be a valid conclusion. Randomized trials comparing two methods of treatment carried out by groups without experience in performing controlled trials raise the anxiety level even higher, since there are examples of apparently well-conducted randomized trials in therapeutic endoscopy for bipolar electrocoagulation, heater probe, and Nd:YAG laser which have not shown significant benefit for any end-point.

Hui et al[42] compared Nd:YAG laser, heater probe, and bipolar probe in a randomized study without a control group. Thirty patients were treated with Nd:YAG laser, 31 with heater probe and 30 with bipolar electrocoagulation. Rebleeding rates were similar (10%, 19.4%, and 10%), as was the duration of hospital stay (4, 4, and 5 d), and the proportion requiring emergency surgery (7%, 13%, and 7%). No significant differences were observed in clinical outcome.

Waring et al[43] compared bipolar electrocoagulation in a randomized study without a control group. Clinical outcome was compared in 29 Bicap-treated men and 31 alcohol-injection-treated men with active bleeding or stigmata of recent haemorrhage. Rebleeding rates were 25% vs. 23%; requirement for urgent surgery, 22% vs. 7%; mortality, 14% vs. 7% for Bicap and alcohol injection, respectively. No significant differences were observed.

In a review[44] of controlled and comparative trials of endoscopic therapy, I have suggested that endoscopists would do well to learn from general surgeons. Injection methods are effective in reducing bleeding from very small blood vessels, and thermal methods are effective in stopping bleeding from medium-sized blood vessels less than 1 mm in diameter, but mechanical methods are usually necessary to secure haemostasis in larger bleeding vessels.

Consensus statement on therapeutic endoscopy and bleeding peptic ulcers

This balanced, authorative view of the current status of therapeutic endoscopy for bleeding peptic ulcer, issued by the Consensus Development

Panel, National Institutes of Health,[45] broadly endorses the use of some promising endoscopic methods, particularly heater probe and bipolar electrocoagulation, but also Nd:YAG laser. The statement emphasizes the value of endoscopic stigmata such as the visible vessel (alliteratively retitled 'pigmented protrusion'), encourages surgical co-operation in patient treatment, and supports the need for randomized controlled trials to assess efficacy and safety.

Meta-analyses

Meta-analyses of published trials of therapeutic endoscopy for bleeding peptic ulcer suggest that overall results show convincing evidence that therapeutic endoscopy is associated with a highly significant reduction in incidence of further bleeding, requirement for urgent surgery, and death. Three recent meta-analyses by Sachs et al,[46] Henry & Cook,[47] and Koelz[48] confirm these comforting conclusions. Meta-analysis (totting up the results of published trials) is still a bit of a cheat, and it is no substitute for an adequately conducted, controlled trial randomizing sufficient numbers. The meta-analyst can choose which trials to include and may also be biased by the increased difficulties of writing and achieving publication of negative trials. The heterogeneity of endoscopic therapeutic trials and the variability of operator expertise make such trials more difficult to subject to meta-analysis than drug trials. The heterogeneity of results from the different trials is surely a healthy feature. The imputation that, since meta-analysis has shown benefit, it is no longer necessary to include a control group in further studies needs to be resisted.

EXPERIMENTAL STUDIES OF THERMAL AND INJECTION METHODS

A study by Whittle et al[49] on severed gastric serosal vessels confirms that injection sclerotherapy performs poorly in experimental animal models of ulcer bleeding. Transected canine serosal gastro-epiploic vessels were injected with various materials and mixtures, including normal and hypertonic saline, adrenaline, old thrombin, cephapirin, tetradecyl, and fresh thrombin. These solutions stopped the bleeding in 0–47% of experiments, with adrenaline mixtures producing the best results.

Experimental studies of injection of adrenaline and alcohol into animal gastric mucosa confirm that these substances produce different effects. Chung et al[50] showed that the vasoconstrictive effect on rat mucosa of injected 1:10 000 adrenaline appears to induce ischaemia without congestion (lower haemoglobin concentration; lower oxygen saturation).

Injection of 3 ml of absolute alcohol into the canine submucosa produced a 2.8-mm mean diameter gastric ulcer. Significant increase in mucosal haemoglobulin saturation, indicating congestion, and decrease in oxygen saturation, suggesting ischaemia, were observed before the development of macroscopic mucosal ulceration. This study by Chung et al[51] indicates the potential for major tissue damage of some injected solutions.

Two in-vitro studies of bipolar electrocoagulation have suggested that more effective coagulation might be achieved by pushing as hard as possible and giving prolonged pulses of diathermy.

The best results, according to Laine[52] (equated with deepest coagulation on beef liver), require: (a) placing the endoscope tip en face, as close as possible to the bleeding lesion, (b) applying maximum force, and (c) using prolonged coagulation times of 14 s (or 7 s × 2) at (3), a low watt setting. The weld strength of vessels treated for prolonged periods (20 s) with bipolar electrocoagulation was double those treated for only 2 s (Bicap).

Excised rabbit arteries were studied and in vessels of 0.5–1.9 mm, the mean weld strength with prolonged coagulation and 500 g force of application was increased from 525 mmHg (2 s) to 1160 (20 s) in this study[53] by Harrison & Morris. Does this hint that this technology is underpowered and might be improved by engineering revision?

Complications of injection scleropathy

Three case reports (Chester & Hurley,[54] Lofperido et al[55] and Levy et al[56]), including one fatality, have indicated the potential of injection methods to cause infarction of the stomach or duodenum. The case histories are outlined below. Thermal methods, like injection methods, have been known to cause perforation (for example, there were two perforations associated with heater probe treatment in Chung et al's study[50] and one in Matthewson et al's study[34]) and to precipitate bleeding if a non-bleeding vessel is disturbed. However, infarction of the bowel is likely to be a complication specific to injection.

A 34-year-old patient with cirrhosis and chronic hypoxia bled from an anterior duodenal ulcer with adherent clot. Five millilitres 1:10 000 adrenaline and 6 ml sodium tetradecylsulphate were injected. He died despite surgery. Necropsy revealed circumferential full-thickness necrosis and severe confluent ulceration of antrum, lesser curve, and duodenum.[56]

Adrenaline 1:10 000 (7–8 cc) and 4 ml of polidocanol, injected into a posterior gastric ulcer in a 48-year-old man, produced extensive gastric ischaemia and gastroparesis requiring intravenous feeding for 2 weeks and subsequent jejunostomy feeding. A Billroth II gastrectomy had to be carried out at 3 months because of gastric stenosis. [55]

Chester & Hurley[54] reported the injection of 12 ml of 5% ethanolamine oleate into an actively bleeding gastric ulcer with a visible vessel in a 79-year-old woman. Following an episode of hypotension and further melaena, she was found to have multiple areas of full-thickness gastric necrosis at urgent gastrectomy.

SURGERY

Surgery remains the only option for the patient with continued, life-threatening bleeding which either cannot be stopped by endoscopic methods or persists in patients in units without these facilities. The role of surgery in the management of GI bleeding has become uncertain. It could be argued that the single most important contribution to the apparently diminishing mortality from GI bleeding in some centres has been the increasing conservatism with which surgery is applied. The paucity of prospective, randomized studies of surgery supporting early surgery, the atrophy of surgical treatment for peptic-ulcer disease in general, and the publication of studies in which two or more recurrent bleeding episodes in individual patients have been treated successfully by repeated endoscopic therapy have been associated with a silent shift towards a more conservative application of surgery.

Wheatley & Dykes[57] in the course of a careful review of the timing of surgery have showed an astonishing variation in rates of surgical intervention. Some groups favouring early surgery achieved operation rates as high as 40–70%, while others favoured a delayed conservative approach with operation rates of 5–10%, without clear advantages for either approach. One series with a 5% operation rate reported an overall mortality rate of 3.5%, while another with a 71% operation rate reported a 3% overall mortality rate. The experience of these authors suggests a role for early surgery in a selected group of patients aged 60 or more with an operation rate of 20% and a mortality rate of 3.8–5.5%,[58] but if patients over 60 could be saved from surgery by endoscopic intervention, the mortality might be even lower. A review of the recent surgical literature by Starlinger & Becker[59] shows that, while in the past several authors have argued that, in particular, the elderly patient with concomitant disease should be operated on early to prevent a rebleed (which increases the likelihood of a fatal outcome especially in this group of patients), this may not be true after endoscopic treatment.

The recent literature supports a trend towards simpler operations for bleeding peptic ulcer, aimed, as with endoscopic therapy, at dealing with the eroded vessel in the ulcer floor, thus reducing the morbidity associated with procedures such as gastrectomy or vagotomy and drainage (procedures designed to prevent ulcer recurrence). A study, in which emergency surgery for bleeding from duodenal ulcer omitted oversewing of the vessel in eight patients, was associated with a 50% rebleeding rate. In this study by Hunt & McIntyre[60] 10 of 81 patients (12%) treated by Billroth I gastrectomy died; 10 of 101 (10%) treated by vagotomy, pyloroplasty and underrunning of the bleeding point died; and one of 16 treated by vagotomy and antrectomy died. Tennan & Murray[61] have suggested that the short- and long-term results of simple undersewing of the vessel in a bleeding gastric ulcer are excellent (9% mortality rate), and that patients subsequently managed on long-term H$_2$-receptor antagonists had no further trouble.

COSTS OF HOSPITALIZATION FOR UGI HAEMORRHAGE

An interesting recent exercise in financial audit by Richter et al[62] identified the average cost of hospitalization for admission of 111 patients with non-cirrhotic UGI bleeding in Massachusetts in 1983. The cost was $3180. Most of the costs incurred were for hospital beds or intensive care (63%) and transfusion of blood products (14%), while costs for physicians' services (9%) and endoscopy (2%) accounted for only a small percentage.

REFERENCES

1 Bloom BS, Fendrick AM, Ramsey SD. Changes in peptic ulcer and gastritis/duodenitis in Great Britain 1970–85. J Clin Gastroenterol 1990; 12: 100–108
2 Turner IB, Jones M, Piper DW. Factors influencing mortality from bleeding peptic ulcers. Scand J Gastroenterol 1991; 26: 661–666
3 Gilbert DA. Epidemiology of upper gastrointestinal bleeding. Gastrointest Endosc 1990; 36: S8–13
4 Kafetz K, Wijesuriya. Causes and mortality in patients aged over 75 years with gastrointestinal haemorrhage. J R Soc Med 1991; 84: 32–34
5 Holman RAE, Davis M, Gough KR, Gartell P, Britton DC, Smith RB. Value of a centralized approach in the management of haematemesis and melaena: experience in a district general hospital. Gut 1990; 31: 504–508
6 Sanderson JD, Taylor RFH, Pugh S, Vicary FR. Specialized gastrointestinal units for the management of upper gastrointestinal haemorrhage. Postgrad Med J 1990; 66: 654–656
7 Jeans PL, Padbury RTA, Toouli J. A prospective evaluation of the management of bleeding peptic ulcer. Aust NZ J Surg 1991; 61: 187–193
8 Branicki FJ, Coleman SY, Tuen HH et al. Acute non-variceal upper gastrointestinal bleeding in Hong Kong: a prospective evaluation in 1049 patients. Eur Gastroenterol Hepatol 1990; 2: 309–314
9 Laporte J-R, Carne X, Vidal X, Moreno V, Juan J. Upper gastrointestinal bleeding in relation to previous use of analgesics and non-steroidal anti-inflammatory drugs. Lancet 1991; 337: 85–89
10 Holvoet J, Terriere L, Van Hee W, Verbist L, Fiercus E, Hautekeefe ML. Relation of upper gastrointestinal bleeding to non-steroidal anti-inflammatory drugs and aspirin: a case-control study. Gut 1991; 32: 730–734
11 Edelson JT, Tosteson ANA, Sax P. Cost-effectiveness of misoprostol for prophylaxis against non-steroidal anti-inflammatory drug-induced gastrointestinal tract bleeding. JAMA 1990; 264: 41–47
12 Cuellar RE, Gavaler JSM, Alexander JA et al. Gastrointestinal tract haemorrhage: the value of a nasogastric aspirate. Arch Intern Med 1990; 150: 1381–1384
13 Olsen LH, Andreassen KH. Stools containing altered blood – plasma urea:creatinine ratio as a simple test for the source of bleeding. Br J Surg 1991; 78: 71–73
14 Johnston JH. Endoscopic risk factors for bleeding peptic ulcer. Gastrointest Endosc 1990; 36: S16–20
15 Stolzing H, Ohmann C, Krick M, Thon K. Diagnostic emergency endoscopy in upper gastrointestinal bleeding – do we have any decision aids for patient selection? Hepatogastroenterology 1991; 38: 224–227
16 Coleman SY, Pritchett CJ, Wong J, Branicki FJ. Risk models for rebleeding and postoperative mortality in bleeding gastric ulcer. Ann R Coll Surg Engl 1991; 73: 179–184

17   Branicki FJ, Boey J, Fok PJ et al. Bleeding duodenal ulcer – a prospective evaluation of
     risk factor for rebleeding and death. Ann Surg 1991; 211: 411–418
18   Konno H, Sakaguchi S, Hachiya T. Bleeding peptic ulcer after abdominal aortic
     aneurysm surgery. Arch Surg 1991; 126: 894–897
19   Lebovics E, Lee SS, Dworkin BM et al. Upper gastrointestinal bleeding following open-
     heart surgery. Dig Dis Sci 1991; 36: 757–760
20   Allum WH, Brearley S, Wheatley KE, Dykes PW, Keighley MRB. Acute haemorrhage
     from gastric malignancy. Br J Surg 1990; 77: 19–20
21   Parente F, Cernuschi M, Valsecchi L et al. Acute upper gastrointestinal bleeding in
     patients with AIDS: a relatively uncommon condition associated with a reduced
     survival. Gut 1991; 32: 987–990
22   Hunt PS, Clarke G. Perforation in patients with bleeding ulcer. Aust NZ J Surg 1991;
     61: 183–185
23   Swain CP. Pathophysiology of bleeding lesions. Gastrointest Endosc 1990; 36: S21–22
24   Allison MC, Fullarton GM, Brown IL, Crean GP, McColl KEL. Enhanced gastric
     mucosal haemostasis after upper gastrointestinal haemorrhage. Gut 1991; 32: 735–739
25   Fullarton GM, Boyd EJS, Crean GP, Hilditch TE, McColl KEL. Effect of simulated
     intragastric haemorrhage on gastric secretion, gastric motility, and serum gastrin. Gut
     1990; 31: 518–521
26   Langman MJS. Problems in assessing pharmacological treatment in acute upper
     gastrointestinal bleeding. Hepatogastroenterology 1990; 37 (suppl 1): 29–30
27   Walt RP, Cottrell J, Mann SG, Freemantle N, Langman MJS. Randomised double-
     blind controlled trial of intravenous famotidine infusion in 1005 patients with peptic
     ulcer bleeding (abstract). Gut 1991; 32: A571
28   Daneshmend TK, Hawkey CJ, Langman MJS, Logan RFA, Long RG, Walt RP.
     Omeprazole vs. placebo for acute upper gastrointestinal bleeding: a randomized double-
     blind controlled trial in 1154 patients. Gut 1990; 31: A1206
29   Fullarton GM, MacDonald AM, Mann SG, McColl KEL. Controlled study of the
     effects of intravenous famotidine on intragastric pH in bleeding peptic ulcers. Aliment
     Pharmacol Therapy 1991; 5: 77–84
30   Arora A, Tandon RK, Achara SK. Letter. Intragastric pH and control of peptic ulcer
     bleeding. Am J Gastroenterol 1991; 86: 116
31   Langman MJS. Letter. Pharmacotherapy of bleeding peptic ulcers – is it time to give up
     the search? Gastroenterology 1990; 98: 1724–1725
32   Rajgopal C, Palmer KR. Endoscopic injection sclerosis: effective treatment for bleeding
     peptic ulcer. Gut 1991; 32: 727–729
33   Lin HJ, Lee FY, Kang WM, Tsai YT, Lee SD, Lee CH. Heat probe thermocoagulation
     and pure alcohol injection in massive peptic ulcer haemorrhage: a prospective
     randomised controlled trial. Gut 1990; 31: 753–757
34   Matthewson K, Swain CP, Bland M, Kirkham JS, Brown SG, Northfield TC.
     Randomized comparison of Nd:YAG laser, heater probe and no endoscopic therapy for
     bleeding peptic ulcers. Gastroenterology 1990; 98: 1239–1244
35   Jensen DM. Heat probe for hemostasis of bleeding peptic ulcers: techniques and results
     of randomized controlled trials (Proceedings of the Consensus Conference on
     Therapeutic Endoscopy in Bleeding Peptic Ulcers). Gastrointest Endosc 1990; 30:
     S42–49
36   Laine L. Bipolar/multipolar electrocoagulation. Gastrointest Endosc 1990; 36: S38–41
37a Chung SCS, Leung JWC, Sung JY, Lo KK, Li AHC. Injection or heat probe for
     bleeding ulcer. Gastroenterology 1991; 100: 33–37
37b Chung SCS, Leung JWC, Steele RJC et al. Endoscopic injection of adrenaline for
     actively bleeding ulcers: a randomized trial. BMJ 1988; 296: 1631–1633
38   Laine L. Multipolar electrocoagulation in the treatment of active upper gastrointestinal
     tract haemorrhage. N Engl J Med 1987; 316: 1613–1617
39   Laine L. Multipolar electrocoagulation versus injection therapy in the treatment of
     bleeding peptic ulcers. A prospective, randomized trial. Gastroenterology 1990; 99:
     1303–1306
40   Balanzo J, Sainz S, Such J et al. Endoscopic hemostasis by local injection of epinephrine
     and polidocanol in bleeding ulcer. A prospective randomized trial. Endoscopy 1988; 20:
     289–291

41   Balanzo J, Villanueva C, Sainz S et al. Injection therapy of bleeding peptic ulcer, a prospective, randomized trial using epinephrine and thrombin. Endoscopy 1990; 22: 157–159

42   Hui WM, Ng MMT, Lok ASF, Lai CL, Lau YN, Lam SK. A randomized comparative study of laser photocoagulation, heater probe, and bipolar electrocoagulation in the treatment of actively bleeding ulcers. Gastrointest Endosc 1991; 7: 295–298

43   Waring JP, Sanowski RA, Sawyer RL, Woods A, Foutch PG. A randomized comparison of multipolar electrocoagulation and injection sclerosis for the treatment of bleeding peptic ulcer. Gastrointest Endosc 1991; 7: 295–298

44   Swain CP. Operative endoscopy in acute upper GI bleeding – indications, techniques, prognosis. Hepatogastroenterology 1991; 38: 201–206

45   Consensus Development Panel, National Institutes of Health. Consensus statement on therapeutic endoscopy and bleeding ulcers. Gastrointest Endosc 1990; 36: S62–63

46   Sacks HS, Chalmers TC, Blum AL, Berrier J, Pagamo D. Endoscopic hemostasis – an effective therapy for bleeding peptic ulcers. JAMA 1990; 264: 494–499

47   Henry D, Cook D. Letter. Meta-analysis workshop in upper gastrointestinal haemorrhage. Gastroenterology 1991; 100: 1481–1482

48   Koelz HR. Die Kurativtherapie des Ulcus ventriculi und des Ulcus duodeni. In: Blum AL, Bauerfeind P, eds. Ulkusalmanach 2. Heidelberg: Springer-Verlag, 1990:

49   Whittle TJ, Sugawa C, Lucas CE et al. Effect of hemostatic agents in canine gastric serosal blood vessels. Gastrointest Endosc 1991; 37: 305–309

50   Chung SCS, Leung JWC, Leung FW. Effect of submucosal epinephrine injection on local gastric blood flow. A study using laser doppler flowmetry and reflectance spectrometry. Dig Dis Sci 1990; 35: 1008–1011

51   Chung SCS, Sung JY, Suen MWM, Leung JWC, Leung FW. Endoscopic assessment of mucosal hemodynamic changes in a canine model of gastric ulcer. Gastrointest Endosc 1991; 37: 310–314

52   Laine L. Determination of the optimal technique for bipolar electrocoagulation treatment. Gastroenterology 1991; 100: 107–112

53   Harrison JD, Morris DL. Does bipolar electrocoagulation time affect vessel weld strength? Gut 1991; 32: 188–190

54   Chester JF, Hurley PR. Gastric necrosis – a complication of endoscopic sclerosis for bleeding peptic ulcer. Endoscopy 22: 287

55   Lopifido S, Patelli G, Latorre L. Extensive necrosis of gastric mucosa following injection therapy of bleeding peptic ulcer. Endoscopy 1990; 22: 285–286

56   Levy J, Khakoo S, Barton R, Vicary R. Fatal injection sclerotherapy of a bleeding peptic ulcer. Lancet 1991; 337: 504

57   Wheatley KE, Dykes PW. Upper gastrointestinal bleeding: when to operate. Postgrad Med J 1990; 66: 926–931

58   Wheatley KE, Snyman JH, Brearley S, Keighley MRB, Dykes PW. Mortality in patients with bleeding peptic ulcer when those aged 60 or over are operated on early. Br Med J 1990; 301: 272

59   Starlinger M, Becker HD. Upper gastrointestinal bleeding – indications and results in surgery. Hepatogastroenterology 1991; 38: 216–219

60   Hunt PS, McIntyre RLE. Choice of operative procedure for bleeding duodenal ulcer. Br J Surg 1990; 77: 1004–1006

61   Tennan RP, Murray WR. Late outcome of undersewing alone for gastric ulcer haemorrhage. Br J Surg 1990; 70: 811–812

62   Richter JM, Wang TC, Fawaz K, Bynum TE, Fallon D, Shapleigh C. Practice patterns and costs of hospitilization for upper gastrointestinal hemorrhage. J Clin Gastroenterol 1991; 13: 268–273

10

Colorectal oncology

H. J. W. Thomas

Gastrointestinal neoplasia is a major cause of morbidity and mortality, accounting for 41 000 deaths in England and Wales each year.[1] Colorectal cancer is the commonest gastrointestinal malignancy (Table 10.1) and is second only to lung cancer as a cause of cancer deaths. The high mortality from colorectal cancer has led to intensive research into its genetics and epidemiology, and into the management of disseminated disease. In the past few years there have been great advances in understanding the genetics and molecular genetics of colorectal cancer. There has also been progress in adjuvant treatment of late stage disease and the treatment of disseminated disease. These advances provide a model for the molecular biology and management of other gastrointestinal malignancies.

Table 10.1 Mortality from gastrointestinal neoplasia in England and Wales in 1988

Site of carcinoma	Number of deaths	
Oesophagus	4884	
Stomach	9425	
Colon	11 494	17 240
Rectum	5746	
Liver and bile duct	1420	
Pancreas	6008	

THE GENETICS OF COLORECTAL CANCER

There are several rare inherited syndromes which predispose to the development of colorectal cancer, the best known of which is familial adenomatous polyposis (FAP). These conditions also provide an insight into the genetic changes which occur during the development of non-familial colorectal cancer. Most colorectal carcinomas are thought to arise from pre-existing benign adenomatous polyps, and this has allowed the analysis of the genetic changes that occur during tumorigenesis.

Inherited predispositions to colorectal cancer

FAP

FAP is a highly penetrant, autosomal-dominant condition in which multiple adenomatous polyps develop throughout the colon and rectum during adolescence. The polyps greatly increase the risk of colorectal cancer, which usually develops by the age of 40 unless prophylactic colectomy is performed.[2]

Patients with FAP who do not develop colorectal cancer, as a result of having had a colectomy, are at increased risk of later developing other malignancies. Duodenal adenomas are found in almost all FAP patients and appear to be premalignant in a manner analogous to that of colonic adenomatous polyps.[3] Intra-abdominal desmoid tumours develop in 4% of FAP patients, and, although non-malignant, they may grow rapidly and be locally invasive.[4] There is also an increased incidence of some extra-intestinal tumours, including primary brain tumours, particularly medulloblastomas,[5, 6] and papillary carcinoma of the thyroid.[7] Hepatoblastoma, a rare childhood tumour, has been reported in the children of FAP patients, some of whom, when successfully treated, have subsequently developed adenomatous polyposis.[8, 9]

The extraintestinal features of FAP have been used to aid presymptomatic diagnosis in individuals at risk. These features include the multiple subcutaneous cysts and osteomas of the Gardner syndrome,[10] and congenital hypertrophy of the retinal pigment epithelium, which is found in a high proportion of FAP patients.[11]

Hereditary non-polyposis colorectal cancer

Hereditary non-polyposis colorectal cancer (HNPCC) is a dominantly inherited predisposition to colorectal cancer in the absence of polyposis. The tumours in these pedigrees show a proximal (right-sided) predominance and an early age of onset. HNPCC is thought to be responsible for approximately 5% of all colorectal cancers.[12-14]

HNPCC has been subdivided into Lynch syndromes I and II. Lynch syndrome I (also known as hereditary site-specific colon cancer) predisposes only to colonic cancer, whereas Lynch syndrome II (also known as cancer family syndrome) predisposes to colorectal cancer, endometrial cancer, ovarian cancer, and stomach cancer.[15, 16] In both syndromes the peak incidence of colorectal cancer is in the fifth decade. Unlike in FAP, the colon is not carpeted in adenomatous polyps, although adenomatous polyps are found in patients with these syndromes.

Common colorectal cancer

There is evidence of the familial clustering of colorectal cancer even after excluding pedigrees with FAP and HNPCC. The first-degree relatives of patients with colorectal cancer have a risk of dying from colorectal cancer 2–3 times greater than that of the general population or of spouse controls.[17-19] These results suggest that there may be an inherited predisposition to common colorectal cancer.

There is also an increased incidence of colorectal cancer in the relatives of both adenoma and carcinoma probands. The prevalence of adenomas in the relatives of adenoma and carcinoma probands is also 2–3 times that in control families. These results are consistent with an inherited predisposition to adenoma formation in common colorectal cancer.[20]

The genetic predispositions to common colorectal cancer has been investigated further. Thirty-five pedigrees, in which there were either multiple cases of colorectal cancer or probands with one or more colonic adenomas, were screened for colonic adenomas and cancers. Polyps were found twice as frequently in the first-degree relatives of probands as in those of spouses, who served as controls.[21]

The pedigrees were analysed to see if there was evidence of an inherited susceptibility to adenomas within the families. A dominant model of inheritance was significantly more likely to explain the observed familial occurrence than was recessive inheritance or sporadic occurrence. The estimated gene frequency was 0.19, with a lifetime penetrance of 0.4 for adenomas or colorectal cancer in gene carriers.

Thus, in addition to the well-known, highly penetrant inherited predispositions to colorectal cancer, such as FAP and the Lynch syndromes, there is also familial clustering of common colorectal cancer. The increased familial incidence of common colorectal cancer may be due to a genetic predisposition to the development of colorectal adenomas which is inherited as a partially penetrant, autosomal-dominant trait.

Screening of patients at high risk of colorectal cancer

The increased risk of colorectal cancer developing among the first-degree relatives of patients with colorectal cancer has led to the establishment of clinics for screening and genetic counselling. At St Mark's Hospital, London, the relatives of patients with colorectal cancer were seen in the family cancer clinic, and their lifetime risk of developing colorectal cancer was calculated.[22] Those with a lifetime risk of 1-in-10 or greater were offered screening every 5 years by colonoscopy, and those with a lifetime risk of between 1-in-10 and 1-in-17 were offered yearly screening for faecal occult blood.

Over 4 years 715 patients were seen, of whom 644 accepted screening. One hundred and fifty-one lower-risk patients were screened for faecal occult blood, and two were found to have polyps. Fifty-nine patients at high risk of colorectal cancer (lifetime risk of 1-in-10 or greater) were screened for faecal occult blood prior to colonoscopy. Of the 57 in whom faecal occult blood was not detected, 13 were found to have adenomatous polyps at colonoscopy. Thus, faecal occult blood appears to be a poor screening test in high-risk patients.

Of 382 high-risk patients screened by colonoscopy, 62 were found to have adenomatous polyps and a further five to have colonic cancer. Of the 715 patients seen, 83 had pedigrees compatible with Lynch syndrome I (hereditary site-specific colon cancer), and 110 pedigrees compatible with Lynch syndrome II (cancer family syndrome). Female patients with Lynch syndrome II were also screened for breast and pelvic malignancy.

This study demonstrates that patients at high risk of developing colorectal cancer can be selected by their family history, and that colonoscopy can detect a high number of premalignant adenomatous polyps.

The *adenomatous polyposis coli* gene

FAP, which is inherited as an autosomal dominant, provides an ideal condition for the rapidly developing techniques of molecular genetics. The *Adenomatous Polyposis Coli (APC)* gene, mutations of which are responsible for FAP, has been cloned and characterized in a remarkably short time.

The location of the *APC* gene was indicated by a case report of a patient with FAP who was found to have a constitutional interstitial deletion of chromosome 5.[23] This location was confirmed by genetic linkage between a polymorphic DNA probe mapped to chromosome 5q21–q22 and the disease in FAP families. No evidence of genetic heterogeneity was found between FAP and the Gardner syndrome, suggesting that the syndromes are allelic.[24, 25] Further polymorphic DNA markers more closely linked and flanking the locus were isolated and have since been used for presymptomatic diagnosis.[26 – 30]

The *APC* gene was isolated simultaneously by two groups.[31 – 34] The precise location of the gene was determined from two patients with FAP, both of whom had submicroscopic deletions of chromosome 5 which overlapped and included the *APC* gene. Mutations of the candidate *APC* gene were then detected in other patients with FAP. The gene is widely expressed in different tissues, and its sequence suggests that it has a coiled-coil structure; its function is, as yet, unknown.

Presymptomatic screening for FAP

The first-degree relative of a FAP patient has a 1-in-2 chance of having inherited the mutant gene and of developing the disease. Individuals at risk have previously been screened for the development of rectal polyps by sigmoidoscopy. The identification of the *APC* gene will allow the specific mutation of the gene in each FAP family to be characterized, and this will permit presymptomatic diagnosis of family members at risk of developing FAP. In families where the specific mutation of the *APC* gene has not been identified, polymorphic DNA markers within the gene will allow accurate presymptomatic diagnosis.

A clinical study, performed before the *APC* gene was identified, has successfully demonstrated the use of linked polymorphic DNA markers for the presymptomatic diagnosis of FAP.[35]

Kindred 353

Leppert et al have reported linkage to markers in the *APC* region of chromosome 5 in an atypical non-FAP kindred with a high incidence of early onset colorectal cancer and a highly variable number of colonic adenomas in affected members.[36] This raises the possibility that different mutant alleles of the *APC* gene may be responsible for other identified predispositions to colorectal cancer.

Genetic alterations in colorectal tumorigenesis

Introduction

The development of malignant tumours in adults involves multiple steps; in colorectal tumorigenesis many of these genetic alterations have been identified and now provide a model for other malignancies. These genetic changes have been shown to include both the activation of dominantly-acting proto-oncogenes and the inactivation of tumour-suppressor genes. The role of these alterations in tumorigenesis has been further clarified by studying their frequency at different stages of tumour development from small adenomatous polyps to metastatic carcinomas.

Activation of proto-oncogenes

Activation of dominantly-acting proto-oncogenes has been shown to play an important role in the development of many different types of human tumour malignancy.[37] Specific mutations leading to the activation of k-*ras*, a cytoplasmic signal transduction protein, occur in up to 60% of sporadic colorectal adenomas and 50% of carcinomas but are present in only 7% of FAP adenomas.[38-41] Increased c-*myc* expression and pp60[c-src] tyrosine kinase activity are also found in colorectal tumours.[42-44] However, no specific mutations have been shown to cause these changes, and it is unclear whether they are associated with, or are the cause of, neoplastic transformation.

Tumour-suppressor genes

Tumour-suppressor genes are a class of genes whose normal function is to suppress cell proliferation. Inactivation of these genes during tumorigenesis results in the loss of normal growth control. De Mars proposed that a mutation of one copy of this type of gene was inherited in conditions such as FAP and that neoplasms resulted from the subsequent somatic mutation of the normal allele.[45] Knudson later proposed that the same germline genes would also be altered somatically in the development of both familial and non-familial cancers.[46]

The inactivation of tumour-suppressor genes during tumorigenesis is often associated with the loss of the tumour-suppressor gene DNA. This may be detected by the loss of restriction fragment length polymorphism alleles in the tumour DNA that are present in normal DNA from the same individual. Thus, the loss of constitutional heterozygosity in tumours may be used to detect the site of tumour-suppressor genes.[47]

Chromosome 5 alterations in colorectal tumorigenesis.   Are mutations of the *APC* gene involved in the development of non-familial colorectal cancer? The mapping of the *APC* gene to chromosome 5 allowed the comparison of normal and tumour DNA from patients with colorectal cancer in order to look for the loss of genetic material on chromosome 5. These experiments demonstrated chromosome-5 allele loss in both common (non-familial) colorectal carcinomas and FAP carcinomas, and also in common adenomatous polyps, but not in FAP polyps.[40, 48–50]

Kinzler et al defined the region of chromosome 5 in which the greatest proportion of colorectal carcinomas showed allele loss.[51] They isolated and characterized a gene from this region which they called *MCC* (mutated in colorectal cancer) and in which they demonstrated mutations in three colorectal carcinomas. The *MCC* gene lies in close proximity to the *APC* gene, and its sequence suggests that the product has a similar coiled-coil structure. It has yet to be determined whether the products of the *APC* and *MCC* genes interact with each other.

De Mars' theory predicted that loss of function of the genes on chromosome 5 would result in tumorigenesis. This has been confirmed by an experiment in which a wild-type chromosome 5 was transferred into a colorectal cancer cell line, resulting in suppression of tumorigenicity.[52]

p53 and DCC *mutations in colorectal neoplasia.*   Two further genes, *p53* and *DCC*, which are mutated during colorectal tumorigenesis have been identified. Frequent karyotypic abnormalities of chromosomes 17 and 18 have been detected in colorectal carcinomas.[53, 54] These cytogenetic abnormalities have been confirmed by molecular studies of paired DNA from normal and tumour tissue which demonstrated allele loss on chromosomes 17 and 18 in a high proportion of colorectal carcinomas.[55, 56]

On chromosome 17 the region in which the greatest proportion of colorectal carcinomas show allele loss was noted to include the gene for the oncoprotein *p53*.[57] Point mutations were found to occur commonly in highly conserved regions of the gene in colorectal cancers but rarely in adenomatous polyps. Inactivation of *p53* thus appears to be associated with the transition from benign to malignant growth.[58]

The transfection of wild-type *p53* into colorectal cancer cell lines has been shown to inhibit their proliferation, whereas the transfection of mutant *p53* does not. This provides further evidence that *p53* acts as a growth suppressor in the human colon.[59]

Fearon et al isolated a gene which they called *deleted in colorectal carcinomas (DCC)* from the common region of genetic loss on chromosome 18.[60] *DCC* has significant sequence homology to neural cell adhesion molecules and other related cell-surface glycoproteins and is expressed in most normal tissue, including colon tissue. Its expression is greatly reduced in most colorectal carcinomas. The precise biological function of *DCC* has yet to be determined.

Other somatic events in colorectal tumorigenesis.   In addition to the genetic alterations on chromosomes 5, 17, and 18, loss of heterozygosity has also been detected on chromosomes 1q, 4p, 6p, 6q, 8p, 9q, and 22q in 25–50% of colorectal carcinomas.[61] These sites of allele loss may represent the location of further tumour-suppressor genes.

A genetic model of colorectal tumorigenesis

Molecular studies have confirmed the clonal nature of colorectal tumours, and they demonstrate the multistep nature of tumorigenesis in the accumulation of genetic changes during the progression from normal mucosa to adenoma to carcinoma.

Fearon & Vogelstein[62] have proposed a genetic model of colorectal tumorigenesis (Figure 10.1). The simplest model of progression from normal mucosa to neoplasia is that chromosome-5 allele loss and k-*ras* mutations are early events, as may also be hypomethylation of DNA, since these changes are frequently seen in adenomas. Chromosome-18 allele loss occurs predominantly in large adenomas, while chromosome-17 loss is usually restricted to carcinomas. There is no rigidity to this sequence of events; allele loss on other chromosome arms is frequently seen. It appears that the net sum of genetic events determines the result rather than the order in which the events occur.

Epidemiology of colorectal cancer

Epidemiological studies have indicated the important role of environmental factors in the aetiology of colorectal cancer, which is predominantly a disease of industrialized, Western countries. Diet has been implicated as the major environmental determinant of risk. Case-control studies have shown a significant association between total fat, and also total energy intake, and the risk of colon cancer. It has been suggested that increased fat in the diet may increase the excretion of bile salts, which in animal studies have been shown to act as tumour promoters. An inverse relationship

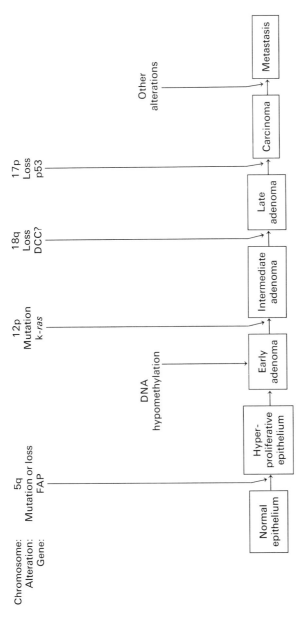

Fig. 10.1   A genetic model for colorectal tumorigenesis. Tumorigenesis proceeds through a series of genetic alterations involving oncogenes (*ras*) and tumour-suppressor genes (particularly those on chromosomes 5q, 17p, and 18q). The three stages of adenomas represent tumours of increasing size, dysplasia, and villous content. (Reproduced with permission from Fearon & Vogelstein 1990.)

between fibre intake and the rates of colon cancer has also been noted (reviewed by Willett[63]).

A prospective study of 120 000 US women was performed to examine the intake of fat and fibre in relation to the incidence of colon cancer over a 6-year follow-up period.[64] The strongest association of individual foods with risk of colon cancer was seen with beef, lamb, and pork intake. There was a significant positive trend for an association between animal fat consumption and risk of colon cancer and an inverse association for dietary fibre. The study concluded that a high consumption of red meat and animal fat increased the incidence of colon cancer independently of total energy intake.

THE MANAGEMENT OF COLORECTAL CANCER

The primary management of colorectal cancer is surgical and the prognosis is closely related to the stage of the disease. The stage is based on Dukes' original classification of rectal carcinomas.[65] Stage A tumours are confined to the intestinal wall and have neither extended beyond the muscularis mucosa nor involved lymph nodes. Stage B tumours have spread beyond the muscularis mucosa but do not involve lymph nodes, and in Stage C tumours there is lymph node spread. This classification has subsequently been extended to colonic carcinomas and modified to subdivide Stage B into those tumours without spread through the serosa (Stage B_1) and those with spread through the serosa (Stage B_2) and a less favourable prognosis.

Most patients have a successful resection of the gross tumour, but 40–50% of patients have invasion of the tumour through the bowel wall or spread to regional lymph nodes (Stage B_2 or Stage C disease) at the time of surgery. The probability of 5-year survival is 70–75% in those with Stage B_2 tumours and 35–60% in those with Stage C disease.

Non-surgical therapy has been aimed at two different groups of patients with colorectal cancer. The first group are those with late-stage disease at the time of surgery for whom the aim of the (adjuvant) therapy is to prevent recurrence. The second group are those with advanced disease for whom the aim of treatment is palliative rather than curative although treatment may result in lengthened survival.

The treatment of advanced colorectal cancer

A variety of treatment modalities have been used to treat metastatic colorectal carcinomas. These include systemic and regional chemotherapy, radiotherapy, and immunotherapy. Recently, the response rates seen in metastatic disease have improved through the use of combinations of fluorouracil and other agents.

Fluorouracil

Fluorouracil remains, after 30 years of use, the most active single agent in the treatment of metastatic colon cancer. Its use is associated with a partial response, a reduction in tumour mass of greater than 50%, in 10–20% of patients. Attempts to improve the response rate by intensifying the regimen, for example, by using both bolus and infusional fluorouracil, have been associated with increased toxicity and little improvement in tumour response.[66]

Fluorouracil has been used in combination with many other cytotoxic drugs in an attempt to improve the response rate of fluorouracil alone. Recently, trials of fluorouracil and etoposide,[67] a combination which has been used successfully in the treatment of gastric carcinoma,[68] and of fluorouracil and cisplatin[69, 70] have failed to improve the response rate above that seen with fluorouracil alone.

Biomodulation of fluorouracil. The combination of fluorouracil and folinic acid has been associated with an increased response rate when compared to fluorouracil alone in randomized trials of the treatment of advanced colorectal cancer.[71] The rationale for this combination depends on biomodulation of the activity of fluorouracil. The active metabolite of fluorouracil is fluorodeoxyuridine monophosphate, which inhibits the action of thymidylate synthase. Supplementation with folinic acid increases the levels of reduced intracellular folate, and this enhances the binding of fluorodeoxyuridine to thymidylate synthetase.[72]

In a recent study 79 patients with metastatic colorectal carcinoma were randomly assigned to either fluorouracil $370 \, mg/m^2$ for 5 d, or the same dosage of fluorouracil with folinic acid $500 \, mg/m^2$ by continuous infusion over 24 hours.[73] The response rate was significantly increased in the folinic acid group as compared to the fluorouracil alone group (44% vs. 13%; $P = 0.0019$). Survival was not significantly improved, but this may have been due to patients who did not respond to fluorouracil alone crossing to the fluorouracil-folinic acid arm.

There remains uncertainty as to the optimal dosage of fluorouracil and folinic acid, and the route of administration. The dosage of fluorouracil used has varied between 370 and $500 \, mg/m^2$, and that of folinic acid between 25 and $500 \, mg/m^2$. Treatment with fluorouracil-folinic acid is associated with dose-limiting gastrointestinal toxicity, and prospective trials of low-dose folinic acid against weekly high-dose folinic acid are in progress.

Recently, two further agents, methotrexate and N-(phosphonacetyl)-L-aspartate (PALA), have been used to enhance the effect of fluorouracil. The use of both agents results in increased conversion of fluorouracil to its active metabolite. In two small randomized trials, treatment with both the combination of methotrexate and fluorouracil and of PALA and fluorouracil compared with fluorouracil alone resulted in a higher response rate than fluorouracil alone.[74, 75] Neither combination appeared to be superior to the response expected with fluorouracil and folinic acid.

Biological response modifiers.   In laboratory studies alpha-interferon enhances the cytotoxic effect of fluorouracil when used in combination on human colon cancer cell lines.[76] This combination was used in an initial study of 30 patients with metastatic colorectal cancer who were treated with fluorouracil 750 mg/m²/d for 5 d and then weekly, and interferon-alpha 9MU subcutaneously three times a week. The researchers reported a response rate of 76% in previously untreated patients. However, this was associated with severe toxicity.[77] Two subsequent trials of the same regimen have failed to reproduce the high response rate and have also been associated with unacceptable toxicity.[78, 79] It is unclear whether alpha-interferon has an immunostimulatory effect or whether its action is due to biochemical modulation of the activity of fluorouracil, as it has been shown to enhance the levels of the active metabolite of fluorouracil.[80]

Regional chemotherapy of metastatic liver disease

The poor response of liver metastases, which are the most common site of advanced colorectal cancer, to systemic chemotherapy has led to trials of intra-arterial chemotherapy. The rationale for this treatment is based on the fact that the blood supply of these secondary deposits is predominantly derived from the hepatic artery. The aim of hepatic intra-arterial chemotherapy has been to improve the response rate and to reduce systemic toxicity as compared to that seen with systemic chemotherapy. Fluorodeoxyuridine has been the drug of choice in these trials as 95% is taken up by the liver when it is administered by intra-arterial infusion.[81]

A recent randomized study comparing intravenous to intra-arterial continuous infusion of fluorodeoxyuridine demonstrated a significantly higher complete and partial response rate in the arterial infusion group as compared to the systemic therapy group (50% vs. 19.6%; $P = 0.001$). There was a trend towards prolonged median survival (17 vs. 12 months) which was not statistically significant. However, 60% of the patients in the systemic therapy group crossed over into the arterial infusion group because of tumour progression, and, of these, 58% had a partial response or stabilization of disease.[82] A similar study has confirmed a significantly higher response rate in patients treated with intrahepatic fluorodeoxyuridine but no improvement in median survival.[83] However, intra-arterial fluorodeoxyuridine therapy has been associated with the development of biliary toxicity in approximately half the patients, whereas dose-limiting diarrhoea developed in a few patients on intravenous therapy.

Combined regional and systemic therapy

Although intra-arterial chemotherapy of hepatic metastases is associated with a higher response rate, survival has not been significantly improved owing to the development of extra-hepatic metastatic disease. In an attempt to overcome this, some small studies have looked at combination therapy with intra-arterial and intravenous chemotherapy as compared to intra-arterial therapy alone. In a study of 44 patients with metastatic colorectal cancer, patients were randomized either to combined intra-arterial and intravenous chemotherapy or to intra-arterial therapy alone. The response rate in the combination arm was similar to that in the arterial-only arm (47% vs. 52%), as was the incidence of toxicity. At a median follow-up of 16 months, extrahepatic metastases had occurred in 61% of the arterial-only group and in 33% of the combined group. Survival at 3 years was 0% in the arterial-only group and 40% in the combined group; the small sample size may account for the lack of statistical significance.[84]

At present the accepted treatment of advanced colorectal cancer is with the combination of fluorouracil and folinic acid.[85] Clinical trials are in progress to assess the value of other combinations of treatment, including either fluorouracil and alpha-interferon, or PALA and regional chemotherapy.

Adjuvant therapy

The high recurrence rate in patients with Stage B_2 and Stage C colorectal cancer following surgical resection has led to trials of adjuvant treatment. Adjuvant treatments of colon and rectal cancer differ, as in colon cancer recurrence is usually manifested by distal spread, with metastatic disease in the liver, whereas in rectal cancer recurrence tends initially to occur locally. Recently trials have demonstrated both an increase in disease-free interval and increased survival with colon and rectal carcinomas in patients receiving adjuvant treatment.

Adjuvant treatment of colon cancer

In colon cancer, following apparently complete surgical resection, metastatic disease may develop later, probably from micrometastases present at the time of surgery. Studies show that adjuvant treatment with fluorouracil following surgery resulted in only a small benefit in the treatment group, as compared to controls managed with surgery alone.[86] The combination of fluorouracil, semustine, and vincristine improved disease-free interval and survival when compared to surgery alone, but the use of semustine was associated with the development of leukaemia in some patients.[87]

More recently, levamisole, an antihelminthic drug, which is thought to have immunomodulatory activity, has been used in combination with fluorouracil as an adjuvant treatment of colon cancer. In an initial study of 401 patients with Stage B_2 or C colon cancer, the combination of fluorouracil and levamisole significantly reduced the recurrence rate, and was

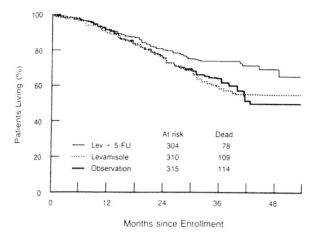

Fig. 10.2   Survival according to study arm. (Reproduced with permission from Moertel et al 1990.)

associated with a significant survival advantage in patients with Stage C disease, when compared to surgery alone. Therapy with levamisole alone produced a borderline advantage.[88]

In a subsequent, larger study 1296 patients with resected Stage B_2 or C colon cancer were randomly assigned to treatment with surgery only or to a combination of fluorouracil and levamisole for a year (Fig. 10.2).[89] Patients with Stage C disease could also be assigned to levamisole treatment alone. At a median follow-up of 3 years, patients with Stage C disease treated with the combination of levamisole and fluorouracil had a 41% reduction ($P = 0.0001$) in the risk of recurrence and a reduction in overall death rate of 33% ($P = 0.006$). Treatment with levamisole alone had no detectable effect. The estimate of survival at 3.5 years was 55% for patients who underwent surgery alone, as compared to 71% in patients treated with the combination of fluorouracil and levamisole. The results were too preliminary to demonstrate any possible effect in patients with Stage B_2 disease.

Adjuvant treatment of rectal cancer

Adjuvant treatment of rectal carcinoma has been primarily aimed at preventing local recurrence, which is seen in 25–45% of patients. Radiotherapy of the pelvis has been shown to be associated with a reduction in local recurrence but with no increase in survival.[90] As a consequence, recent trials have looked at the combination of chemotherapy and radiotherapy as adjuvant therapy for Stage B_2 and C rectal carcinomas.

A study was performed comparing surgery alone, surgery and radiotherapy, and surgery combined with chemotherapy and radiotherapy in 202 patients with Stage B_2 or C rectal carcinoma.[91] A significant reduction in

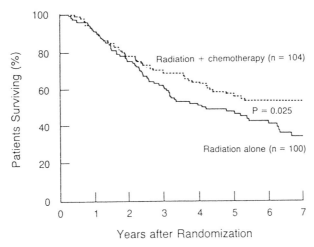

Fig. 10.3   Survival according to treatment group. The *P* value has been adjusted for imbalances in prognostic variables. (Reproduced with permission from Krook et al 1991.)

the recurrence rate at 80 months was seen in the patients receiving combination radio- and chemotherapy, and there was a survival benefit. However, eight patients developed acute leukaemia or myelodysplastic syndrome, a development which was attributed to the prolonged treatment with semustine.

A study was performed to determine whether a less prolonged course of chemotherapy would be as effective without causing haematological toxicity (Fig. 10.3).[92] Two hundred and four patients with Stage B_2 or C rectal carcinoma were randomized to postoperative radiation therapy alone (4500–5040 cGy), or to radiation therapy combined with fluorouracil which was preceded and followed by a cycle of systemic therapy with fluorouracil and semustine. At a median follow-up of more than 7 years, the combined treatment had reduced the recurrence of rectal cancer by 34% ($P = 0.0016$). Initial local recurrence was reduced by 46% ($P = 0.036$) and distal recurrence by 37% ($P = 0.011$). Combined chemotherapy reduced the rate of cancer-related deaths by 36% ($P = 0.0071$) and the overall death rate by 29% ($P = 0.025$). Side-effects from the chemotherapy were seldom severe. Severe side-effects occurred equally in both groups and were usually due to small-bowel obstruction as a consequence of radiation therapy.

This study demonstrates a significant improvement in survival with combined treatment of radiotherapy and chemotherapy after surgery for late-stage rectal carcinoma. Further studies are in progress to assess whether chemotherapy alone would be as effective as combination therapy. In patients who may receive radiotherapy, the importance of closing the pelvis at operation to avoid irradiation of the small bowel has been emphasized.

OTHER GASTROINTESTINAL TUMOURS

The understanding of the genetics and molecular biology of other gastro-intestinal tumours is less advanced than that of colorectal cancer. Colorectal cancer is the only gastrointestinal tumour in which there are highly pen-etrant inherited predispositions. However, multiple genetic changes during tumorigenesis have also been demonstrated in other tumours such as hepatocellular carcinoma.[93] As yet, the treatment of other advanced gastro-intestinal malignancies, except, possibly, for gastric cancer,[94] remains con-fined to clinical trials and is, in general, less successful than that of colorectal cancer.[85]

CONCLUSION

Great progress has been made in understanding the genetics of colorectal cancer. The *adenomatous polyposis coli (APC)* gene has been identified, allowing the presymptomatic diagnosis of FAP and the investigation of other, possibly related, inherited predispositions to colorectal cancer. Several of the somatic genetic alterations that lead to the development of colorectal cancer have been identified and an understanding has been reached of the multiple steps that are involved in tumorigenesis. These developments may allow the identification of individuals at risk of colo-rectal cancer in the population and lead to effective prevention by screening and to novel therapeutic approaches in the management of colorectal cancer.

Adjuvant chemotherapy of late-stage colonic and rectal carcinomas has been shown to improve disease-free interval and survival. Improved re-sponse rates have been seen with the palliative chemotherapy of advanced colorectal cancer using combinations of fluorouracil and folinic acid. The role of regional chemotherapy and other agents which modulate the action of fluorouracil is under active investigation. More speculative treatments for the future include the use of autologous tumour vaccines and of monoclonal antibodies to tumour antigens.

REFERENCES

1 Office of Population Censuses and Surveys. 1988 Mortality Statistics, England and Wales. HMSO 1990
2 Northover JMA, Murday V. Familial colorectal cancer and familial adenomatous polyposis. Baillière's Clinical Gastroenterology 1990; Vol 3, No 3: 593–613
3 Domizio P, Talbot IC, Spigelman AD, Williams CB, Phillips RKS. Upper gastrointestinal pathology in familial adenomatous polyposis: results from a prospective study of 102 patients. J Clin Pathol 1990; 43: 738–743
4 Bussey HJR. Familial polyposis coli. Baltimore: Johns Hopkins University Press, 1975
5 Turcot J, Despres J-P, St Pierre F. Malignant tumors of the central nervous system associated with familial polyposis of the colon: a report of two cases. Dis Colon Rectum 1959; 2: 465–468

6 Kropilak M, Jagelman DG, Fazio VW, Lavery IL, McGannon E. Brain tumours in familial adenomatous polyposis. Dis Colon Rectum 1989; 32: 778–782
7 Plail RO, Glazer G, Thomson JPS, Bussey HJR. Adenomatous polyposis: an association with carcinoma of the thyroid? Br J Surg 1985; 72: 138S
8 Kingston JE, Herbert A, Draper GJ, Mann JR. Association between hepatoblastoma and polyposis coli. Arch Dis Child 1983; 58: 959–962
9 Li FP, Thurber WA, Seddon J, Holmes GE. Hepatoblastoma in families with polyposis coli. J Am Med Assoc 1987; 257: 2475–2477
10 Gardner EJ, Richards RC. Multiple cutaneous and subcutaneous lesions occurring simultaneously with heriditary polyposis and osteomatosis. Am. J Hum Genet 1953; 5: 139–148
11 Polkinghorne PJ, Ritchie S, Neale K, Schoeppner G, Thomson JPS, Jay BS. Pigmented lesions of the retinal pigment epithelium and familial adenomatous polyposis. Eye 1990; 4: 216–217
12 Lynch HT, Watson P, Lanspa SJ et al. Natural history of colorectal cancer in hereditary nonpolyposis colorectal cancer (Lynch syndromes I and II). Dis Colon Rectum 1988; 31: 439–444
13 Mecklin J-P. Frequency of hereditary colorectal carcinoma. Gastroenterology 1987; 93: 1021–1025
14 Westlake P, Sutherland LR, Lafreniere R, Huchcroft S, Bryant H. The frequency of hereditary nonpolyposis cancer. Gastroenterology 1990; 98: A318
15 Lynch HT, Kimberling W, Albano WA et al. Hereditary nonpolyposis colorectal cancer (Lynch syndromes I and II) 1. Clinical description of resource. Cancer 1985; 56: 934–938
16 Mecklin JP, Jarvinen HJ. Clinical features of colorectal cancer in cancer family syndrome. Dis Colon Rectum 1986; 29: 160–164
17 Woolf CM. A genetic study of carcinoma of the large intestine. Am J Hum Genet 1958; 10: 42–47
18 Macklin MT. Inheritance of cancer of the stomach and large intestine in man. J Natl Cancer Inst 1960; 24: 551–571
19 Lovett E. Family studies in cancer of the colon and rectum. Br J Surg 1976; 63: 13–18
20 Bishop DT, Burt RW. Genetic epidemiology and molecular genetics of colorectal adenomas and cancer. In: Roger P, Reich CB, Winauer SJ, eds. Large bowel cancer policy, prevention, research and treatment (Frontiers in gastrointestinal research). Basel: Karger, 1991: Vol. 18, pp 99–114
21 Cannon-Albright LA, Skolnick MH, Bishop DT, Lee RG, Burt RW. Common inheritance of susceptibility to colonic adenomatous polyps and associated colorectal cancers. New Engl J Med 1988; 319: 533–537
22 Houlston RS, Murday V, Harocopos C, Williams CB, Slack J. Screening and genetic counselling for relatives of patients with colorectal cancer in a family cancer clinic. Br Med J 1990; 301: 366–368
23 Herrera L, Katati S, Gibas L, Pietrzak E, Sandberg AA. Gardner syndrome in a man with an interstitial deletion of 5q. Am J Med Genet 1986; 25: 473–476
24 Bodmer WF, Bailey CJ, Bodmer J et al. Localization of the gene for familial adenomatous polyposis on chromosome 5. Nature 1987; 328: 614–616
25 Leppert M, Dobbs M, Scambler P et al. The gene for familial polyposis coli maps to the long arm of chromosome 5. Science 1987; 238: 1411–1413
26 Nakamura K, Lathrop M, Leppert M et al. Localization of the genetic defect in familial adenomatous polyposis within a small region of chromosome 5. Am J Hum Genet 1988; 43: 638–644
27 Varesco L, Thomas HJW, Cottrell S et al. CpG island clones from a deletion encompassing the gene for adenomatous polyposis coli. Proc Natl Acad Sci USA 1989; 86: 10 118–10 122
28 Tops CMJ, Wijnen JT, Griffioen G et al. Presymptomatic diagnosis of familial adenomatous polyposis by bridging DNA markers. Lancet 1989; 2: 1361–1363
29 Meera Khan P, Tops CMJ, vd Broek M et al. Close linkage of a highly polymorphic marker (D5S37) to familial adenomatous polyposis (FAP) and confirmation of FAP localization on chromosome 5q21–22. Hum Genet 1988; 79: 183–185
30 Dunlop MG, Wyllie AH, Nakamura Y et al. Genetic linkage map of six polymorphic DNA markers around the gene for familial adenomatous polyposis on chromosome 5. Am J Hum Genet 1990; 47: 982–987

31 Kinzler KW, Nilbert MC, Su L-K et al. Identification of FAP locus genes from chromosome 5q21. Science 1991; 253: 661–665

32 Nishisho I, Nakamura Y, Miyoshi Y et al. Mutations of chromosome 5q21 genes in FAP and colorectal cancer patients. Science 1991; 253: 661–665

33 Groden J, Thliveris A, Samovitz W et al. Identification and characterization of the familial adenomatous polyposis coli gene. Cell 1991; 66: 589–600

34 Joslyn G, Carlson M, Thliveris A et al. Identification of deletion mutations and three new genes at the familial polyposis locus. Cell 1991; 66: 601–613

35 Dunlop MG, Wyllie AH, Steel CM, Piris J, Evans HJ. Linked DNA markers for presymptomatic diagnosis of familial adenomatous polyposis. Lancet 1991; 337: 313–316

36 Leppert M, Burt R, Hughes JP et al. Genetic analysis of an inherited predisposition to colon cancer in a family with a variable number of adenomatous polyps. N Engl J Med 1990; 322: 904–908

37 Bishop JM. The molecular genetics of cancer. Science 1987; 235: 305–311

38 Bos JL, Fearon ER, Hamilton SR et al. Prevalence of *ras* gene mutations in human colorectal cancers. Nature 1987; 327: 293–297

39 Forrester K, Almoguera C, Han K, Grizzle WE, Perucho M. Detection of high incidence of K-*ras* oncogenes during human colon tumorigenesis. Nature 1987; 327: 298–303

40 Vogelstein B, Fearon ER, Hamilton SR et al. Genetic alterations during colorectal tumour development. N Engl J Med 1988; 319: 525–532

41 Farr CJ, Marshall CJ, Easty DJ, Wright NA, Powell SC, Paraskeva C. A study of *ras* mutations in colonic adenomas from familial polyposis coli patients. Oncogene 1988; 3: 673–678

42 Rothberg PG, Spandorfer JM, Erisman MD et al. Evidence that c-*myc* expression defines two genetically distinct forms of colorectal adenocarcinoma. Br J Cancer 1985; 52: 629–632

43 Bolen JB, Veillette A, Schwartz AM, DeSeau V, Rosen N. Activation of the pp60$^{c\text{-}src}$ protein kinase activity in human colon carcinoma. Proc Natl Acad Sci USA 1987; 84: 2251–2255

44 Cartwright CA, Meisler AI, Eckhart W. Activation of the pp60$^{c\text{-}src}$ protein kinase is an early event in colonic carcinogenesis. Proc Natl Acad Sci USA 1990; 87: 558–562

45 De Mars R. In: 23rd Annual Symposium Fundamental Cancer Research 1969, 105–106 (Baltimore, Md: Williams and Wilkins, 1970)

46 Knudson AG. Mutation and cancer: statistical study of retinoblastoma. Proc Natl Acad Sci USA 1971; 68: 820–823

47 Hansen MF, Cavenee WK. Genetics of cancer predisposition. Cancer Res 1987; 47: 5518–5527

48 Solomon E, Voss R, Hall V et al. Chromosome 5 allele loss in human colorectal carcinomas. Nature 1987; 328: 616–619

49 Rees M, Leigh SEA, Delhanty JDA, Jass JR. Chromosome 5 allele loss in familial and sporadic colorectal adenomas. Br J Cancer 1989; 59: 361–365

50 Sasaki M, Okamoto M, Sato C et al. Loss of constitutional heterozygosity in colorectal tumours from patients with a familial polyposis coli and those with nonpolyposis colorectal carcinoma. Cancer Res 1989; 49: 4402–4406

51 Kinzler KW, Nilbert MC, Vogelstein B et al. Identification of a gene located at chromosome 5q21 that is mutated in colorectal cancers. Science 1991; 251: 1366–1370

52 Tanaka K, Oshimura M, Kikuchi R, Seki M, Hayashi T, Miyaki M. Suppression of tumorigenicity in human colon carcinoma cells by introduction of normal chromosome 5 or 18. Nature 1991; 349: 340–342

53 Reichmann A, Martin P, Levin B. Chromosomal banding patterns in human large bowel cancer. Int J Cancer 1981; 28: 431–440

54 Muleris M, Salmon RJ, Zafrani B, Girodet J, Dutrillaux B. Consistent deficiencies of chromosome 18 and of the short arm of chromosome 17 in eleven cases of human large bowel cancer: a possible recessive determinism. Ann Genet (Paris) 1985; 28: 206–213

55 Fearon ER, Hamilton SR, Vogelstein B. Clonal analysis of human colorectal tumours. Science 1987; 238: 193–197

56 Monpezat J-Ph, Delattre O, Bernard A et al. Loss of alleles on chromosome 18 and on the short arm of chromosome 17 in polypoid colorectal carcinomas. Int J Cancer 1988; 41: 404–408

57 Baker SJ, Fearon ER, Nigro JM et al. Chromosome 17 deletions and *p53* gene mutations in colorectal carcinomas. Science 1989; 244: 217–221

58 Baker SJ, Preisinger AC, Jessup JM et al. *p53* mutations occur in combination with 17p allelic deletions as late events in colorectal tumorigenesis. Cancer Res 1990; 50: 7717–7122

59 Baker SJ, Markowitz S, Fearon ER, Willson JKV, Vogelstein B. Suppression of human colorectal carcinoma cell growth by wild-type *p53*. Science 1990; 249: 912–915

60 Fearon ER, Cho KR, Nigro JM et al. Identification of a chromosome 18q gene that is altered in colorectal cancers. Science 1990; 247: 49–56

61 Vogelstein B, Fearon ER, Kern SE et al. Allelotypes of colorectal carcinomas. Science 1989; 244: 207–211

62 Fearon ER, Vogelstein B. A genetic model of colorectal tumorigenesis. Cell 1990; 61: 759–767

63 Willett W. The search for the causes of breast and colon cancer. Nature 1989; 338: 389–394

64 Willett WC, Stampfer MJ, Colditz GA, Rosner BA, Speizer FF. Relation of meat, fat, and fibre intake to the risk of colon cancer in a prospective study among women. N Engl J Med 1990; 323: 1644–1672

65 Dukes CE. The classification of cancer of the rectum. J Path Bacteriol 1932; 35: 323–332

66 Poplin EA, Kraut M, Baker L, Brodfuehrer J, Vaitkevicius V. A dose-intensive regimen of 5-fluorouracil for the treatment of metastatic colorectal cancer. Cancer 1991; 67: 367–371

67 Zelkowitz RS, Posner MR, Cummings F et al. A phase I/II trial of 5-fluorouracil and etoposide in metastatic colorectal carcinoma. Proc Am Soc Clin Oncol 1989; 8: 125

68 Wilke H, Preusser P, Fink U et al. New developments in the treatment of gastric cancer. Semin Oncol 1990; 17: 61–70

69 Kemeny N, Israel K, Niedzwiecki D et al. Randomised study of continuous infusion fluorouracil plus cisplatin in patients with metastatic colorectal cancer. J Clin Oncol 1990; 8: 313–318

70 Lokich JJ, Ahlgren JD, Cantrell J et al. A prospective randomised comparison of protracted infusional 5-fluorouracil with or without weekly bolus cisplatin in metastatic colorectal carcinoma. Cancer 1991; 67: 14–19

71 Arbuck SG. Overview of the clinical trials using 5-FU and leucovorin for the treatment of colorectal cancer. Cancer 1989; 63 (suppl 6): 1036–1044

72 Houghton JA, Maroda SJ, Phillips JO. Biochemical determinants of responsiveness to 5-fluorouracil and its derivatives in xenografts of human colorectal adenocarcinomas in mice. Cancer Res 1981; 48: 3062–3069

73 Doroshaw JH, Multhauf P, Leong L et al. Prospective randomized comparison of fluorouracil versus fluorouracil and high dose continuous infusion leucovorin calcium for the treatment of advanced measurable colorectal cancer in patients previously unexposed to chemotherapy. J Clin Oncol 1990; 8: 491–501

74 Nordic Gastrointestinal Tumour Adjuvant Therapy Group. Superiority of sequential methotrexate, fluorouracil, and leucovorin to fluorouracil alone in advanced symptomatic colorectal carcinoma: a randomised trial. J Clin Oncol 1989; 7: 1437–1446

75 O'Dwyer PJ, Paul AR, Walczak J, Weiner LM, Litwin S, Conus RL. Phase II study of biochemical modulation by low-dose PALA in patients with colorectal cancer. J Clin Oncol 1990; 8: 1497–1503

76 Wadler S, Wersto R, Weinberg V, Thompson D, Schwartz EL. Interaction of fluorouracil and interferon in human colon cancer cell lines: cytotoxic and cytokinetic effects. Cancer Res 1990; 50: 5735–5739

77 Wadler S, Schwartz EL, Goldman M et al. Fluorouracil and recombinant alfa-2a-interferon: an active regimen against advanced colorectal carcinoma. J Clin Oncol 1989; 7: 1769–1775

78 Pazdur R, Ajani JA, Patt YZ et al. Phase II study of fluorouracil and recombinant interferon alfa-2a in previously untreated advanced colorectal carcinoma. J Clin Oncol 1990; 8: 2027–2031

79 Kemeny N, Younes A, Seiter K et al. Interferon alfa-2a and 5-fluorouracil for advanced colorectal carcinoma. Cancer 1990; 66: 2470–2475

80 Elias L, Sandoval JM. Interferon effects upon fluorouracil metabolism by HL-60 cells. Biochem Biophys Res Commun 1989; 163: 867–874

81 Ensminger W, Rosowsky A, Raso V et al. A clinical-pharmacological evaluation of hepatic

arterial infusions of 5-fluoro-2'deoxyuridine and 5-fluorouracil. Cancer Res 1978; 38: 3784–3792

82 Kemeny N, Daly J, Reichman B et al. Intrahepatic or systemic infusion of fluorodeoxyuridine in patients with liver metastases from colorectal carcinoma. Ann Intern Med 1987; 107: 459–465

83 Hohn DC, Stagg RJ, Friedman MA et al. A randomized trial of continuous intravenous versus intraarterial floxuridine in patients with colorectal cancer metastatic to the liver (The Northern California Oncology Group Trial). J Clin Oncol 1989; 7: 1646–1654

84 Safi F, Bittner R, Roscher R, Schuhmacher K, Gaus W, Beger GH. Regional chemotherapy for hepatic metastases of colorectal carcinoma. Cancer 1989; 64: 379–387

85 Rubens RD, Towlson KE, Ramirez AJ et al. Appropriate chemotherapy for palliating advanced cancer. Br Med J 1992; 304: 35–40

86 Buyse M, Zeleniuch-Jacquotte A, Chalmers TC. Adjuvant therapy of colorectal cancer: why we still don't know. J Am Med Assoc 1988; 259: 3571–3578

87 Wolmark N, Fisher B, Rockette H et al. Postoperative adjuvant chemotherapy or BCG for colon cancer: results from NSABP protocol C-01. J Natl Cancer Inst 1988; 80: 30–36

88 Laurie JA, Moertel CG, Fleming TR et al. Surgical adjuvant therapy of large-bowel carcinoma: an evaluation of levamisole and the combination of levamisole and fluorouracil. J Clin Oncol 1989; 7: 1447–1456

89 Moertel CG, Fleming TR, Macdonald JS et al. Levamisole and fluorouracil for adjuvant therapy of resected colon carcinoma. N Engl J Med 1990; 322: 352–358

90 Rosenthal SA, Trock BJ, Cola LR. Randomized trials of adjuvant radiation therapy for rectal carcinoma: a review. Dis Colon Rectum 1990; 33: 335–343

91 Gastrointestinal Tumor Study Group. Prolongation of disease-free interval in surgically treated rectal carcinoma. N Engl J Med 1985; 312: 1465–1472

92 Krook JE, Moertel CG, Gunderson LL et al. Effective surgical adjuvant therapy for high risk rectal carcinoma. N Engl J Med 1991; 324: 709–715

93 Fujimori M, Tokino T, Hino O et al. Allelotype study of primary hepatocellular carcinoma. Cancer Res 1991; 51: 89–93

94 Findlay M, Mansi JL, Ford HT et al. Epirubicin, cisplatin and 5-fluorouracil (ECF) is highly effective in advanced gastric cancer. Eur J Cancer 1991; 27 (suppl 2): 571

11

The pharmacotherapy of portal hypertension

A. K. Burroughs   P. A. McCormick

Bleeding from oesophageal varices, gastric varices, and portal hypertensive gastropathy is a major cause of morbidity and mortality in cirrhotic patients. The risk of first gastrointestinal bleeding in cirrhotics with varices is approximately 30%.[1] This risk depends on several risk factors, which include the size of varices, endoscopic red signs on varices, and the degree of liver dysfunction,[2] but statistical models which include these variables still lack sufficient specificity for use with individual patients.[3] In contrast, once a patient has bled from varices the risk of rebleeding is 70% or more. Mortality from bleeding is related to the severity of liver disease; it is less than 10% in Pugh's grade A, approximately 25% in grade B, and 50% or more in grade C disease. The tension on the variceal wall, which is related to the radius of the varix, as well as the intravariceal pressure, is believed to be critical in the pathogenesis of rupture.[4] Thus, any reduction in intravariceal pressure by reducing portal pressure and/or increasing resistance in the collateral blood vessels feeding the varices should diminish the risk of bleeding.

DRUGS FOR ACUTE VARICEAL BLEEDING

In the emergency setting, vasoconstrictor drugs have been used for many years to diminish portal pressure, but only recently have randomized clinical trials confirmed some efficacy.

Somatostatin and octreotide

The most recent interest in this area has been in the use of somatostatin and octreotide. Both drugs have been shown to induce modest reductions in wedge hepatic venous pressure (WHVP) in some studies, but no effect in others.[5] WHVP is the same as portal pressure if the major site of resistance is sinusoidal, as in alcoholic cirrhosis and to a variable degree in most other forms of cirrhosis. The variability in pressure reduction had led most clinicians to consider somatostatin or octreotide as unlikely therapeutic agents for variceal bleeding. However, all studies have shown that azygous blood flow (a measure of collateral blood flow, including that through varices) is reduced, so that there may be a therapeutic effect by means of the decreased collateral blood flow. The variability of pressure reduction has also been shown with other agents (for example, vasopressin or propranolol), so that this probably reflects normal biological variability among patients. More importantly, there is the possibility that the haemodynamic effects of vasoactive agents during variceal bleeding may be qualitatively or quantitatively different from those in stable patients, in whom haemodynamic studies are normally performed. Furthermore, the optimal dosage and duration of treatment of these agents have been largely empirical. It is the authors' view that if a vasoactive drug is to be used in acute variceal bleeding, it should have few side-effects (which tends to exclude vasopressin). In addition the therapeutic agent should be used as soon as possible, not only before sclerotherapy, but also in combination with sclerotherapy over several days. This is because the maximum risk of early bleeding with or without emergency sclerotherapy is within the first 5 d following admission for variceal bleeding.[1]

Many trials have been conducted with somatostatin against various therapies, including placebo, other vasoconstrictor agents, and tamponade or sclerotherapy (Table 11.1). Thus, it is difficult to perform a meta-analysis because of the range of different therapies, but evaluation of the crude efficacy rates shows encouraging results. A definite advantage of somatostatin or octreotide is the lack of side-effects, which were, statistically, significantly lower in nearly all trials, as compared with other active therapies, and which were not different from that of placebo. There is also some evidence that somatostatin may control postsclerotherapy bleeding.[6]

The two largest trials of somatostatin are placebo-controlled trials,[7,8] but they provide contrasting results as to the efficacy of somatostatin. Although they show a similar efficacy of somatostatin, 64% and 65%, the evaluation was made over different intervals: 30 h[7] and 5 d.[8] In contrast, there was a marked contrast in the placebo response rates: 86%[7] and 41%.[8] The differences might be explained by the selection of patients in the US study: only 84 evaluable patients were reported, recruited from 11 centres over 14 months.

One issue raised by these results is the difficulty in comparing results in acute trials of variceal bleeding because of varying and nebulous definitions of therapeutic end-points. This was addressed by a Working Team Report at the 1992 World Congress of Gastroenterology in Athens. In some trials, despite the increased efficacy of one treatment as compared to another, there is no difference in transfusion requirements,[9-11] suggesting that the end-points chosen may not be clinically important or, indeed, relevant. In the Royal Free Hospital somatostatin trial,[8] the increased efficacy of somatostatin as compared to placebo was mirrored by a halving of transfusion requirement ($P = 0.025$), and a reduction of the use of balloon tamponade and/or emergency sclerotherapy or surgery. As with other trials of vaso-

Table 11.1 Somatostatin and octreotide[a] for variceal bleeding

Author	Date	Patient admissions	Maximal duration of treatment	Efficacy Somatostatin: other therapy
Kravetz et al[80]	1984	61	48 h	53%: 58% (vasopressin)
Jenkins et al[81]	1985	22	24 h	100%: 33% (vasopressin)
Bagarani et al[82]	1987	50	48 h	67%: 32% (vasopressin)
Saari et al[83]	1990	54	72 h	66%: 52% (vasopressin)
Walker et al[84]	1991	50	24 h	68%: 80% (glypressin)
Cardona et al[85]	1989	38	24 h	45%: 55% (vasopressin/nitroglycerin)
Rguez-Moreno et al[86]	1991	31	?	40%: 67% (vasopressin/nitroglycerin)
Silvain[a] et al[87]	1991	50	24 h	55%: 48% (vasopressin/nitroglycerin)
McKee[a88]	1990	40	48 h	50%: 70% (tamponade)
Averginos[b] et al[9]	1991	92	24 h	71%: 80% (tamponade)
Jaramillo et al[89]	1991	39	<24 h	58%: 50% (tamponade)
Jenkins et al[90]	1988	80	5 d	77%: 80% (sclerotherapy)
Valenzuela et al[7]	1989	84	30 h	65%: 83% (placebo)
Burroughs et al[8]	1990	120	5 d	64%: 41% (placebo)

[a] Octreotide.
[b] Efficacy was also assessed in a third group given the combination of somatostatin and balloon tamponade.

active drugs, no study of somatostatin or octreotide has shown a reduction in mortality.

In summary, somatostatin and octreotide remain the best candidates for the 'optimal' drug treatment for acute variceal bleeding because of their simplicity of administration and lack of side-effects. However, further trials are needed to establish their value as adjuvant therapy to emergency sclerotherapy. If they could reduce transfusion requirements before endoscopy, or reduce the chance of active bleeding at the time of diagnostic endoscopy (thus facilitating sclerotherapy), and/or reduce the chance of rebleeding following a single session of injection, then these drugs could become established as routine adjunctive treatment for variceal bleeding – even if mortality was not reduced.

Glypressin

Glypressin has been in use for over a decade, but all the initial clinical studies were not randomized trials, and the haemodynamic data were poorly documented. This triglycyl analogue of vasopressin has a longer duration of action by slow breakdown to lysine vasopressin, allowing bolus administration, as well as intrinsic vasoconstrictive activity. The best haemodynamic data[12] showed that a bolus of 2 mg reduced the hepatic pressure venous gradient (the difference between the wedged and free hepatic venous pressure) by an average of 15% and azygous blood flow by 27%. In addition, a second study has shown that intravariceal pressure was significantly reduced by a 2-mg bolus of glypressin, as compared to placebo, by an average of 25%.[13] Three of 11 (27%) patients did not respond – as with somatostatin there are some non-responders. The effects of glypressin on the systemic circulation are similar to those of vasopressin, and thus potentially deleterious.[12, 14] There is a reduction in cardiac output and elevation of right atrial pressure and pulmonary capillary wedge pressure, as well as an increase in systemic vascular resistance and mean arterial pressure. As with vasopressin, the addition of nitroglycerin (0.6 mg sublingual) abolished these effects on the systemic circulation, but did not further decrease the hepatic venous pressure gradient (HVPG).[14] Thus, it would be prudent to administer nitroglycerin with glypressin, as has been advocated with vasopressin.[15] However, clinical reports of adverse events of glypressin caused by these effects on the systemic circulation are less frequent than with vasopressin. This may be because fewer vasopressor units are given: 2 mg glypressin every 4 h is less than the standard 0.4 u/min vasopressin infusion.

A trial of the combination of glypressin and nitroglycerin versus balloon tamponade showed that no patient needed to stop the combined therapy because of complications. Evaluation at 12 h showed that the therapies seemed equivalent,[16] although a similar study using vasopressin and nitroglycerin showed that tamponade was more effective.[17] Two placebo-controlled studies both show that glypressin is more effective,[18,19] although in one[18] this was not statistically significant, but significant differences in efficacy and reduced blood transfusion requirement were shown in the other.[19]

Vasopressin and the combination of vasopressin with nitroglycerin

Vasopressin has been used for the emergency treatment of bleeding varices for approximately 40 years. It has serious side-effects resulting from vasoconstriction of cardiac, skin, and splanchnic arterioles. Many centres no longer use vasopressin unless it is combined with nitrovasodilators, which remove the systemic side-effects without affecting efficacy.[10,11,15] It has been known for some time that the portal pressure reduction by vasopressin is very variable, some patients not responding. Following administration of vasopressin, intra-variceal pressure falls to the same extent as WHVP, a mean of 14% versus 16%,[20] whereas the reduction in HVPG is greater (mean -23%) but is similar to the intravariceal pressure – superior vena cava gradient (-26%); this greater reduction is due to decreases in free hepatic venous pressure (FHVP) and superior vena cava pressures. Thus, the effect of vasopressin on intravariceal pressure, which influences variceal wall tension, is only modest, and may explain the frequent clinical failures of vasopressin. Duplex ultrasonography shows that left gastric venous flow, the major feeding vein of oesophageal varices, is reduced by 54% following vasopressin infusion.[21]

Vasopressin has been administered traditionally as an infusion of 0.4 u/min for at least 12 h or more, although in the earliest clinical studies it was given as a short infusion of 20 u over 20 min. Neither haemodynamic nor therapeutic comparisons have been made between the two regimens. It is of interest that a recent study has shown abnormal systemic pressor responses to prolonged administration of vasopressin in cirrhotics.[22] In cirrhotics as compared to controls, 0.4 u/min of vasopressin induced similar peak increases in arterial pressure, followed by a similar heart-rate and cardiac output reduction. However, in control subjects after 30 min from the start of infusion, blood pressure and systemic vascular resistance had returned to normal, and systemic oxygen consumption had fallen significantly. In contrast, in the cirrhotic group, the blood pressure and systemic vascular resistance remained significantly higher than baseline values, with no reduction in systemic oxygen consumption. There was no significant difference in the heart-rate reduction between controls and cirrhotics. Thus, the vasopressor effect of vasopressin is maintained abnormally in cirrhotic patients, probably because of an insufficient buffering of the arteriolar vasoconstrictor responses (as heart-rate changes were no different). In addition, the absence of a reduction in systemic oxygen consumption implies that the persistent arteriolar constriction might be related to an abnormally sustained sympathetic vascular tone in cirrhotic patients.

As mentioned above, the effect of vasoactive drugs may be different during variceal haemorrhage, and may provide an explanation for the variability in clinical efficacy. An elegant study has addressed this question.[23] At a dose of 0.2 u/min of vasopressin, there was a significant decrease in WHVP (-13%), which did not decrease further with a doubling of the vasopressin dose, or even at a dose of 0.8 u/min in one patient. There was no tachyphylaxis over 24 h, and no rebound pressure increase after stopping the drug abruptly. All the patients included in this report had remained stable and had received similar volumes of blood products during the 24-h infusion. Interestingly, no effect was noted on systemic blood pressure. This may mean that the systemic vasoconstrictor effect may be blunted during haemorrhage as compared to that in the stable cirrhotic patients. There was no difference in HVPG between those who remained stable, or continued to bleed or rebleed during vasopressin, so that it was not possible to correlate the haemodynamic response of vasopressin with its clinical efficacy. Larger studies with continuous hepatic venous pressure monitoring would be needed. In another study from the same group,[24] 22 alcoholic cirrhotics were evaluated, with continuous portal pressure monitoring who had not received other specific treatments to stop bleeding. The WHVP was the same on the first day in the group that remained stable ($n = 13$), and in the combined group that continued to bleed ($n = 2$) or re-bled within 5 d ($n = 7$). However, the initial HVPG was lower in the stable group because of a higher FHVP. On day 2, the WHVP rose by a mean of 4 mmHg in the group that eventually bled. There was a mean increase of only 2 mmHg in both FHVP and HVPG. The lowest HVPG in the group that bled was 16 mmHg; a patient with an HVPG greater than 16 mmHg had a 50% chance of either continuing to bleed or suffering early rebleeding. Five of the patients who bled had catheters in position – in all, the HVPG was higher immediately preceding bleeding as compared to baseline values (mean 23 mmHg vs. 18 mmHg). Fluid balance did not correlate with any haemodynamic index but was higher on the first day in the group that had early rebleeding; it may have been responsible for the WHVP rise, as there is a linear relationship between blood volume and portal pressure.[25] This can be evaluated in future studies.

DRUGS TO PREVENT FIRST BLEEDING AND REBLEEDING FROM VARICES

Among the various treatments for portal hypertension for either primary or secondary prevention of variceal bleeding, medical treatment is the most recent and is by its nature simpler and cheaper to administer than long-term sclerotherapy or surgery. Thus, there has been a great deal of research and clinical interest in the long-term pharmacotherapy of portal hypertension, initiated by the seminal paper of Lebrec et al.[26]

Table 11.2   Classes of drugs that lower portal pressure

Non-selective beta blockers
Cardioselective beta blockers
Alpha and beta blocker (labetalol)
Alpha antagonists (including clonidine, a central alpha-2 agonist)
Alpha, agonists (methoxamine)
$5HT_2$ antagonists
Vasoconstrictors (vasopressin and analogues)
Somatostatin and octreotide
Nitrate vasodilators
Vasodilators (molsidomine, pentoxifylline)
Diuretics (loop and potassium sparing)
Beta-2 antagonist (experimental drug)
Anti-platelet-activation factor (experimental drug)
Anti-glucagon

The aim of long-term medical treatment of portal hypertension is to reduce portal pressure, and thus prevent bleeding. Portal pressure could be reduced in three ways: diminishing the portal inflow, and/or reducing the intrahepatic vascular resistance, and/or reducing the resistance in the collateral circulation. Theoretically, controlling portal pressure might prevent the development of portal hypertension and varices. This has been shown in animal models of schistosomal portal hypertension.[27]

Many drugs have been evaluated in cirrhotics with portal hypertension, whereas patients with non-cirrhotic portal hypertension have rarely been studied. The types of drugs that lower portal pressure are shown in Table 11.2.

Virtually all clinical trials and long-term treatment studies have been conducted with non-selective beta blockers, particularly propranolol. Recently the combination of propranolol and isosorbide mononitrate has been used in a short-term clinical study.[28]

Haemodynamic changes in systemic and portal circulations with beta blockers

In 1980, Lebrec et al[26] showed that twice daily oral propranolol (80 to 360 mg daily), given to reduce the resting pulse rate by 25%, produced a sustained mean decrease in WHVP of 25% (4.5 mmHg) in alcoholic cirrhotics without jaundice, ascites, or encephalopathy. The WHVP closely reflects portal pressure in alcoholic cirrhosis, in which the site of resistance is sinusoidal and postsinusoidal.[29] There was also a mean decrease in cardiac output of 31% and in hepatic blood flow of 24%. These haemodynamic changes could be maintained at 3 and 9 months with prolonged administration.[30] There was no correlation between the decrease in HVPG and cardiac output, so that the latter could not be the sole reason for the fall in WHVP.

Hillon et al[31] later showed that for a similar decrease in cardiac output, there was a significantly more marked decrease in HVPG following oral propranolol (40 mg) than following oral atenolol (100 mg). This suggested that extracardiac mechanisms (beta-2 receptor blockade) were also responsible for the reduction in HVPG following propranolol. This reduction is, in part, due to unopposed alpha-adrenergic activity in the splanchnic bed causing vasoconstriction, during beta-2 receptor blockade.[32] In man, an experimental beta-2 blocker (ICI 118551) caused a 12% drop in WHVP without changing cardiac output.[33]

In the early reports propranolol was always found to reduce HVPG, but the extent was very variable. The patients studied were nearly all categorized as modified Child's grade A or B, that is, with good or moderate liver function. However, later reports[34-36] found that acute administration of oral propranolol, even with adequate plasma concentrations, did not reduce the HVPG in some decompensated cirrhotics,[35] or had a less marked effect. In one study[36] one-third of patients showed no HVPG change with 40 mg of oral propranolol, and only 43% of a group of these non-responders showed a fall in HVPG with incremental doses of propranolol. The percentage reduction in resting heart rate correlated only with plasma propranolol concentrations and not with HVPG reduction. Even if severity of liver disease was taken into account, neither the percentage reduction in resting heart rate nor the plasma propranolol concentrations correlated with the percentage reduction in HVPG. Other workers have also found that pulse-rate reduction was not related to severity of liver disease or to propranolol concentration.[37] This suggests that a 25% reduction in resting pulse rate is not a reliable index of HVPG reduction and should not be used as such.

The variable effect of propranolol on HVPG reduction and its possible relationship to a reduction in the frequency of variceal bleeding (the therapeutic response) are further complicated by other haemodynamic indices. Valla et al[38] found that the reduction in WHVP in alcoholic cirrhotics was not paralleled by a similar reduction in portal pressure reduction when this is measured directly. Other authors[39,40] have found no fall in portal pressure with direct measurement. The discrepancies between WHVP and direct portal pressure measurement in alcoholic cirrhotics following propranolol administration may be due to an increase in portal collateral resistance and/or intrahepatic vascular resistance that offsets a reduction in portal pressure caused by a decrease in portal outflow. Using Doppler ultrasound, Ohnishi et al[39] have shown a reduction in portal flow that is greater than the fall in portal pressure.

It is now clear that there are non-responders to propranolol in terms of portal pressure. Bendtsen et al[41] have defined non-responders as those exhibiting less than 10% reduction in portal pressure following an oral dose of 80 mg propranolol. They compared the haemodynamic indices between responders and non-responders. All patients showed evidence of adequate beta blockade with plasma levels above 50 ng/ml, and a fall in cardiac output. The non-responders had a lower baseline cardiac index and a higher systemic vascular resistance – that is, their circulations were less hyperdynamic. There was no relationship between the effect of propranolol and the height of portal pressure, severity of liver disease, or presence of ascites.

Compared to placebo, propranolol reduces intravariceal pressure.[42] It is clear, therefore, that pressure at the site of rupture can be reduced. Unfortunately, the study establishing this was not designed to assess any correlation between variceal pressure and WHVP reduction, and it may be that if collateral resistance is usually increased by propranolol, then intra-variceal pressure would fall, and portal pressure would not.

Azygous blood flow is an indirect measure of collateral blood flow in cirrhotics that includes blood flowing through oesophageal varices.[34, 43] In all studies, it is reduced in every patient given propranolol. The percentage reduction in azygous blood flow averages 32%, much greater than the average HVPG reduction. The reduction in azygous blood flow appears to be a specific effect of beta-2 blockade in the splanchnic bed, because it is not blocked by alpha-adrenergic blockade; that is, it is not caused by un-opposed alpha-adrenergic vasoconstriction.[44] The magnitude of the de-crease in azygous blood flow following administration of propranolol was not related to the degree of hepatic decompensation in one study.[43] How-ever, in another study intravenous propranolol reduced azygous blood flow less markedly in decompensated cirrhotics.[45] Despite these discrepancies, azygous blood flow appears to be a good index to assess a haemodynamic response to propranolol. However, as for pressure measurements,[40] no direct correlation has been found between azygous blood flow and risk of variceal haemorrhage.[46]

Therefore, we do not have a reliable baseline haemodynamic index with which to assess the probability of a therapeutic response to propranolol, that is, the reduction in frequency of variceal bleeding.[47, 48] There is only one preliminary report[49] which has analysed the factors which might predict an absolute reduction of HVPG to 12 mmHg or less in a group of cirrhotics some of whom had bled: 18 of 150 (12%) reduced their HVPG to this extent. The only variables which were independently predictive of this HVPG reduction were a lower baseline HVPG (mean 14.7 mmHg vs. 20 mmHg) and a higher arterial pressure (mean 97 mmHg vs. 88 mmHg). A marked acute response to propranolol (> 20% reduction from baseline HVPG – in 36 [24%] patients) was predicted by the absence of previous episodes of bleeding (36% vs. 8% of those who had previously bled) and the absence of ascites (32% vs. 15% with ascites). When neither previous bleeding nor ascites were present, 42% of these patients had a marked response. This is the first study which has attempted to look at predictive factors for a haemodynamic response to propranolol. Unfortunately, the correlation with the therapeutic response was not made. However, recently there has been evidence of such an index predicting bleeding in *response* to

propranolol: in the Barcelona, Boston, and New Haven primary propranolol prophylaxis trial,[50] bleeding did not occur in patients whose HVPG fell
to 12 mmHg or less.[51] In addition, a haemodynamic index which might
predict rebleeding from varices has been suggested by Sacerdoti et al.[52]
Patients who had a percentage reduction of HVPG of greater than 12% at 1
month following nadolol administration did not rebleed.

Nitrovasodilators and combinations with beta blockers

Nitroglycerin, isosorbide mononitrate, and dinitrate are vasodilators which
act via nitric oxide in vascular smooth-muscle cells.[53] Several groups have
found that these vasodilators decrease WHVP, portal pressure, or intravariceal pressure,[54, 55] but, as for propranolol, other groups have not
detected any pressure reduction.[56] There is a theoretical possibility that
WHVP is reduced by vasodilators whereas portal pressure is not, as WHVP
is dependent on hepatic arterial blood flow and arterial pressure, as well as
portal blood flow and intrahepatic portal resistance. In normal persons, low
doses of vasodilators decrease venous return by inducing venous pooling,
while the arterial pressure remains unchanged. The decreased venous
return induces constriction in the splanchnic arteriolar bed secondary to
reduction in cardiac filling pressure. In turn, this causes unloading of the
cardiopulmonary baroreceptors[57]. However, in cirrhotic patients the same
low dose of vasodilators has no splanchnic haemodynamic effects.

Vasodilators in high doses lower arterial pressure as well as reducing
venous return. This activates arterial baroreceptors, causing constriction of
splanchnic arterioles. In cirrhotics this could reduce both portal inflow and
pressure, but this has been little studied, although it is known that arterial
baroreflexes are abnormal in cirrhotics.[58] Rector et al[56] suggest that the
response to vasodilators is dependent on the pulmonary wedged pressure
(PWP). In those patients whose PWP was lower than 12 mmHg, there was a
reduction in WHVP. However, those with a PWP higher than 12 mmHg
had an increase in WHVP. Presumably, in the latter group, the secondary
decrease in PWP was not sufficient to cause cardiopulmonary baroreceptor
unloading to trigger splanchnic arteriolar vasoconstriction. Finally, vasodilators may act by reducing intrahepatic or collateral vascular resistance,
as has been demonstrated in man.[59]

Thus, as single agents, nitrovasodilators are not optimal hypotensive
agents in cirrhotics. In high doses they induce arterial hypotension, and
may decrease systemic oxygen consumption and increase plasma lactate
concentrations if the reduction in blood pressure is of the order of 20% or
more[60] – this would suggest hypoxia of tissues. Tolerance of vasodilators
could be a problem, and one study has shown an antiaggregative platelet
effect. Moreover, there is some evidence that isosorbide 5-mononitrate
(ISMN) may impair the renal function.[61]

However, the combination of nitrovasodilators with other drugs could theoretically enhance portal pressure reduction. In a short-term haemo-dynamic study,[62] the addition of ISMN to propranolol caused a further reduction in mean HVPG: from 21.5 mmHg ± 3.9 to 18.6 mmHg ± 4.2 with propranolol, and to 15.7 mmHg ± 3.1 mmHg following ISMN without a further decrease in azygous venous blood flow. However, mean arterial pressure fell by 22% and hepatic blood flow by 15.5%. In the long-term part of the study ISMN also caused a further reduction in HVPG in comparison to propranolol alone, with only a 12% reduction in mean arterial blood pressure.

Although FHVP increased in this study, the additional fall in HVPG was entirely due to a further decrease in WHVP. A further interesting observa-tion was that the propranolol 'non-responders' became 'responders' follow-ing the addition of ISMN, and this subgroup of patients was the one which had the greatest pharmacological response. The same researchers[28] have furthered their evaluation by comparing the effects of oral propranolol alone and the combination of propranolol and ISMN in a randomized controlled trial over 3 months. The HPVG decreased by more than 20% of the baseline values in only 10% of propranolol-treated patients but in 50% of the combined therapy group. ISMN did not further reduce hepatic blood flow or intrinsic clearance of indocyanine green, as compared to propranolol alone.

ISMN has no first-pass effect (unlike isosorbide dinitrate), making dosage easier to determine in cirrhotic patients, and it appears to maintain its effect over time – that is, tolerance was not induced.

Molsidomine

This vasodilator does not induce tolerance and has little effect on arterial pressure in normal persons. However, it is metabolized to its active form in the liver. Three groups have now published data. In the first[63] the mean WHVP (−11%) and porto-hepatic venous gradient (−15%) were reduced by molsidomine, as were arterial pressure (−13.5%) and hepatic blood flow (−17.4%). Free hepatic venous pressure was not affected, nor was the intrinsic hepatic clearance of indocyanine green. Interestingly, heart rate did not change, suggesting that baroreceptor constricting reflexes were not involved. Therefore, the action of molsidomine may be that of a direct portal vasodilator. However, three of 13 (24%) patients did not respond. In a German study 28% had no reduction in HVPG.[64]

In the third study,[65] reductions similar to those of the other studies in WHVP and HPVG were found with 2 mg or 4 mg orally, and these effects could also be shown at 2 h. Only 13% of patients did not respond (one of eight) in terms of HVPG reduction. Mean azygous blood flow did not change (with wide variation between patients), despite reduction in cardiac output and liver blood flow, suggesting a reduction in resistance in the collateral vessels. Thus, the action of molsidomine may be due to both portal-collateral and hepatic vasodilation, and reduced portal inflow secondary to reflex arteriolar vasoconstrictor in splanchnic organs. However, hepatic blood flow and intrinsic clearance of indocyanine green were also significantly reduced, contrary to the first study, but to a similar degree to propranolol combined with 40 mg ISMN. Care should be taken in long-term studies, regarding the severity of liver disease, particularly as hepatic metabolism is crucial to the action of the drug.

Diuretics

In 1985 Klein[66] reported that long-term spironolactone reduced WHVP. This observation passed unnoticed for some time, as did the original reports of the 1960s.

Volume contraction might theoretically induce a reduction in portal inflow because of reflex vasoconstrictor secondary to baroreceptor reflexes. Okumura et al[67] evaluated the haemodynamic effects of a 4-week oral administration of 100 mg spironolactone ($n = 15$) or 40 mg frusemide ($n = 10$) in cirrhotics with ascites. They showed a mean reduction of HVPG of 22% and of WHVP of 16% in the spironolactone group but none in the frusemide group. The circulating volume did not fall in the frusemide group but did fall in the spironolactone group, but there was no correlation with HVPG reduction. However, there was a negative correlation with the posttreatment aldosterone concentrations. In neither group was there a change in the estimated hepatic blood flow; but, in both groups, the cardiac output and mean arterial pressure fell, without change in heart rate. The systemic vascular resistance did not change in the spironolactone group but fell in the frusemide group. It is not clear if these differences between spironolactone and frusemide are real, as, theoretically, volume contraction should occur with both, following chronic administration. It is not known if similar effects could be induced in cirrhotics without ascites who have increased plasma volumes, nor whether the combination with beta blockers enhances the portal pressure reduction.

RANDOMIZED CLINICAL TRIALS OF BETA BLOCKERS

Prevention of the first gastrointestinal haemorrhage

The randomized clinical trials of beta blockers comprise eight trials involving 951 patients – six with propranolol and two with nadolol (Table 11.3). A comprehensive meta-analysis[68a] and an update[68b] show that the incidence of first bleeding was significantly reduced without evidence of statistical heterogeneity. The pooled relative risk of bleeding in patients taking beta blockers was almost half that of those taking placebo: 0.51 (95% confidence interval, 0.4–0.7), $P < 0.001$. The mortality rate was also reduced but not significantly: 0.8 (95% confidence interval, 0.6–1.0).[68b] Using individual patient data, rather than trial outcomes, a meta-analysis[70]

Table 11.3 Randomized trials of beta blockers for the primary prevention of variceal bleeding

Trial (author)	Sample size	Mean or median follow-up (months)	Bleeding rate %		Death rate %	
			Controls	Beta blocker	Controls	Beta blocker
Pascal*	230	16	27	17	36	21
IMPP*	174	28	35	21	31	44
Ideo*[a]	79	23	22	3	18	10
Lebrec*[a]	106	12	19	13	19	19
Conn et al[50]	102	34	22	4	22	16
Strauss*	36	16	25	20	44	35
Andreani[b] et al[91]	84	c. 20	32	5	41	30
PROVA[a][92]	140	15	18	18	22	15

* See references in Pagliaro et al 1989. [68a]
[a] Nadolol.
[b] Also had a prophylactic sclerotherapy group.

of four of the trials involving 589 patients has shown that after 2 years (taking age and severity of cirrhosis into account, as these factors affected mortality) the survival rate was only slightly better in the beta-blocker group ($P = 0.09$). However, prevention of fatal bleeding by beta blockers was highly significant ($P = 0.004$) – a saving of eight lives among 100 patients followed for 2 years. This was also true for the prevention of bleeding: a mean of 78% of patients free of rebleeding in the propranolol group versus 65% in the control group ($P = 0.002$). These differences remained after adjustment for the cause and severity of cirrhosis, ascites and size of varices. The first two factors were associated with bleeding and death in both the beta-blocker and control groups. The advantage of analysing individual patient data (the first such meta-analysis in hepatology or gastroenterology) is that censored data and prognostic data can all be taken into account. Secondly, data can be combined after the same period of follow-up. Comparison between proportional hazard models and adjusted log rank tests can be made for several subgroups of interest, for example, alcoholics versus non-alcoholics, ascitic versus non-ascitic, and nadolol versus propranolol, as was done in this meta-analysis. None of these analyses affected the overall difference between treatment groups.

The data from prophylactic trials suggest that screening for moderate and large varices in cirrhotics should become part of routine clinical practice, and, if such varices are found, beta blockers should be given to reduce the incidence of bleeding and death from bleeding.

Prevention of bleeding from portal hypertensive gastropathy

In the first propranolol trial, patients who had gastric mucosal bleeding were also included, and propranolol was shown to protect from rebleeding from this source, but the numbers were too small to establish statistical significance. Portal hypertensive gastropathy is now a recognized entity, also known as congestive gastropathy. It may lead to chronic anaemia as well as upper-gastrointestinal bleeding.[71] In animal models the mucosa has a microvasculopathy which results in reduced oxygenation of the surface gastric mucosa and is more susceptible to injurious agents.[72] Whatever the triggering agent for occult or frank blood loss, propranolol has been shown to prevent both acute and chronic bleeding in a single-blind randomized study.[73] Thus, the actuarial percentages of patients free of rebleeding from portal hypertensive gastropathy at 12 months were 65% versus 38% ($P < 0.05$), and at 30 months 52% versus 7% ($P < 0.05$). There were also fewer episodes of acute rebleeding (mean episodes/patient/month: 0.01 vs. 0.12).

Prevention of rebleeding from varices: beta blockers compared to no treatment

There were 11 trials involving 637 patients (Table 11.4). The same meta-

Table 11.4 Randomized trials of beta blockers for the prevention of rebleeding from varices

Trial (author)	Sample size	Mean or median follow-up (months)	Bleeding rate %		Death rate %	
			Controls	Beta blocker	Controls	Beta blocker
Poynard et al[69]	74	29	64	16	22	8
Burroughs et al[93]	48	21	59	54	23	15
Villeneuve*	79	23	81	76	38	45
Queuniet*	99	25	65	57	21	24
Gatta*	24	14	67	25	25	8
Colombo*	62	12	47	25	23	12
Colombo*	62	12	47	31	23	10
Chiu et al[94]	36	12	56	28	11	0
Garden et al[95]	81	16	77	47	44	37
Cerebelaud et al[96]	84	16	66	34	—	—
Von Kobe*	54	—	46	38	32	23
Colman et al[97]	100	—	50	35	4	4

* See references in Pagliaro et al 1989.[68a]

analyses[68a,b] show that the risk of rebleeding is significantly reduced by beta blockers. The pooled relative risk is 0.4 (95% confidence interval, 0.3–0.5), $P < 0.001$ with no statistical heterogeneity. However, there is no significant effect on mortality, the pooled relative risk being 0.7 (95% confidence interval, 0.5–1.04). The difference in mortality is far less than in the primary prevention trials. Clinical factors which might predict the therapeutic response for rebleeding with propranolol are not yet known, but non-compliance, presence of a hepatocellular carcinoma, and non-reduction of resting heart rate have been suggested by Lebrec's group.[69] Some haemodynamic criteria may be shown to be useful in the future,[52] but their measurement remains invasive and impractical. A partial solution to this problem may be the correlation of intravariceal pressure reduction, measured endoscopically, and the incidence of rebleeding.

Prevention of rebleeding from varices: beta blockers compared to sclerotherapy

There were eight trials involving 644 patients (Table 11.5). The same meta-analyses[68a] showed that the two therapies are equivalent, with a relative risk of 1 (95% confidence interval, 0.7–1.7) for mortality, and 0.7 (95% confidence interval, 0.5–1.1) for rebleeding. Thus, on this basis, beta blockers would be the treatment of first choice for the prevention of rebleeding, barring contraindications, as they are less expensive and invasive than sclerotherapy, and do not increase the endoscopy workload. However, many groups still use long-term sclerotherapy despite this evidence. In future, combination drug therapy should make the pharmacological approach more effective.

Prevention of rebleeding from varices: addition of beta blockers to sclerotherapy versus sclerotherapy alone, or versus beta blockers alone

There were seven trials of sclerotherapy and beta blockers versus sclerotherapy alone involving 347 patients (Table 11.6). There was no advantage in combining beta blockers with long-term sclerotherapy: relative risk 0.7, (95% confidence interval, 0.45–1.2). Theoretically, the drug might prevent rebleeding before variceal obliteration. Only one group[74,75] showed rebleeding to be significantly decreased both before and after eradication, and only one other trial showed a significant advantage in adding a beta blocker[76]. Mortality was unchanged: relative risk 0.95, (95% confidence interval, 0.5–1.75).

There were two trials of sclerotherapy and beta blockers versus beta blockers alone.[77,78] Both showed a significant advantage in adding sclerotherapy to beta blockers in terms of rebleeding: beta blockers alone, rebleeding 65% – in combination, 45%;[77] beta blockers alone, 60% – in

Table 11.5 Randomized trials of beta blockers *vs.* sclerotherapy for the prevention of variceal bleeding

Trial (author)	Sample size	Mean or median follow-up (months)	Bleeding rate %		Death rate %	
			Beta blockers	Sclerotherapy	Beta blockers	Sclerotherapy
Alexandrino*	65	29	74	55	32	29
Fleig*	105	26	48	31	32	36
Dollet*	51	36	44	64	32	29
Westaby et al[73a]	108	24	52	42	77	64
Teres et al[17]	72	11	49	21	31	21
Liu et al[99]	118	?	75	35	41	53
Rossi et al[100]	53	19	48	50	26	23
Martin et al[101]	76	36	53	55	23	31

* See references in Pagliaro et al 1989.[68a]

Table 11.6 Randomized trials of beta blockers combined with sclerotherapy *vs.* sclerotherapy alone

Trial (author)	Sample size	Mean or median follow-up (months)	Bleeding rate %		Death rate %	
			Beta blockers and sclerotherapy	Sclerotherapy	Beta blockers and sclerotherapy	Sclerotherapy
Westaby et al[98]	53	6	27	30	35	26
Vickers et al[99]	69	24	51	44	37	26
Vinel et al[76]	65	12	21	38	12	19
Jensen et al[74]	31	–	20	75	7	6
Gerunda et al[103]	60	6	20	17	–	–
Lundell et al[104]	41	–	12e	11e	5	26
Bertoni et al[105]	28	–	7	29	7	21

e = episodes.

* See references in Pagliaro et al 1989.[68a]

combination, 39%.[78] There was no improvement in mortality. The results of all nine trials do not justify a routine use of the combination of beta blockers and sclerotherapy.

COMPLICATIONS OF BETA BLOCKERS: EFFECTS ON KIDNEY AND LIVER FUNCTION AND HEPATIC ENCEPHALOPATHY

There are no reports of fatal complications of beta blockers in cirrhotic patients. Withdrawal caused by the expected side-effects – for example, heart failure and asthma – is infrequent. A recent review has the references for the effects reported on kidney, liver, and brain (encephalopathy) in cirrhotic patients.[79] Occasionally hepatic encephalopathy may be precipitated by propranolol, but the effect is reversible.

SUMMARY

Drug therapy for acute variceal bleeding should be viewed as an adjunct to emergency sclerotherapy. Its role in preventing very early rebleeding (within days) following sclerotherapy needs to be established. The best candidates for such a role are somatostatin and octreotide, but combinations of glypressin or vasopressin with nitroglycerin have therapeutic effect in the short term. Propranolol is the drug for long-term prevention of rebleeding and prevention of the first variceal bleed. For primary prophylaxis, it significantly reduces the rate of bleeding, and there is a trend towards reduced mortality. It should be used in cirrhotic patients with large varices. For secondary prophylaxis, propranolol significantly reduces rebleeding but does not improve survival. The reduction in rebleeding is similar to that of long-term sclerotherapy when compared in randomized studies. There is no value in adding beta blockers to sclerotherapy; beta blockers can be used as the first-line therapy to prevent variceal rebleeding. They also have been shown to reduce the frequency of rebleeding from congestive gastropathy.

Many patients do not show a decrease of portal pressure during treatment with propranolol. The addition of ISMN converts many 'non-responders' to responders. Current clinical trials are evaluating whether therapeutic efficacy is improved by this drug combination.

REFERENCES

1 Burroughs AK, Mezzanotte G, Phillips A et al. Cirrhotics with variceal haemorrhage: the importance of the time interval between admission and the start of analysis for survival and rebleeding rates. Hepatology 1989; 9: 801–807
2 North Italian Endoscopic Club (NIEC) for the Study and Treatment of Oesophageal Varices. Prediction of the first variceal haemorrhage in patients with cirrhosis of the liver and oesophageal varices: a prospective study. N Engl J Med 1988; 319: 983–989

3   Merkel C, Gatta A. Correspondence. Can we predict the first variceal bleeding in the individual patient with cirrhosis and esophageal varices? J Hepatol 1991; 13: 378

4   Polio J, Groszmann RJ. Haemodynamic factors involved in the development and rupture of esophageal varices. A pathophysiological approach to treatment. Semin Liv Dis 1986; 6: 318–328

5   Burroughs AK. Leader. Somatostatin and octreotide for variceal bleeding. J Hepatol 1991; 13: 1–4

6   Jenkins SA, Ellenbogen S, Jaser N, Baxter JN, Shields R. Abstract. Efficacy of somatostatin in controlling post-injection sclerotherapy bleeding from varices per se, oesophageal ulcers and oesophagitis. Gut 1990; 31: A628

7   Valenzuela JE, Schubert T, Fogel MR et al. A multicentre, randomised double-blind trial of somatostatin in the management of acute haemorrhage from oesophageal varices. Hepatology 1989; 10: 958–961

8   Burroughs AK, McCormick PA, Hughes MD, Sprengers D, D'Heygere F, McIntyre N. Randomised double-blind placebo-controlled trial of somatostatin for variceal bleeding. Emergency control and prevention of early variceal rebleeding. Gastroenterology 1990; 99: 1388–1395

9   Avgerinos A, Klonis C, Rekoumis G, Gouma P, Papadimitriou N, Raptis S. A prospective randomised trial comparing somatostatin, balloon tamponade, and the combination of both methods in the management of acute variceal haemorrhage. J Hepatol 1991; 13: 78–83

10 Tsai Y-T, Lay C-S, Lai K-H et al. Controlled trial of vasopressin plus nitroglycerin versus vasopressin alone in the treatment of bleeding oesophageal varices. Hepatology 1986; 6: 406–409

11 Gimson AES, Westaby D, Hegarty J et al. A randomised trial of vasopressin and vasopressin plus nitroglycerin in the control of acute variceal haemorrhage. Hepatology 1986; 6: 410–413

12 Valla D, Lees S, Moreau R et al. Effects de la glypressine sur le circulations splanchnique et systèmique des malades atteints de cirrhose. Gastroenterol Clin Biol 1985; 9: 877–880

13 Cestari R, Braga M, Missale G, Ravelli P, Burroughs AK. Haemodynamic effect of triglycyl-lysine vasopressin (glypressin) on intravascular oesophageal variceal pressure in patients with cirrhosis. A randomized placebo-controlled trial. J Hepatol 1990; 10: 205–210

14 Lin H-C, Tsai Y-T, Chang T-T et al. Systemic and portal haemodynamic changes following triglycyl-lysine vasopressin plus nitroglycerin administration in patients with hepatitis B related cirrhosis. J Hepatol 1990; 10: 370–374

15 Bosch J, Groszmann RJ, Garcia-Pagan JC et al. Association of transdermal nitroglycerin to vasopressin infusion in the treatment of variceal haemorrhage; a placebo-controlled clinical trial. Hepatology 1989; 10: 962–968

16 Fort E, Sautereau D, Silvain C, Ingrand P, Pillegand B, Beauchant M. A randomised trial of terlipressin plus nitroglycerin vs. balloon tamponade in the control of acute variceal haemorrhage. Hepatology 1990; 11: 678–681

17 Teres J, Planas R, Panes J et al. Vasopressin/nitroglycerin infusion vs. esophageal tamponade in the treatment of acute variceal bleeding. A randomized control trial. Hepatology 1990; 11: 964–968

18 Freeman JG, Cobden I, Record C. Placebo-controlled trial of terlipressin (glypressin) in the management of acute variceal bleeding. J Clin Gastroenterol 1989; 11: 58–60

19 Soderlund C, Magnusson I, Torngren S, Lundell L. Terlipressin (triglycyl-lysine vasopressin) controls acute bleeding oesophageal varices. A double-blind randomised placebo-controlled trial. Scand J Gastroenterol 1990; 25: 622–630

20 Bosch J, Bordas J, Mastai R et al. Effects of vasopressin on the intravariceal pressure in patients with cirrhosis: comparison with the effects on portal pressure. Hepatology 1988; 18: 861–865

21 Ohnishi K, Sato S. Effects of vasopressin on left gastric venous flow in cirrhotic patients with esophageal varices. Am J Gastroenterol 1990; 85: 293–297

22 Moreau R, Hadengue A, Soupison T et al. Abnormal pressor response to vasopressin in patients with cirrhosis: evidence for impaired buffering mechanisms. Hepatology 1990; 12: 7–12

23   Ready J, Robertson A, Rector W. Effects of vasopressin on portal pressure during haemorrhage from esophageal varices. Gastroenterology 1991; 100: 1411–1416
24   Ready J, Robertson A, Goff JS, Rector W. Assessment of the risk of bleeding from esophageal varices by continuous monitoring of portal pressure. Gastroenterology 1991; 100: 1403–1410
25   Zimmon DS, Kessler RE. The portal pressure–blood volume relationship in cirrhosis. Gut 1974; 15: 99–101
26   Lebrec D, Novel O, Corbic M et al. Propranolol – a medical treatment for portal hypertension. Lancet 1980; 2: 180–182
27   Sarin SK, Groszmann RJ, Mosca PG et al. Propranolol ameliorates the development of portal-systemic shunting in a chronic murine schistosomiasis model of portal hypertension. J Clin Invest 1991; 87: 1032–1036
28   Garcia-Pagan JC, Feu F, Bosch J, Rodes J. Propranolol compared with propranolol plus isosorbide mononitrate for portal hypertension in cirrhosis. A randomised controlled study. Ann Intern Med 1991; 114: 869–873
29   Boyer TD, Triger DR, Horisawa M et al. Direct transhepatic measurement of portal vein pressure using a thin needle. Comparison with wedged hepatic vein pressure. Gastroenterology 1977; 72: 584–589
30   Lebrec D, Hillon P, Munoz C et al. The effect of propranolol on portal hypertension in patients with cirrhosis. A haemodynamic study. Hepatology 1982; 2: 523–527
31   Hillon P, Lebrec D, Munoz C et al. Comparison of the effects of a cardioselective and non-selective beta-blocker on portal hypertension in patients with cirrhosis. Hepatology 1982; 28: 528–533
32   Price HL, Cooperman LH, Warden JC. Control of the splanchnic circulation in man. Role of beta-adrenergic receptors. Circ Res 1967; 21: 333–340
33   Bihari D, Westaby D, Grimson AES et al. Reductions in portal pressure by selective beta-2 adrenoceptor blockade in patients with cirrhosis and portal hypertension. Br J Clin Pharmacol 1984; 17: 753–757
34   Bosch J, Mastai R, Kravetz D et al. Effects of propranolol on azygous venous blood flow and hepatic and systemic haemodynamics in cirrhosis. Hepatology 1984; 4: 1200–1205
35   Colman JC, Jennings GL, McLean AJ et al. Letter. Propranolol in decompensated alcoholic cirrhosis. Lancet 1982; 2: 1040–1041
36   Garcia-Tsao G, Grace ND, Groszmann RJ et al. Short-term effects of propranolol on portal venous pressure. Hepatology 1986; 6: 101–106
37   Caujolle B, Ballet F, Poupon R. Relationship among beta-adrenergic blockade, propranolol concentration and liver function in patients with cirrhosis. Scand J Gastroenterol 1988; 23: 925–930
38   Valla D, Bercoff E, Menu Y et al. Discrepancy between wedged hepatic venous pressure and portal venous pressure after acute propranolol administration in patients with alcoholic cirrhosis. Gastroenterology 1984; 86: 1400–1403
39   Ohnishi K, Nakayama T, Saito M et al. Effects of propranolol on portal haemodynamics in patients with chronic liver disease. Am J Gastroenterol 1985; 80: 132–135
40   Rector WG. Propranolol for portal hypertension. Evaluation of therapeutic response by direct measurement of portal vein pressure. Arch Intern Med 1985; 145: 648–650
41   Bendtsen F, Henriksen JH, Sorensen TIA. Propranolol and haemodynamic response in cirrhosis. J Hepatol 1991; 13: 144–148
42   Feu F, Bordas JM, Garcia-Pagan J, Bosch J, Rodes J. Double-blind investigation of the effects of propranolol and placebo on the pressure of oesophageal varices in patients with portal hypertension. Hepatology 1991; 13: 917–922
43   Cales P, Braillon A, Hiron MI et al. Superior portosystemic collateral circulation estimated by azygous blood flow in patients with cirrhosis. Hepatology 1984; 1: 37–46
44   Mastai R, Bosch J, Navasa M. Abstract. Reduction in azygous blood flow is an intrinsic effect of beta-adrenergic blockade in patients with cirrhosis. Hepatology 1985; 2 (suppl): S282
45   Brallion A, Cales P, Valla D et al. Influence of the degree of liver failure on systemic and splanchnic haemodynamics and on the response to propranolol in patients with cirrhosis. Gut 1986; 27: 1204–1209

46 Bosch J, Mastai R, Kravetz D et al. Measurements of azygous venous blood flow in the evaluation of portal hypertension in patients with cirrhosis. Clinical and haemodynamic correlations in 100 patients. J Hepatol 1985; 1: 125–139

47 Valla D, Jiron I, Poynard T et al. Failure of haemodynamic measurements to prevent recurrent gastro-intestinal bleeding in cirrhotic patients receiving propranolol. J Hepatol 1987; 5: 144–148

48 Vorobioff J, Picabea E, Villavicencio R et al. Acute and chronic haemodynamic effect of propranolol in unselected cirrhotic patients. Hepatology 1987; 7: 648–653

49 Pereira O, Garcia-Pagan J, Feu F et al. Abstract. Factors influencing the portal pressure response to propranolol administration in patients with cirrhosis. Hepatology 1991; 14: 133A

50 Conn HO, Grace ND, Bosch J et al. Propranolol in the prevention of the first haemorrhage from esophagogastric varices: a multicentre randomized clinical trial. Hepatology 1991; 13: 902–912

51 Groszmann RJ, Bosch J, Grace ND et al. Haemodynamic events in a prospective randomized trial of propranolol versus placebo in the prevention of a first variceal haemorrhage. Gastroenterology 1990; 99: 1401–1407

52 Sacerdoti D, Merkel C, Gatta A. Correspondence of the 1-month effect of nadolol on portal pressure in predicting failure of prevention of rebleeding in cirrhosis. J Hepatol 1991; 12: 124–125

53 Waldman SA, Murad F. Cyclic GMP synthesis and function. Pharmacol Rev 1987; 39: 163–196

54 Moreau R, Lebrec D. Leader. Nitrovasodilators and portal hypertension. J Hepatol 1990; 10: 263–267

55 Iwao T, Toyonaga A, Sumino M et al. Hemodynamic study during transdermal application of nitroglycerin tape in patients with cirrhosis. Hepatology 1991; 13: 124–128

56 Rector WG, Hossack KF, Ready JB. Nitroglycerin for portal hypertension. A controlled comparison of the haemodynamic effects of graded doses. J Hepatol 1990; 10: 375–380

57 Hirsch AT, Levenson DJ, Cutler SS, Dzau VJ, Creager MA. Regional vascular responses to prolonged lower body negative pressure in normal subjects. Am J Physiol 1989; 257: H219–H225

58 Koshy A, Moreau R, Cerini R et al. Effects of oxygen inhalation on tissue oxygenation in patients with cirrhosis. Evidence for an impaired arterial baroreflex control. J Hepatol 1989; 9: 240–245

59 Navasa M, Bosch J, Chesta J, Rodes J. Isosorbide 5-mononitrate reduces hepatic vascular resistance and portal pressure in patients with cirrhosis. Gastroenterology 1988; 96: 1110–1118

60 Moreau R, Roulot D, Braillon A et al. Low dose of nitroglycerin failed to improve splanchnic haemodynamics in patients with cirrhosis: evidence for an impaired cardiopulmonary baroreflex function. Hepatology 1989; 10: 93–97

61 Salmeron JM, Del Arbol L, Gines A et al. Abstract. Isosorbide 5-mononitrate increases plasma renin activity and aldosterone and impairs renal function in cirrhosis with ascites. J Hepatol 1991; 13 (suppl 2): S67

62 Garcia-Pagan JC, Navasa M, Bosch J, Bru C, Pizcueta P, Rodes J. Enhancement of portal pressure reduction by the association of isosorbide 5-mononitrate to propranolol administration in patients with cirrhosis. Hepatology 1990; 11: 230–238

63 Vinel JP, Monnin J-L, Combis J-M, Cales P, Desmorat H, Pascal J-P. Haemodynamic evaluation of molsidomine: a vasodilator with antianginal properties in patients with alcoholic cirrhosis. Hepatology 1990; 11: 239–242

64 Huppe D, Jäger D, Tromm A, Tunn S, Barmeyer J, May B. Einflub von Molsidomin auf die portale und kardiale Haemodynamik bei Leberzirrhose. Dtsch Med Wochenschr 1991; 116: 841–845

65 Del Arbol L, Garcia-Pagan J, Feu F, Pizueta M, Bosch J, Rodes J. Effects of molsidomine, a long-acting venous dilator, on portal hypertension. J Hepatol 1991; 13: 179–186

66 Klein CP. Spironolactone in der Behandlung der portalen Hypertonie bei Leberzirrhoses. Dtsch Med Wochenschr 1985; 110: 1774–1776

67   Okumura H, Aramaki T, Katsuta Y et al. Reduction in hepatic venous pressure gradient as a consequence of volume contraction due to chronic administration of spironolactone in patients with cirrhosis and no ascites. Am J Gastroenterol 1991; 86: 46–52

68a Pagliaro L, Burroughs AK, Sorensen T et al. Therapeutic controversies and randomised controlled trials (RCTs): prevention of bleeding and rebleeding in cirrhosis. Gastroenterol Int 1989; 2:71–84

68b Pagliaro L, Burroughs AK, Sorensen TIA et al. Correspondence. Beta blockers for preventing variceal bleeding. Lancet 1990; 336: 1001–1002

69   Poynard T, Lebrec D, Hillon P et al. Propranolol for prevention of recurrent gastrointestinal bleeding in patients with cirrhosis: a prospective study of factors associated with rebleeding. Hepatology 1987; 7: 447–451

70   Poynard T, Cales P, Pasta L et al. Beta-adrenergic antagonist drugs in the prevention of gastro-intestinal bleeding in patients with cirrhosis and esophageal varices. N Engl J Med 1991; 324: 1532–1538

71   D'Amico G, Montalbano L, Traina M et al. Natural history of congestive gastropathy in cirrhosis. Gastroenterology 1990; 99: 1558–1564

72   Sarfeh IJ, Tarnawski A. Increased susceptibility of the portal hypertensive gastric mucosa to damage. J Clin Gastroenterol 1991; 13 (suppl): S18–S21

73   Perez-Ayuso R, Pique J, Bosch J et al. Propranolol in prevention of recurrent bleeding from severe portal hypertensive gastropathy in cirrhosis. Lancet 1991; 337: 1431–1434

73a Westaby D, Polson RJ, Gimson AE et al. A controlled trial of oral propranolol compared with injection sclerotherapy for the long-term management of variceal bleeding. Hepatology 1990; 11: 353–359

74   Jensen LS, Krarup N. Propranolol in prevention of rebleeding from esophageal varices during the course of endoscopic sclerotherapy. Scand J Gastroenterol 1989; 24: 239–245

75   Jensen LS, Krarup N. Propranolol may prevent recurrence of oesophageal varices after obliteration by endoscopic sclerotherapy. Scand J Gastroenterol 1990; 25: 352–356

76   Venel JP, Lamouliliette H, Cales P et al. Abstract. Propranolol reduced the rebleeding rate during injection sclerotherapy: results of a randomized study. Gastroenterology 1990; 98: A644

77   O'Connor KW, Lehman G, Yune H et al. Comparison of three non-surgical treatments for bleeding esophageal varices. Gastroenterology 1989; 96: 899–906

78   Ink O, Martin T, Poynard et al. Abstract. Does chronic sclerotherapy improve the efficacy of long-term propranolol for prevention of recurrent bleeding in patients with severe cirrhosis? A prospective multicenter randomized trial. J Hepatol 1991; 13 (suppl 2): S37

79   Burroughs AK, McCormick PA. Long-term pharmacologic therapy of portal hypertension. In: Rikkers L, ed. Management of variceal haemorrhage. Surg Clin N Am 1990; 70: 319–339

80   Kravetz D, Bosch J, Teres J et al. Comparison of intravenous somatostatin and vasopressin infusions in the treatment of acute variceal haemorrhage. Hepatology 1984; 4: 422–446

81   Jenkins SA, Baxter JN, Corbett WA et al. A prospective randomised controlled clinical trial comparing somatostatin and vasopressin in controlling acute variceal haemorrhage. Br Med J 1985; 290: 270–278

82   Bagarani M, Albertini V, Anza M et al. Effect of somatostatin in controlling bleeding from oesophageal varices. Ital J Surg Sci 1987; 17: 121–126

83   Saari A, Elvilaakso E, Inberg M et al. Comparison of somatostatin and vasopressin in bleeding oesophageal varices. Am J Gastroenterol 1990; 85: 804–807

84   Walker S, Kreichgauer H-P, Bode JC. Abstract. Terlipressin versus somatostatin in bleeding esophageal varices. Controlled, double-blind study. J Hepatol 1991; 13 (suppl 2): S180

85   Cardona C, Vida F, Balanzo J, Cusso X, Farre A, Guarner C. Eficacia terapeutica de la somatostatina versus vasopresina mas nitroglicerina en la haemorragia activa por varices esofagogastrica. Gastroenterol Hepatol 1989; 12: 30–34

86   Rguez-Moreno F, Santolaria F, Glez-Reimers E et al. Abstract. A randomised trial of somatostatin versus vasopressin plus nitroglycerin in the treatment of acute variceal bleeding. J Hepatol 1991; 13 (suppl 2): S162

87   Silvain C, Carpentier S, Sautereau D et al. Abstract. A randomised trial of glypressin plus transdermal nitroglycerin versus octreotide in the control of acute variceal haemorrhage. Hepatology 1991; 14: 133A

88   McKee R. A study of octreotide in oesophageal varices. Digestion 1990; 45 (suppl 1): 60–65

89   Jaramillo JL, de la Mata M, Mino G, Costan G, Gomez-Camacho F. Somatostatin versus Sengstaken balloon tamponade for primary haemostasis of bleeding oesophageal varices. J Hepatol 1991; 12: 100–105

90   Jenkins SA, Baxter JN, Ellenbogen S, Shields R. Abstract. A prospective randomised controlled clinical trial comparing somatostatin and injection sclerotherapy in the control of acute variceal haemorrhage: preliminary results. Gut 1988; 29: A1431

91   Andreani T, Poupon R, Balkau B et al. Preventive therapy of first gastrointestinal bleeding in patients with cirrhosis: results of a controlled trial comparing propranolol, endoscopic sclerotherapy and placebo. Hepatology 1990; 12: 1413–1419

92   PROVA Study Group. Prophylaxis of first haemorrhage from esophageal varices by sclerotherapy, propranolol or both in cirrhotic patients, a randomized multicentre trial. Hepatology 1991; 14: 1016–1024

93   Burroughs AK, D'Heygere F, McIntyre N. Pitfalls in studies of prophylactic therapy for variceal bleeding in cirrhotics. Hepatology 1986; 6: 1407–1413

94   Chiu K-W, Sheen I-S, Liaw Y-F. A controlled study of glypressin versus vasopressin in the control of bleeding from oesophageal varices. J Gastroenterol Hepatol 1990; 5: 549–553

95   Garden OJ, Mills PR, Birnie GG, Murray GD, Carter DC. Propranolol in the prevention of recurrent variceal haemorrhage in cirrhotic patients: a controlled trial. Gastroenterology 1990; 98: 1985–1990

96   Cerebelaud J, Roulot D, Braillon A et al. Reduction of portal pressure by acute administration of frusemide in patients with alcoholic cirrhosis. J Hepatol 1989; 9: 246–251

97   Colman J, Jones P, Finch C, Dudley F. Abstract. Propranolol in the prevention of variceal haemorrhage in alcoholic cirrhotic patients. Hepatology 1990; 12: 851

98   Westaby D, Melia E, Hegarty J et al. Use of propranolol to reduce the rebleeding rate during injection sclerotherapy prior to variceal obliteration. Hepatology 1986; 6: 673–675

99   Liu JD, Yeng YS, Chen PH et al. Abstract. Endoscopic injection sclerotherapy and propranolol in the prevention of recurrent variceal bleeding. World Congress of Gastroenterology, Sydney 1990: FP118

100   Rossi V, Cales P, Burtin P et al. Prevention of recurrent variceal bleeding in alcoholic cirrhotic patients: prospective controlled trial of propranolol and sclerotherapy. J Hepatol 1991; 12: 283–289

101   Martin T, Taupignon A, Lavignolle A, Perrin D, LeBodic L. Prévention des récidives hémorragiques chez des malades, atteints de cirrhose. Resultats d'une étude controlée comparant propranolol et sclerose endoscopique. Gastroenterol Clin Biol 1991; 15: 833–837

102   Vickers C, Rodes J, Hillenbrand P et al. Abstract. Prospective controlled trial of propranolol and sclerotherapy for prevention of rebleeding from esophageal varices. Gut 1987; 28: A1359

103   Gerunda GE, Neri D, Cangrandi F et al. Abstract. Nadolol does not reduce early rebleeding in cirrhotics undergoing endoscopic variceal sclerotherapy: a multicenter randomized controlled trial. Hepatology 1990; 12: 988

104   Lundell L, Leth R, Lind T et al. Evaluation of propranolol for prevention of recurrent bleeding from esophageal varices between sclerotherapy sessions. Acta Chir Scand 1990; 156: 711–715

105   Bertoni G, Fornaciari G, Beltrami M et al. Nadolol for prevention of variceal rebleeding during the course of endoscopic injection sclerotherapy: a randomised pilot study. J Clin Gastroenterol 1990; 12: 364–365 (letter)

12

Hepatitis C virus

G. M. Dusheiko

After serological tests for hepatitis A and hepatitis B viruses had become available by 1974, it became clear that most cases of post-transfusion hepatitis were not caused by either type A or B hepatitis.[1] The enigmatic name of non-A, non-B (NANB) hepatitis was assigned to this form of hepatitis. Although in the ensuing years many groups of investigators subsequently claimed to have identified the aetiological agent of NANB hepatitis or to have developed serological tests, none of the claims or tests could be validated.[2] Despite this difficulty, however, a considerable body of information on NANB hepatitis in human beings and chimpanzees was compiled. Finally, in 1989, taking advantage of new biotechnological techniques and of the fact that infectious material could be obtained from chimpanzees, Houghton et al succeeded in isolating the genome of the major NANB agent by recombinant DNA technology.[3-5] A viral protein (5-1-1) was expressed to enable detection of the circulating antibody to HCV in patients with chronic NANB hepatitis. The cloning and sequencing of the genome, of what is now rightfully called the hepatitis C virus (HCV), was accordingly a major breakthrough in the long search for a causative agent of NANB hepatitis. The timely identification of this agent and the development of specific tests for the diagnosis of HCV have provided tools for studying the molecular virology, epidemiology, and natural history of type C hepatitis, and have improved the treatment of this disease. The advent of serological tests also allows us to distinguish hepatitis C from the recently cloned hepatitis E virus, which causes enteric or epidemic NANB hepatitis.[6]

Preliminary epidemiological assessment suggests that there are approximately 100 million type C hepatitis carriers globally. About 175 000 new cases are said to occur annually in the US and in Europe, and 350 000 cases per year in Japan. HCV is the major viral cause of chronic liver disease in Europe, and an important cause of chronic liver disease in Africa and Asia.

VIROLOGY OF HCV

The putative NANB virus was previously thought to possess a lipid envelope, and to be approximately 50–80 nm in diameter. HCV is now

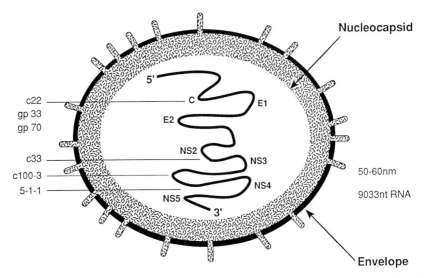

Fig. 12.1 A stylized depiction of the hepatitis C virus, showing an artistic representation of the viral particle, RNA genome, non-coding 5′ region, coding region, and proteins expressed from the viral genome and used in serological assays.
C = nucleocapsid protein coding region
E = envelope protein coding region
NS = Non-structural region

believed to be an enveloped virus, approximately 50 nm in size, and is known to possess an RNA genome of approximately 9000 nucleotides (Fig. 12.1). There are preliminary reports of viral particles which have been visualized by electron microscopy. The genomic organization suggests some homology with Flavi- or Pestiviruses, but HCV may be sufficiently individualized to be placed in its own genus.[7] Genomic sequences have been published for the prototype strain isolated in the US (HCV 1), and two strains isolated in Japan (HCV-J and HCV-JH). Partial sequences of other isolates are being reported from other geographical regions.[8]

The viral genomic RNA is a single-stranded plus sense RNA, with a single long open reading frame. The gene product is a viral polyprotein precursor of 3011 amino acids, which undergoes proteolytic posttranslational cleavage to yield structural (core, and envelope) and non-structural (proteases, helicases, RNA-dependent RNA polymerase) proteins. To some extent, knowledge of the nature of HCV proteins is based on predictions made from nucleotide sequences, but an increasing number of proteins are being recombinantly expressed.

The structural proteins are derived from the 5′ third of the genome,[9] and the non-structural proteins from the 3′ (NS1 to NS5) regions. The 5′ end begins with a non-coding region of at least 341 bases. This sequence of HCV appears to be highly conserved, with a high degree of sequence homology among most isolates so far sequenced.[10, 11] Two glycosylated proteins, gp35 and gp70, may be coded by the E1 and E2 regions of the genome, analogous to the NS1 region of flaviviruses, and could be envelope proteins of the hepatitis C virus.[12] Variable and hypervariable regions within the putative envelope glycoproteins have been described.[13, 14] These regions may code for important antigenic sites, and are probably involved in escape from host immunity, perhaps accounting for the fact that HCV infections are frequently persistent. This genomic diversity has important implications in vaccine development and immunodiagnostic testing. The first commercially available diagnostic tests were based on antibodies to an expressed protein (c100-3) derived from the NS3/NS4 region.

DIAGNOSIS OF HCV

HCV antibodies

There are no tests for antigens of HCV in serum, as the virus circulates in serum at a concentration below the level of detection of antigen by standard immunoassays. Most of the seroepidemiological and diagnostic studies of hepatitis C were initially based on the prevalence of antibodies to c100-3, an antibody to an antigen which represents only 4% of total viral protein. More recently, other antigens have been expressed, including a 22-kDa structural protein of HCV, whose coding region has been mapped to the aminoterminal region of the HCV polyprotein, and which is ostensibly a nucleocapsid (core) antigen of HCV.[15] A second series of non-structural antigens, including c33, and c200, have been derived from the NS3 and NS4 regions and expressed in yeast or *E. coli*. Together these antigens are the basis for solid phase enzyme linked immunoassays (Ortho Laboratories, New Jersey, and Abbott Laboratories, Chicago) for antibodies to HCV, which considerably improve the sensitivity of diagnosis.

An immunodominant epitope within the capsid antigen has been identified,[16] and antibodies to the core antigen, anti-c22, usually appear earlier than those to c100-3. Anti-c22 has been identified in blood donors who were previously involved in transmitting hepatitis C, but in whose serum anti-c100-3 was not detectable;[17] antibodies to core epitopes have also been detected in patients with chronic NANB hepatitis who were previously negative for anti-c100-3. The antibodies detected are probably not neutralizing as they are found in chronic carriers. In contrast, it is suspected, but unproven, that antibodies to the E (envelope) glycoproteins are neutralizing. Assays based on antibodies to synthetic peptides derived from immunodominant regions of both core and non-structural antigens are being developed.[18] IgM antibody tests have also been developed. The clearance of IgM anti-HCV may distinguish between acute, resolving disease and chronic disease.[19]

Supplemental antibody tests

Initial surveys of antibody to hepatitis C in blood donors indicated a high rate of false positive tests. This has necessitated the development of 'supplemental' assays for confirmation of a positive anti-HCV result. The most widely used supplemental test is the recombinant immunoblot assay (RIBA) in which four HCV antigens are fixed to a nitrocellulose filter, along with control proteins. The four antigens comprise one structural (c22) and three non-structural antigens (c33, c100-3, 5-1-1). The strips are incubated with serum specimens, and antibodies, if present, bind to the antigens. Serum samples are scored as positive if antibodies to two antigens are present.

A close correlation has been found between 4-RIBA positive samples and viraemia, enabling discrimination between infective and non-infective donors.[20] The proportion of RIBA-positive donors varies from region to region. In Western Europe 20–40% of ELISA-reactive donors are RIBA-reactive, and about the same proportion have detectable HCV RNA by polymerase chain reaction (PCR). RIBA tests are a valuable adjunct to donor testing. Unfortunately, the tests are expensive (£15.00 per test), are relatively insensitive, may give indeterminate results, and are not ideally configured for verification of a positive ELISA test. Several other assays for verification of a positive ELISA test are available, including neutralization assays and automated recombinant immunoblot assays ('matrix' assays).

HCV RNA testing

Since the antigens of HCV are present in very low titres, direct tests for viraemia in HCV have relied on the detection of HCV RNA in serum. RNA detection necessitates an amplification of the circulating HCV RNA, and thus sensitive assays for HCV RNA have been developed, based on PCR. In this test, HCV RNA is extracted from virus-infected serum or plasma, reversely transcribed to DNA, and amplified by appropriate primers homologous to HCV RNA by the enzyme TAQ polymerase in a programmable thermal cycler. RNA can then be detected by ethidium bromide staining of a gel, or by autoradiography. RNA is detected in most (60–80%) anti-HCV-positive patients, and is also detectable in some anti-HCV-negative patients with chronic NANB hepatitis.[21]

The plasma concentration of virions has been estimated to range from 10^2 to 5×10^7/ml.[22] The sensitivity of the test is improved by using an internal (nested) set of primers, and by using primers derived from the 5' untranslated region of the genome, which is highly conserved. There is little standardization of the PCR assay at present.[23] None the less, assays for HCV RNA are proving valuable in establishing the presence of HCV RNA in clinical samples, in the diagnosis of HCV in acute and chronic antibody-negative patients, and in monitoring antiviral therapy.[24] Three basic temporal patterns of viraemia have been observed: transient viraemia in acute resolving non-A, non-B hepatitis (NANBH); viraemia lasting for several years in chronic NANBH; and intermittent viraemia in chronic NANBH, with an initial transient phase followed by recurrence after many months.[25]

HCV RNA can also be detected in formalin-fixed, paraffin-embedded liver biopsies by PCR, and has been detected by in-situ hybridization.

Serological diagnosis: acute hepatitis C

Anti-c100-3 appears in the circulation after a mean interval of 15 weeks from the acute illness and first elevations of the aminotransferase (ALT)[26] (Fig. 12.2). Although roughly one-third of seroconversions take place early in the acute phase of the disease, sometimes as early as 2 weeks,[27] sero-conversion can be delayed for a year or longer. Anti-c33 or anti-c22 not infrequently appears a week or two earlier than anti-c100-3. Antibodies to HCV are found in a varying proportion of patients with acute sporadic NANB hepatitis, depending upon the geographical location, mode of acquisition of hepatitis, and severity of the disease. Seroconversion occurs much less frequently, and in lower titre, in acute self-limiting infections as compared with those that progress to become chronic.[28–30] The presence of anti-HCV antibodies therefore seems largely to reflect active replication of HCV. A substantial proportion of patients with sporadically acquired NANBH remain anti-HCV seronegative, however, and it will be important

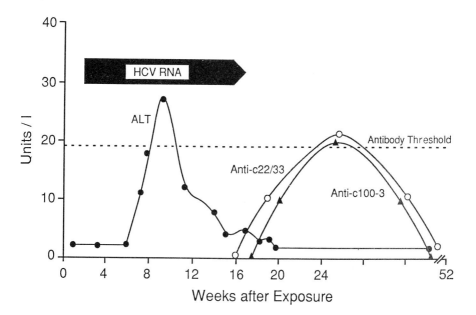

Fig. 12.2   Serological course in acute resolving HCV infection.

to determine whether these patients represent HCV infection with poor serological response, or are due to other unclassified NANB agents.

During the early phase of primary HCV infection, serum HCV RNA is the only diagnostic marker of infection, and RNA testing therefore remains the only means of diagnosis in seronegative patients. Unfortunately, the test is available only in research laboratories. Serum HCV RNA has been detected within 1–3 weeks of transfusion in patients with hepatitis C, and usually lasts less than 4 months in patients with acute self-limited hepatitis C, but it may persist for decades in patients with chronic disease.[24] Patients without a history of transfusion are just as likely to be positive for anti-HCV as patients with transfusion-associated hepatitis.[31]

A suitable immunodiagnostic test for resolved infection and immunity is not available, but antibodies to the envelope region are being sought.

Serological diagnosis: chronic hepatitis C

Anti-HCV antibodies persist in most patients with chronic posttransfusion NANB hepatitis (Fig. 12.3). In studies in chimpanzees, anti-HCV (that is, anti-c100-3) was not neutralizing, because primates with high levels of this antibody were also shown to have high titres of circulating hepatitis C virus.[32] The development and maintenance of current diagnostic antibodies to hepatitis C virus therefore appears to reflect concomitant virus replication, and consequently a high potential for infectivity.

Some patients may improve spontaneously, but the number of patients who do so is unclear. These patients lose the antibody after a follow-up of at

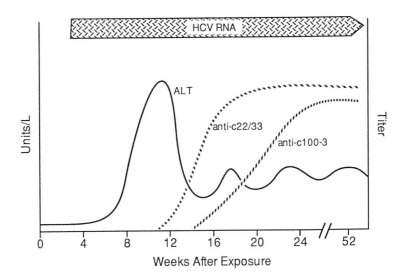

Fig. 12.3   Serological course in chronic hepatitis C infection.

least 5 years, and usually develop normal serum aminotransferases.[33] Other patients may have a decline in anti-HCV titre with time.[28]

HCV RNA usually persists in patients with abnormal serum aminotransferases and anti-HCV. However, HCV RNA, and hence viraemia, can also be found in patients with normal liver function tests. Isolates of HCV in individual patients may show nucleotide substitutions with time, suggesting that the HCV RNA mutates at a rate similar to those of other RNA viruses.[34] Preliminary, but unconfirmed, reports have suggested that the HCV antigens can be detected in liver biopsy preparations in chronic carriers.

EPIDEMIOLOGY AND TRANSMISSION OF HEPATITIS C

Transmission

Hepatitis C is known to be transmitted by parenteral or unapparent parenteral routes. The virus circulates in relatively low titres in blood, but transmission by blood transfusion and blood products, including factor VII, factor IX, fibrinogen, and cryoglobulin, has been well documented. Similarly, transmission among intravenous drug abusers through shared needles accounts for the high prevalence of infection in this group. Transmission after needle-stick injury may also occur.

The precise mechanism of most cases of transmission of community-acquired disease is uncertain, but sexual transmission seems possible, albeit a relatively inefficient and infrequent means. Several studies suggest that sexual transmission may occur: anti-HCV has been found in 11% of sexual partners of anti-HCV-positive intravenous drug abusers, and may correlate with the presence of HIV.[35] The overall HCV infection rate is also higher in sexually promiscuous groups (prostitutes [8.9%], clients of prostitutes [16.3%], and homosexual men [5.4%]) than in voluntary blood donors (0.4%) in Spain.[36] Significantly more homosexual than heterosexual subjects attending a sexually transmitted disease clinic were positive for anti-HCV, and the prevalence of anti-HCV antibody correlates with the lifetime number of sexually transmitted diseases.[37] Other studies, however, have not found a high prevalence of sexual transmission in partners of anti-HCV-positive haemophiliacs.[38]

Transmission by saliva (or saliva-containing blood) and by a human bite has been reported.[39–41] Dentists in New York, particularly those practising oral surgery, have a higher prevalence of anti-HCV antibody as compared to blood donors.

Intrafamilial transmission

The role of intrafamilial transmission requires clarification. Although household transmission appears to be relatively infrequent, the true attack rate may be underestimated, since the prevalence of HCV infection in family members is based on the current diagnostic tests, which usually reflect chronic infection rather than resolved disease. In Japan, up to 8% of family members of an index patient with HCV have been found to be anti-HCV positive, but no specific relative could be linked to HCV positivity, making it difficult to identify the route of infection.[42]

Maternal–infant transmission

Mother-to-infant transmission has been observed, but the importance of this route remains controversial. Wejstal[43] showed that children born to anti-HCV-positive mothers acquired passively transferred antibodies that were present transiently in serum and disappeared within 7 months. Giovannini et al studied 49 children born to HIV-positive mothers and found 25 mother–children pairs anti-HCV positive. Although maternal anti-HCV antibodies fell to undetectable levels in all 25 infants by 2–4 months of age, in 11 infants, active production of antibody was observed between 6–12 months. Six of these had abnormal serum enzymes.[44] A disturbing finding, however, has been the detection of persistent HCV RNA in serum in the absence of anti-HCV in newborn babies delivered by women who were anti-HCV positive, suggesting silent transmission of HCV.[45] Thus, the current evidence seems to suggest that perinatal transmission may occur, particularly in highly viraemic and anti-HIV-positive mothers. It is not clear, however, how important this route is in perpetuating the reservoir of human infection, and the natural history of the carrier state in children is unknown.

Population studies

The prevalence of type C hepatitis in blood donors has now been ascertained in many countries. The positive immunoassay rate ranges from 0.81 to 1.4%: in most Western countries, the prevalence ranges from 0.3 to 0.7%; in Japan and southern Europe, the range is 0.9–1.2%. A higher prevalence has been found in southern Italy and eastern Europe than in northern Europe.[46] The prevalence in commercial (paid) donors is higher (10–15%).[47] There remains considerable controversy regarding the specificity of the screening ELISA assay,[48] as the ELISA tests are poorly specific in low-risk blood donors, and only 20–60% of donors have a positive supplemental test (RIBA II). Supplemental RIBA testing is highly predictive of infectivity, and correlates with the intensity of the ELISA result. A higher prevalence has been found in Africans; for example, in South Africa up to 4.2% of men are anti-HCV positive.[49, 50] False positive results can occur in stored serum from tropical areas. Most anti-HCV-positive donors give no history of blood transfusion, but some admit to previous drug use. Clustering of HCV infections has been reported in Japan.[51]

Posttransfusion hepatitis C

Prior to the introduction of HCV screening, the incidence of post-transfusion hepatitis (PTH) NANB, ranged from 2 to 19%.[52] The incidence of NANB hepatitis has declined since 1985 to 2–4% as a result of the interdiction of high-risk blood donors, and, in some countries, serum aminotransferase and antibody to hepatitis B core antigen screening.

Serological testing now indicates that seroconversion to anti-HCV occurs in 85–100% of patients with chronic post-transfusion NANB hepatitis.[53] Retrospective studies have shown a higher prevalence of anti-HCV at onset in those developing chronic disease (83%) than those who recover from PTH. Anti-HCV persists for years and even decades in chronic hepatitis C but may decline in titre or disappear with resolution.

Anti-HCV testing should effect at least a further 50% reduction in the incidence of posttransfusion hepatitis. In both Spain and Japan, the incidence has already been reduced from 9.6% and 4.6% to 1.6% and 1.9%, respectively.[53, 54] A low incidence of posttransfusion hepatitis C still occurs after transfusion of blood negative for anti-HCV.[55] Although the cost-effectiveness of screening is unknown, screening is demanded by countries willing and able to pay for health care. Blood banks in the US voluntarily began testing donations for anti-HCV in 1990.[56] In the UK, despite the demonstrable imprecision of donor screening, and the relatively low incidence of post transfusion NANB hepatitis, the number of cases per year necessitates screening,[57] and this was initiated in September 1991. Since 2 000 000 donor units are administered yearly in the UK, and approximately 0.1% of these are infectious, 2000 cases of hepatitis C transmission could result annually.

Community-acquired transmission

Surveillance data had suggested that sporadic NANB hepatitis represents between 20 and 42% of all diagnosed cases of hepatitis. The majority of cases of NANB hepatitis cannot be accounted for by past blood transfusion, or, indeed, an identifiable source of parenteral exposure to this virus. In the US, the proportion of patients with type C hepatitis with a history of blood transfusion has declined in the past 7 years, whereas, in contrast, the proportion with a history of parenteral drug use has increased. By 1987, only 5% of cases of NANB in the US were transfusion associated, whereas 42% were related to drug abuse. Approximately 40% were of unknown source.[58, 59] The advent of serological testing has shown that most community-acquired NANB hepatitis is also due to hepatitis C, and anti-HCV is detectable in 28–58% of community-acquired NANB hepatitis. The rate of positivity is higher in patients who progress to chronicity: for example, Bortolotti et al found a prevalence of 71% in patients who progressed to chronicity, as compared with 25% of those who recovered.[60] It would appear that patients with no history of transfusion are just as likely to go on to chronic hepatitis. A substantial proportion of acute community-acquired cases remain unclassified, and studies using PCR to detect HCV RNA remain the only diagnostic test to exclude another virus.

Fulminant hepatitis is more common in sporadic NANB hepatitis. Although most cases of NANB fulminant hepatitis in Japan are due to hepatitis C, this may not be true in the West.

Hepatitis C in high-risk populations

A high prevalence of anti-HCV is found in many risk groups exposed to blood or blood components. The highest prevalences worldwide are found in haemophiliacs, 50–90% of whom are anti-HCV positive, depending upon age, the duration of infection, factor VIII requirement, and the source of factor VIII. The high prevalence in haemophiliacs reflects the contamination by HCV of factor VIII, which is derived from thousands of donors. In the US, source plasma for these pools is still derived from paid donors. Haemophiliacs may also be HCV RNA positive without detectable anti-HCV, particularly if also infected with HIV.[61] Solvent detergent inactivation and pasteurization have been shown to reduce the risk of transmitting HCV infection.

The prevalence of anti-HCV is high in multiply transfused patients with thalassaemia major, but varies geographically according to the source of the blood administered to patients.[62] The prevalence in intravenous drug users is extremely high (70–92%), because of repeated exposure to carriers of HCV through shared, contaminated needles.

Several other groups have been shown to be at risk. These include haemodialysed patients, particularly in areas such as the Middle East. Anti-HCV is apparently also common in transplant patients requiring frequent blood transfusions, including renal, liver, and bone-marrow transplant recipients.[63–65] Liver transplantation is a relatively common therapeutic necessity for patients with cirrhosis which is due to hepatitis C, and recurrent hepatitis C disease is apparently common in these patients posttransplant. In all these groups, previously positive patients may lose the antibody after the procedure because of immunosuppression.[66] The role of immunosuppression in the expression of liver disease caused by HCV remains to be determined.[67] Hepatitis C has also been transmitted by organ transplantation, and may cause severe post-organ-transplantation liver disease.[68]

Nosocomial and occupational exposure is being evaluated. Health care workers appear to be at comparably low risk.[69, 70] However, there are well-documented instances of needlestick transmission of HCV, and of NANB hepatitis after surgery without transfusion. Human immunoglobulin is generally regarded as a safe product, but there are occasional reports of transmission by inadequately prepared intravenous immunoglobulin batches.[71]

Prevalence of anti-HCV in chronic liver disease

Serological testing has shown a high prevalence of anti-HCV in patients with chronic active hepatitis and/or cirrhosis considered to be due to NANB hepatitis.[28] The disease in these persons may or may not be associated with a history of blood transfusion. The prevalence varies according to the background endemicity of hepatitis C in the population.[72] Tests for anti-HCV are now important in establishing a diagnosis of what was formerly considered cryptogenic cirrhosis.

Autoimmune hepatitis

There are conflicting reports regarding the occurrence of hepatitis C antibodies in patients with autoimmune liver disease. Clearly, the ELISA assay for anti-HCV is prone to false positive results in patients with high concentrations of immunoglobulins in serum.[73] These false reactive anti-HCV antibodies in patients with anti-smooth-muscle antibody may actually disappear with immunosuppressive treatment.[74] However, Italian patients with autoimmune chronic active hepatitis (CAH) appear to have a high frequency of genuine exposure to HCV, whereas seropositivity in UK patients usually represents a false positive result. It is therefore not certain whether anti-HCV in patients with chronic active hepatitis represents persistent anti-HCV from earlier disease, whether the autoimmune disease is induced by HCV,[75] or whether autoantibodies in autoimmune hepatitis patients cross-react with HCV-related antigens.[76] In Japan, 80% of patients with chronic NANB hepatitis have circulating antibodies to a pentadecapeptide (GOR), an epitope of normal hepatocytes; this phenomenon may represent an autoimmune response peculiar to type C hepatitis.[77]

Up to 50% of patients with type II autoimmune hepatitis (anti-liver kidney microsomal [LKM], antibody positive) are anti-HCV positive, and anti-HCV and anti-LKM in association may also represent another example of molecular mimicry. Anti-HCV-positive patients with anti-LKM autoimmune CAH are usually older males, and have lower titres of anti-LKM than patients without anti-HCV. The target antigen of antibodies to LKM is a portion of the cytochrome P450 II D6 molecule; anti-LKM not directed to a c100-3 epitope, but some sequence homology between HCV and cytochrome P450 may exist.[78] This association has some therapeutic implications, as the autoimmune disease is responsive to corticosteroids, and may be aggravated by alpha interferon.

Hepatitis B and HIV

HCV may cause disease concurrently with hepatitis B, particularly in risk groups such as haemophiliacs and drug abusers, or where these diseases are endemic in the same environment: the combination may cause aggravated disease;[79, 80] likewise, in drug abusers and haemophiliacs, HIV and HCV may coexist and cause severe, accelerated liver disease.

Alcoholic liver disease

In several countries, a higher prevalence of anti-HCV has been found in patients with alcoholic liver disease. The prevalence of hepatitis C antibodies correlates with the severity of liver injury, and is higher in patients with cirrhosis than in those with only fatty change.[81] The relationship is a complex one,[82] apparently reflecting in part, the higher rate of transfusions in alcoholics with decompensated liver disease and a common environmental risk.

Hepatocellular carcinoma

Serological analysis of patients with hepatocellular carcinoma (HCC) has shown a high prevalence of anti-HCV in them; several case-control studies in Europe have suggested that up to 70% of male patients with HCC are anti-HCV positive.[83, 84] The highest prevalence of HCV in HCC is found in Italian, Japanese, and Spanish patients; the prevalence is lower in Chinese and African patients, in whom the disease is more commonly associated with chronic hepatitis B. Since HCV is an RNA virus, it is believed that chronic HCV infection induces necroinflammatory change which progresses to cirrhosis and eventual malignant transformation.[85] In Japan, at least, a history of transfusion has been documented in 42% of anti-HCV-positive patients with HCC. The mean interval between the date of transfusion and the diagnosis of cirrhosis and HCC is usually long: 21 and 29 years, respectively.[86]

Other diseases

Although NANB hepatitis has been thought to be associated with aplastic anaemia, to date there is no conclusive evidence to link HCV infection with aplastic anaemia.[87]

Cryoglobulinaemia has been associated with hepatitis C, and up to 54% of patients with mixed cryoglobulinaemia are anti-HCV positive (verified by RIBA). The surprising role of HCV in the pathogenesis of this disease is unknown.[88, 89]

CLINICAL FEATURES

Acute hepatitis C

The mean incubation period of hepatitis C is 6–12 weeks. However, with a large inoculum, as in cases following administration of factor VIII, the incubation period is reduced to 4 weeks or less.[27,90] The acute course of HCV infection is clinically mild, and the peak serum-ALT elevations are less than those encountered in acute hepatitis A or B. Only 25% of cases are icteric. Subclinical disease is common; such patients may first present decades later with sequelae such as cirrhosis or HCC. During the early clinical phase the serum-ALT levels may fluctuate, and may become normal or near normal, making the determination of true convalescence difficult. Severe or fulminant hepatitis C may occur but is rare. The diagnosis of such cases requires confirmation by HCV RNA testing. Arthritis, rashes, glomerulonephritis, vasculitis, neurological syndromes, and aplastic anaemia have been reported. The histological features of acute hepatitis C are similar to those of hepatitis A or B, except that sinusoidal cell activation is marked. The distinction from evolving chronic hepatitis C can be difficult.

Chronic hepatitis C

The clinical and epidemiological features of transfusion-associated and sporadic NANB hepatitis have been well documented, although the disease previously required identification by prospective biochemical monitoring. The disease has a disturbing propensity to progress to chronic hepatitis (Fig. 12.4). From 50 to 75% of patients with type C posttransfusion hepatitis continue to have abnormal serum aminotransferase levels after 12

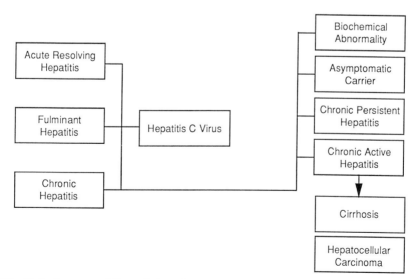

Fig. 12.4   Spectrum of disease in hepatitis C infection.

months, and chronic hepatitis histologically.[26] The risk of chronic infection after sporadic hepatitis C is probably similar.

Most patients with chronic hepatitis C are asymptomatic, or only mildly symptomatic. In symptomatic patients, fatigue is the most common complaint, and is variously described as lack of energy, increased need for sleep, or fatiguability. Many patients do not give a history of acute hepatitis or jaundice. Physical findings are generally mild and variable, and there may be no abnormalities. With more severe disease, spider angiomata and hepatosplenomegaly may be found. Serum aminotransferases decline from the peak values encountered in the acute phase of the disease, but remain 2–8-fold abnormal. The serum-ALT concentrations may fluctuate over time, and may even, intermittently, be normal. Many patients have a sustained elevation of the serum aminotransferases. The relationship between HCV RNA in serum and serum aminotransferases is complex, and although most patients with raised serum ALT are HCV RNA positive, the converse is not always true.

The spectrum of chronic disease varies. Most patients appear to have an indolent, only slowly progressive course with little increase in mortality after 20 years. However, cirrhosis develops in 20% of patients with chronic disease within 10 years, although the cirrhosis remains indolent and only slowly progressive for a prolonged period.[91] The disease is not necessarily benign, however, and rapidly progressive cirrhosis can occur. Older age of infection, concomitant alcohol abuse, and concurrent HBV or HIV infection may be important aggravating cofactors. With the development of cirrhosis, weakness, wasting, oedema, and ascites become progressive problems. Older patients may present with complications of cirrhosis, or even HCC. With progressive disease, the laboratory values become progressively more abnormal. The finding of aspartate aminotransferase (AST) greater than ALT, low albumin, and prolonged prothrombin time suggest cirrhosis. Low levels of autoantibodies may also become detectable.

Two main pathological forms of chronic hepatitis, chronic active hepatitis (CAH) and chronic persistent hepatitis (CPH), occur in hepatitis C; these terms require reassessment in the light of new information of the evolution of the hepatitis.[92] A characteristic histological pattern of mild chronic hepatitis with portal lymphoid follicles and varying degrees of lobular activity is found in many patients.[93]

Interestingly, routine screening of blood donors for anti-HCV indicates that a significant proportion of asymptomatic anti-HCV-positive blood donors do indeed have progressive liver disease: several histological studies in asymptomatic anti-HCV-positive donors have shown that 45–62% had chronic active hepatitis, and 7–15% had active cirrhosis.[94] Progression to HCC is also well documented, and despite the indolent and slowly progressive nature of the disease in many, it is apparent from serological testing for anti-HCV that HCV is a leading cause of morbidity from liver disease in the West.

MANAGEMENT

Acute hepatitis C

The management of acute sporadic or transfusion-related hepatitis C is along conventional lines, and is largely non-specific and supportive. The diagnosis remains one of exclusion in most, although if the patient is seen early enough, HCV RNA in serum may be detectable at the time that the serum aminotransferases are elevated. Anti-HCV may be detectable, particularly in severe, icteric cases, and in most of those patients destined to go on to chronic disease. Many patients will not be jaundiced. The serum aminotransferases should be measured at weekly intervals; during the recovery phase, these levels should be measured periodically (1–3-month intervals), as the determination of true convalescence in this illness can be difficult.

Approximately 50% of patients will still have elevated serum aminotransferases 6 months after diagnosis. Patients should be encouraged to rest during the acute, severe phase of the illness. Most patients can be effectively cared for at home. A gradual return to normal activity is encouraged. The diet should be as palatable as possible. Potentially hepatotoxic medications may aggravate the hepatic injury. Oral contraceptives can probably be continued. Exhausting exercise should be discouraged until the serum aminotransferases are normal. Hospitalization is indicated for patients with more severe symptoms, a serum bilirubin level greater than 200 mmol/L, or a prothrombin time that is prolonged for more than 3 s, neuropsychiatric symptoms, spontaneous bleeding, or persistent vomiting.

Therapeutic trials of alpha interferon have been undertaken. Most have not reduced the rate of chronic disease, but might indicate an amelioration of the severity of the chronic hepatitis lesion. A trial of beta interferon in Japan, given intravenously for 1–3 months, did significantly reduce the risk of chronic hepatitis.[95] Until these findings can be reproduced, however, the routine administration of interferon for acute hepatitis C cannot be advised. Liver transplantation is necessary for the treatment of fulminant hepatitis C where indices indicate a high probability of a fatal outcome.

Chronic hepatitis C

Asymptomatic patients detected through blood screening require a supplemental test to verify their HCV status, as the rate of false positive anti-HCV tests in low-risk donors is high. Ideally, HCV RNA should be measured in all patients to confirm viraemia, but the test is not generally available for routine diagnosis. If the test is reproducibly positive, serum aminotransferases, bilirubin, alkaline phosphatase, and prothrombin time should be measured. In patients whose lifestyle or geographical origin suggests that they are at risk of other forms of viral hepatitis, HBsAg and HIV infection need also be considered. In equivocal cases, the diagnosis of chronic hepatitis C may still require confirmation, and careful exclusion of all other forms of chronic hepatitis, including alcoholism, inborn errors of metabolism, hepatoxicity, and disease of the biliary tract. Because auto-immune hepatitis is treated differently, it is particularly advisable to exclude this diagnosis by measuring the titres of anti-smooth-muscle and anti-LKM antibodies even in those with a positive anti-HCV test, and to measure HCV RNA in anti-HCV-positive patients for whom interferon is contemplated.

In patients with more than 2-fold elevations in serum aminotransferases, a liver biopsy to ascertain the degree of inflammatory activity and fibrosis in the liver should be considered. The patient should be monitored for 1–3 months to assess the trend in serum aminotransferases.

Relapses and remissions can occur. Prospective studies have suggested that 10–20% of patients with chronic NANB hepatitis develop cirrhosis within a 10-year period. However, in many patients the disease is silently and insidiously progressive, even after cirrhosis is present. None the less, morbidity from cirrhosis and HCC is well established; patients with chronic hepatitis C, with elevated ALT and chronic hepatitis histologically, should be considered for antiviral therapy.

Major restrictions need not be placed on the lifestyle of the patient with compensated hepatitis C. The drinking of excess spirits is discouraged, as there is evidence that the combination of type C hepatitis and alcohol abuse may be detrimental. Small quantities of beer and wine are permissible. The patient should be counselled and advised not to donate blood. It is not yet clear how efficiently hepatitis C may be transmitted by sexual contact. This can apparently occur, however, in highly viraemic individuals after pro-longed contact. It is prudent therefore to test regular sexual partners for anti-HCV.

Alpha interferon

Preliminary therapeutic trials of alpha interferon indicated that a pro-portion of patients may respond to treatment with this agent. Larger, placebo-controlled studies have indicated that approximately 50% of patients have normal serum aminotransferases after treatment courses of alpha interferon of approximately 3 million units three times a week for 6 months (Fig. 12.5).[96, 97]

Both anti-c100-3-positive and -negative patients respond, presumably reflecting the insensitivity of the anti-c100-3 test.[98, 99] Serum HCV RNA may become undetectable in patients after 4–8 weeks of alpha interferon treatment in patients who respond, but an undetectable HCV RNA at the end of treatment does not preclude relapse in patients.

However, after stopping treatment for 6 months, one-half of the respon-sive patients promptly relapse. Serum aminotransferases usually increase in patients who are HCV RNA positive at the end of therapy.[100] Our studies at

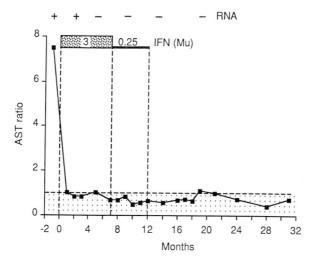

Fig. 12.5 Clinical course in a patient responding to 3 MU three times weekly alpha interferon for 6 months, followed by 0.25 Mu three times weekly for 6 months, showing normalization of aminotransferases and disappearance of HCV RNA.

the Royal Free Hospital, London, indicate that 20% of patients have a prolonged response to therapy and do not develop elevated serum amino-transferases. These patients also become negative for HCV RNA. Other regimens are being evaluated.[101] Initiating therapy with a dose of 15–20 million units per week, and prolonging therapy for a year may result in lower relapse rates. However, relapses still occur after higher doses, and patients have more side-effects at higher doses.

The cost of 6 months of treatment is at least £1500. Treatment should not be continued beyond 3 months in patients who do not have reduced levels of serum ALT. Responsive patients usually exhibit histological improvement, and may have a decrease in collagen III propeptide concentrations.[102]

Unfortunately, responsiveness to alpha interferon remains somewhat unpredictable; patients with cirrhosis respond less well, however. Most patients tolerate the treatment quite well; however, many develop flu-like symptoms, some develop severe psychological side-effects, and patients with cirrhosis may develop significant thrombocytopaenia, leucopaenia, and therefore infections.[103] Thyroid abnormalities occur in approximately 3% of treated patients.

Some patients may actually worsen on treatment with interferon, and develop increased serum aminotransferases. A positive anti-HCV antibody in patients with autoimmune disease remains a pitfall in diagnosis which has implications for treatment.[104] Such patients require confirmation by immunoblot assay or HCV RNA, as they may optimally require corticosteroid therapy rather than alpha interferon.[105]

It is possible that such patients have an underlying autoimmune status associated with hepatitis C and exacerbated by interferon treatment. For such patients, and for patients who do not respond to treatment, ribavirin may be an alternative.[106] This nucleoside analogue has been shown to suppress HCV, but it is weakly efficacious, and doses above 1.2 g per d are associated with mild haemolytic anaemia. A multicentre trial of ribavirin for hepatitis C is now in progress.

SUMMARY

In 1989, taking advantage of new recombinant DNA technology, the major agent of NANB hepatitis was isolated, and serological tests developed. Preliminary epidemiological assessment indicates that hepatitis C is an important cause of chronic liver disease, cirrhosis, and HCC worldwide. The molecular virology of HCV has identified differences between the prototype strain and other isolates. Serological assays have been developed which enable the diagnosis of chronic hepatitis C. Assays for HCV RNA are being used to study viraemia. The availability of markers of hepatitis C has facilitated the study of the epidemiology and natural history of the disease, and has improved its treatment.

REFERENCES

1 Feinstone SM, Kapikian AZ, Purcell RH, Alter HJ, Holland PV. Transfusion associated hepatitis not due to viral hepatitis type A or B. N Engl J Med 1975; 292: 767–770
2 Dienstag JL. Non-A, Non-B hepatitis. II. Experimental transmission, putative virus agents and markers, and prevention. Gastroenterology 1983; 85: 743–768
3 Kuo G, Choo QL, Alter HJ et al. An assay for circulating antibodies to a major etiologic virus of human non-A, non-B hepatitis. Science 1989; 244: 362–364
4 Choo QL, Kuo G, Weiner AJ, Overby LR, Bradley DW, Houghton M. Isolation of a cDNA clone derived from a blood-borne non-A, non-B viral hepatitis genome. Science 1989; 244: 359–362
5 Choo QL, Weiner AJ, Overby LR, Kuo G, Houghton M, Bradley DW. Hepatitis C virus: the major causative agent of viral non-A, non-B hepatitis. Br Med Bull 1990; 46: 423–441
6 Reyes GR, Purdy MA, Kim JP et al. Isolation of a cDNA from the virus responsible for enterically transmitted non-A, non-B hepatitis. Science 1990; 247: 1335–1339
7 Takamizawa A, Mori C, Fuke I et al. Structure and organization of the hepatitis C virus genome isolated from human carriers. J Virol 1991; 65: 1105–1113
8 Chen P-J, Lin M-H, Tu S-J, Chen D-S. Isolation of a complementary DNA fragment of hepatitis C virus in Taiwan revealed significant sequence variations compared with other isolates. Hepatology 1991; 14: 73–78
9 Okamoto H, Okada S, Sugiyama Y et al. The 5'-terminal sequence of the hepatitis C virus genome. Jpn J Exp Med 1990; 60: 167–177
10 Han JH, Shyamala V, Richman KH et al. Characterization of the terminal regions of hepatitis C viral RNA: identification of conserved sequences in the 5' untranslated region and poly(A) tails at the 3' end. Proc Natl Acad Sci USA 1991; 88: 1711–1715
11 Choo QL, Richman KH, Han JH et al. Genetic organization and diversity of the hepatitis C virus. Proc Natl Acad Sci USA 1991; 88: 2451–2455
12 Hijikata M, Kato N, Ootsuyama Y, Nakagawa M, Shimotohno K. Gene mapping of the putative structural region of the hepatitis C virus genome by in vitro processing analysis. Proc Natl Acad Sci USA 1991; 88: 5547–5551

13 Hijikata M, Kato N, Ootsuyama Y, Nakagawa M, Ohkoshi S, Shimotohno K. Hypervariable regions in the putative glycoprotein of hepatitis C virus. Biochem Biophys Res Commun 1991; 175: 220–228

14 Weiner AJ, Brauer MJ, Rosenblatt J et al. Variable and hypervariable domains are found in the regions of HCV corresponding to the flavivirus envelope and NS1 proteins and the pestivirus envelope of glycoproteins. Virology 1991; 180: 842–848

15 Harada S, Watanabe Y, Takeuchi K et al. Expression of processed core protein of hepatitis C virus in mammalian cells. J Virol 1991; 65: 3015–3021

16 Nasoff MS, Zebedee SL, Inchauspé G, Prince AM. Identification of an immunodominant epitope within the capsid protein of hepatitis C virus. Proc Natl Acad Sci USA 1991; 88: 5462–5466

17 Chiba J, Ohba H, Matsuura Y et al. Serodiagnosis of hepatitis C virus (HCV) infection with an HCV core protein molecularly expressed by a recombinant baculovirus. Proc Natl Acad Sci USA 1991; 88: 4641–4645

18 Hosein B, Fang CT, Popovsky MA, Ye J, Zhang M, Wang CY. Improved serodiagnosis of hepatitis C virus infection with synthetic peptide antigen from capsid protein. Proc Natl Acad Sci USA 1991; 88: 3647–3651

19 Quiroga JA, Campillo ML, Catillo I, Bartolomé J, Porres JC, Carreño V. IgM antibody to hepatitis C virus in acute and chronic hepatitis C. Hepatology 1991; 14: 38–43

20 Van der Poel CL, Cuypers HTM. Reesink HW et al. Confirmation of hepatitis C virus infection by new four-antigen recombinant immunoblot assay. Lancet 1991; 337: 317–319

21 Kato N, Yokosuka O, Omata M, Hosoda K, Ohto M. Detection of hepatitis C virus ribonucleic acid in the serum by amplification with polymerase chain reaction. J Clin Invest 1990; 86: 1764–1767

22 Ulrich PP, Romeo JM, Lane PK, Kelly I, Daniel LJ, Vyas GN. Detection, semiquantitation, and genetic variation in hepatitis C virus sequences amplified from the plasma of blood donors with elevated alanine aminotransferase. J Clin Invest 1990; 86: 1609–1614

23 Cristiano K, Di Bisceglie AM, Hoofnagle JH, Feinstone SM. Hepatitis C viral RNA in serum of patients with chronic non-A, non-B hepatitis: detection by the polymerase chain reaction using multiple primer sets. Hepatology 1991; 14: 51–55

24 Farci P, Alter HJ, Wong D et al. A long-term study of hepatitis C virus replication in non-A, non-B hepatitis. N Engl J Med 1991; 325: 98–104

25 Garson JA, Ring C, Tuke P, Tedder RS. Enhanced detection by PCR of hepatitis C virus RNA. Lancet 1990; 336: 878–879

26 Lee S-D, Hwang S-J, Lu R-H, Lai K-H, Tsai Y-T, Lo K-J. Antibodies to hepatitis C virus in prospectively followed patients with posttransfusion hepatitis. J Infect Dis 1991; 163: 1354–1357

27 Lim SG, Lee CA, Charman H, Tilsed G, Griffiths PD, Kernoff PBA. Hepatitis C antibody assay in a longitudinal study of haemophiliacs. Br J Haematol 1991; 78: 398–402

28 Alter HJ, Purcell RH, Shih JW et al. Detection of antibody to hepatitis C virus in prospectively followed transfusion recipients with acute and chronic non-A, non-B hepatitis. N Engl J Med 1989; 321: 1494–1500

29 Alter MJ, Sampliner RE. Editorial. Hepatitis C: and miles to go before we sleep. N Engl J Med 1989; 321: 1538–1540

30 Nishioka K, Watanabe J, Furuta S et al. Antibody to the hepatitis C virus in acute hepatitis and chronic liver diseases in Japan. Liver 1991; 11: 65–70

31 Alter MJ, Hadler SC, Judson FN et al. Risk factors for acute non-A, non-B hepatitis in the United States and association with hepatitis C virus infection. JAMA 1990; 264: 2231–2235

32 Bradley DW, Krawczynski E, Ebert JW et al. Parenterally transmitted non-A, non-B hepatitis: virus-specific antibody response patterns in hepatitis C virus-infected chimpanzees. Gastroenterology 1990; 99: 1054–1060

33 Tanaka E, Kiyosawa K, Sodeyama T et al. Significance of antibody to hepatitis C virus in Japanese patients with viral hepatitis: relationship between anti-HCV antibody and the prognosis of non-A, non-B post-transfusion hepatitis. J Med Virol 1991; 33: 117–122

34 Ogata N, Alter HJ, Miller RH, Purcell RH. Nucleotide sequence and mutation rate of the H strain of hepatitis C virus. Proc Natl Acad Sci USA 1991; 88: 3392–3396

35 Tor J, Llibre JM, Carbonell M et al. Sexual transmission of hepatitis C virus and its relation with hepatitis B virus and HIV. BMJ 1990; 301: 1130–1133
36 Sanchez-Quijano A, Rey C, Aguado I et al. Hepatitis C virus infection in sexually promiscuous groups. Eur J Clin Microbiol Infect Dis 1990; 9: 610–612
37 Tedder RS, Gilson RJ, Briggs M et al. Hepatitis C virus: evidence for sexual transmission. BMJ 1991; 302: 1299–1302
38 Schulman S, Grillner L. Antibodies against hepatitis C in a population of Swedish haemophiliacs and heterosexual partners. Scand J Infect Dis 1990; 22: 393–397
39 Abe K, Inchauspé G. Transmission of hepatitis C by saliva. Lancet 1991; 337: 248
40 Wang J-T, Wang T-H, Lin J-T, Sheu J-C, Lin S-M, Chen D-S. Hepatitis C virus RNA in saliva of patients with post-transfusion hepatitis C infection. Lancet 1991; 337: 48
41 Dusheiko GM, Smith M, Scheuer PJ. Hepatitis C transmitted by a human bite. Lancet 1990; 336: 503–504
42 Kiyosawa K, Sodeyama T, Tanaka E et al. Intrafamilial transmission of hepatitis C virus in Japan. J Med Virol 1991; 33: 114–116
43 Wejstal R, Hermodsson S, Iwarson S, Norkrans G. Mother to infant transmission of hepatitis C virus infection. J Med Virol 1990; 30: 178–180
44 Giovannini M, Tagger A, Ribero ML et al. Letter. Maternal-infant transmission of hepatitis C virus and HIV infections: a possible interaction. Lancet 1990; 335: 1166
45 Thaler MM, Park C-K, Landers DV et al. Vertical transmission of hepatitis C virus. Lancet 1991; 338: 17–18
46 Rassam SW, Dusheiko GM. Epidemiology and transmission of hepatitis C infection. Eur J Gastroenterol 1991; 3: 585–591
47 Dawson GJ, Lesniewski RR, Stewart JL et al. Detection of antibodies to hepatitis C virus in US blood donors. J Clin Microbiol 1991; 29: 551–556
48 Barbara JA, Contreras M. Non-A, non-B hepatitis and the anti-HCV assay. Vox Sang 1991; 60: 1–7
49 Coursaget P, Bourdil C, Kastally R et al. Prevalence of hepatitis C virus infection in Africa: anti-HCV antibodies in the general population and in patients suffering from cirrhosis or primary liver cancer. Res Virol 1990; 141: 449–454
50 Ellis LA, Brown D, Conradie JD et al. Prevalence of hepatitis C in South Africa: detection of anti-HCV in recent and stored serum. J Med Virol 1990; 32: 249–251
51 Ito S, Ito M, Cho MJ, Shimotohno K, Tajima K. Massive sero-epidemiological survey of hepatitis C virus: clustering of carriers on the southwest coast of Tsushima, Japan. Jpn J Cancer Res 1991; 82: 1–3
52 Dienstag JL. Non-A, non-B hepatitis. I. Recognition, epidemiology, and clinical features. Gastroenterology 1983; 85: 439–462
53 Esteban JI, Gonzalez A, Hernandez JM et al. Evaluation of antibodies to hepatitis C virus in a study of transfusion-associated hepatitis. N Engl J Med 1990; 323: 1107–1112
54 Japanese Red Cross Non-A Non-B Hepatitis Research Group. Effect of screening for hepatitis C virus antibody and hepatitis B virus core antibody on incidence of post-transfusion hepatitis. Lancet 1991; 338: 1040–1041
55 Widell A, Sundstrom G, Hansson BG, Moestrup T, Nordenfelt E. Antibody to hepatitis-C-virus-related proteins in sera from alanine-aminotransferase-screened blood donors and prospectively studied recipients. Vox Sang 1991; 60: 28–33
56 Public Health Service. Inter-agency guidelines for screening donors of blood, plasma, organs, tissues and semen for evidence of hepatitis B and hepatitis C. MMWR 1991; 40: 1–17
57 Contreras M, Barbara JA, Anderson CC et al. Low incidence of non-A, non-B post-transfusion hepatitis in London confirmed by hepatitis C virus serology. Lancet 1991; 337: 753–757
58 Alter MJ. Inapparent transmission of hepatitis C: footprints in the sand. Hepatology 1991; 14: 389–391
59 Alter MJ. Hepatitis C: a sleeping giant. Am J Med 1991; 91 (suppl 3B): 112S–115S
60 Bortolotti F, Tagger A, Cadrobbi P et al. Antibodies to hepatitis C virus in community-acquired acute non-A, non-B hepatitis. J Hepatol 1991; 12: 176–180
61 Simmonds P, Zhang LQ, Watson HG et al. Hepatitis C quantification and sequencing in blood products, haemophiliacs, and drug users. Lancet 1990; 336: 1469–1472

62 Wonke B, Hoffbrand AV, Brown D, Dusheiko G. Antibody to hepatitis C virus in multiply transfused patients with thalassaemia major. J Clin Pathol 1990; 43: 638–640

63 Baur P, Daniel V, Pomer S, Scheurlen H, Opelz G, Roelcke D. Hepatitis C-virus (HCV) antibodies in patients after kidney transplantation. Ann Hematol 1991; 62: 68–73

64 Poterucha JJ, Rakela J, Ludwig J, Taswell HF, Wiesner RH. Hepatitis C antibodies in patients with chronic hepatitis of unknown etiology after orthotopic liver transplantation. Transplant Proc 1991; 23: 1495–1497

65 Ponz E, Campistol JM, Barrera JM et al. Hepatitis C virus antibodies in patients on hemodialysis and after kidney transplantation. Transplant Proc 1991; 23: 1371–1372

66 Read AE, Donegan E, Lake J et al. Hepatitis C in patients undergoing liver transplantation. Ann Intern Med 1991; 114: 282–284

67 Read AE, Donegan E, Lake J et al. Hepatitis C in liver transplant recipients. Transplant Proc 1991; 23: 1504–1505

68 Pereira BJG, Milford EL, Kirkman RL, Levey AS. Transmission of hepatitis C virus by organ transplantation. N Engl J Med 1991; 325: 454–460

69 Polywka S, Laufs R. Hepatitis C virus antibodies among different groups at risk and patients with suspected non-A, non-B hepatitis. Infection 1991; 19: 81–84

70 Hofmann H, Kunz C. Low risk of health care workers for infection with hepatitis C virus. Infection 1990; 18: 286–288

71 Lever AML, Webster ADB, Brown D, Thomas HC. Non-A, non-B hepatitis occurring in agammaglobulinaemic patients after intravenous immunoglobulin. Lancet 1984; 2: 1062–1064

72 Pohjanpelto P, Tallgren M, Farkkila M et al. Low prevalence of hepatitis C antibodies in chronic liver disease in Finland. Scand J Infect Dis 1991; 23: 139–142

73 McFarlane IG, Smith HM, Johnson PJ, Bray GP, Vergani D, Williams R. Hepatitis C virus antibodies in chronic active hepatitis: pathogenetic factor or false-positive result? Lancet 1990; 335: 754–757

74 Schvarcz R, von-Sydow M, Weiland O. Autoimmune chronic active hepatitis: changing reactivity for antibodies to hepatitis C virus after immunosuppressive treatment. Scand J Gastroenterol 1990; 25: 1175–1180

75 Lenzi M, Johnson PJ, McFarlane IG et al. Antibodies to hepatitis C virus in autoimmune liver disease: evidence for geographical heterogeneity. Lancet 1991; 338: 277–280

76 Onji M, Kikuchi T, Michitaka K, Saito I, Miyamura T, Ohta Y. Detection of hepatitis C virus antibody in patients with autoimmune hepatitis and other chronic liver diseases. Gastroenterol Jpn 1991; 26: 182–186

77 Mishiro S, Hoshi Y, Takeda K et al. Non-A, non-B hepatitis specific antibodies directed at host-derived epitope: implication for an autoimmune process. Lancet 1990; 336: 1400–1403

78 Manns MP, Griffin KJ, Sullivan KF, Johnson EF. LKM-1 autoantibodies recognize a short linear sequence in P450IID6, a cytochrome P-450 monooxygenase. J Clin Invest 1991; 88: 1370–1378

79 Fong T-L, Di Bisceglie AM, Waggoner JG, Banks SM, Hoofnagle JH. The significance of antibody to hepatitis C virus in patients with chronic hepatitis B. Hepatology 1991; 14: 64–67

80 Fattovich G, Tagger A, Brollo L et al. Hepatitis C virus infection in chronic hepatitis B virus carriers. J Infect Dis 1991; 163: 400–402

81 Pares A, Barrera JM, Caballeria J et al. Hepatitis C virus antibodies in chronic alcoholic patients: association with severity of liver injury. Hepatology 1990; 12: 1295–1299

82 Mendenhall CL, Seeff L, Diehl AM et al. Antibodies to hepatitis B virus and hepatitis C virus in alcoholic hepatitis and cirrhosis: their prevalence and clinical relevance. Hepatology 1991; 14: 581–589

83 Tanaka K, Hirohata T, Koga S et al. Hepatitis C and hepatitis B in the etiology of hepatocellular carcinoma in the Japanese population. Cancer Res 1991; 51: 2842–2847

84 Bruix J, Barrera JM, Calvet X et al. Prevalence of antibodies to hepatitis C virus in Spanish patients with hepatocellular carcinoma and hepatic cirrhosis. Lancet 1989; 2: 1004–1006

85 Levrero M, Tagger A, Balsano C et al. Antibodies to hepatitis C virus in patients with hepatocellular carcinoma. J Hepatol 1991; 12: 60–63

86 Kiyosawa K, Sodeyama T, Tanaka E et al. Interrelationship of blood transfusion, non-A, non-B hepatitis and hepatocellular carcinoma: analysis by detection of antibody to hepatitis C virus. Hepatology 1990; 12: 671–675

87 Pol S, Driss F, Devergie A, Brechot C, Berthelot P, Gluckman E. Is hepatitis C virus involved in hepatitis-associated aplastic anemia? Ann Intern Med 1990; 113: 435–437

88 Ferri C, Greco F, Longombardo G et al. Antibodies to hepatitis C virus in patients with mixed cryoglobulinemia. Arthritis Rheum 1991; 34: 1606–1610

89 Durand JM, Lefevre P, Harle JR, Boucrat J, Vitvitski L, Soubeyrand J. Cutaneous vasculitis and cryoglobulinaemia type II associated with hepatitis C virus infection. Lancet 1991; 337: 499–500

90 Bamber M, Murray A, Arborgh BAM et al. Short incubation non-A, non-B hepatitis transmitted by factor VIII concentrates in patients with congenital coagulation disorders. Gut 1981; 22: 854–859

91 Patel A, Sherlock S, Dusheiko G, Scheuer PJ, Ellis LA, Ashrafzadeh P. Clinical course and histological correlations in post-transfusion hepatitis C: the Royal Free Hospital experience. Eur J Gastroenterol Hepatol 1991; 3: 491–495

92 Scheuer PJ. Classification of chronic viral hepatitis: a need for reassessment. J Hepatol 1991; 13: 372–374

93 Scheuer PJ, Ashrafzadeh P, Sherlock S, Brown D, Dusheiko GM. The pathology of hepatitis C. Hepatology 1992 (in press)

94 Alberti A, Chemello L, Cavalletto D et al. Antibody to hepatitis C virus and liver disease in volunteer blood donors. Ann Intern Med 1991; 114: 1010–1012

95 Omata M, Yokosuka O, Takano S et al. Resolution of acute hepatitis C after therapy with natural beta interferon. Lancet 1991; 338: 914–915

96 Davis GL, Balart LA, Schiff ER et al. Treatment of chronic hepatitis C with recombinant interferon alfa. A multicenter randomized, controlled trial (Hepatitis Interventional Therapy Group). N Engl J Med 1989; 321: 1501–1506

97 Di-Bisceglie AM, Martin P, Kassianides C et al. Recombinant interferon alfa therapy for chronic hepatitis C. A randomized, double-blind, placebo-controlled trial. N Engl J Med 1989; 321: 1506–1510

98 Ohnishi K, Nomura F, Nakano M. Interferon therapy for acute posttransfusion non-A, non-B hepatitis: response with respect to anti-hepatitis C virus antibody status. Am J Gastroenterol 1991; 86: 1041–1049

99 Marcellin P, Giostra E, Boyer N, Loriot MA, Martinot-Peignoux M, Benhamou JP. Is the response to recombinant alpha interferon related to the presence of antibodies to hepatitis C virus in patients with chronic non-A, non-B hepatitis? J Hepatol 1990; 11: 77–79

100 Chayama K, Saitoh S, Arase Y et al. Effect of interferon administration on serum hepatitis C virus RNA in patients with chronic hepatitis C. Hepatology 1991; 13: 1040–1043

101 Kakumu S, Arao M, Yoshioka K et al. Recombinant human alpha-interferon therapy for chronic non-A, non-B hepatitis: second report. Am J Gastroenterol 1990; 85: 655–659

102 Schvarcz R, Glaumann H, Weiland O, Norkrans G, Wejstal R, Fryden A. Histological outcome in interferon alpha-2b treated patients with chronic posttransfusion non-A, non-B hepatitis. Liver 1991; 11: 30–38

103 Renault PF, Hoofnagle JH. Side-effects of alpha interferon. Semin Liver Dis 1989; 9: 273–277

104 Davis GL. Editorial; comment. Hepatitis C virus antibody in patients with chronic autoimmune hepatitis: pitfalls in diagnosis and implications for treatment. Mayo Clin Proc 1991; 66: 647–650

105 Czaja AJ, Taswell HF, Rakela J, Schimek CM. Frequency and significance of antibody to hepatitis C virus in severe corticosteroid-treated autoimmune chronic active hepatitis [see comments]. Mayo Clin Proc 1991; 66: 572–582

106 Reichard O, Andersson J, Schvarcz R, Weiland O. Ribavirin treatment for chronic hepatitis C. Lancet 1991; 337: 1058–1061

13

Variants of hepatitis B virus

W. F. Carman

Hepatitis B virus (HBV), like all viruses to a greater or lesser degree, mutates continuously and randomly during its many replication cycles. Not all such new 'strains' are infectious or able to replicate. For example, mutations that occur in vital regions such as receptor molecules are unlikely to lead to viable virions. Such constraints thus limit the range of mutants that can be selected. It is clear that one of the functions of this process is to generate variants that outmanoeuvre the host immune response: these variants are termed escape mutants.

Most escape mutants are selected by pressure from antibodies, the effector molecules of the humoral immune response. However, there is some evidence from other viral systems that selection of mutated epitopes that no longer act as targets for helper[1] or cytotoxic T cells[2,3] can occur. This mechanism is considered to be one way in which chronic viral infections arise.

In this review, previous work on the subject of variants of HBV will be briefly outlined, and I will attempt to bring the subject up to date. This work attempts to build on other reviews that have appeared recently in gastroenterological[4] and virological[5] journals.

THE IMMUNE RESPONSE AGAINST HBV

Antibodies are produced against all the proteins of HBV (core, HBeAg, polymerase, surface, pre-S1, pre-S2, and HBx). Some of these are protective (for example, anti-pre-S1,[6] -S2,[7] and anti-HBs [and perhaps anti-HBc[8]]), some arise as part of the natural response but seem to play no role in clearance of the virus (for example, anti-HBc and anti-pre-S1/2[9]), and others play an as yet undefined role in clearance of the infection and pathogenesis (for example, anti-HBe). Anti-HBe appears at the same time as clearance of HBeAg, often with a peak of serum transaminases. As the immune response is believed to play a vital role in the pathogenesis of hepatitis caused by HBV, it is no surprise that clearance of an antigen should occur at the same time as an increased intensity of liver damage. This situation is seen most clearly in patients treated with interferon (an immune-enhancing agent), in whom clearance occurs after a rise in trans-

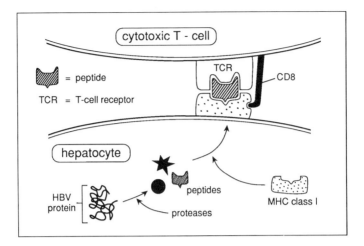

Fig. 13.1   Interaction between the hepatocyte and cytotoxic T cell. A peptide, shown as a range of different sized or shaped digestion products of a native protein, is presented to an appropriate major histocompatibility complex (MHC) class 1 HLA antigen. This complex is presented on the surface of the hepatocyte, where it is recognized by the T cell. The T-cell receptor (TCR), in association with the CD8 molecule, binds, and a process is set off that results in the destruction of the infected cell.

aminases. What was unexplained until recently is how HBeAg production alone can be switched off, yet the virus continues to circulate. This process is discussed below.

Although antibodies may play a role in clearance of infected cells through complement activation or the recruitment of killer cells, the major response against infected hepatocytes is believed to be T-cell based.[10] The exact target is not known, but could, in theory, be any of the viral proteins. Cytotoxic T cells respond to short peptides that are presented on the surface in association with major histocompatibility complex (MHC) class 1 antigens. This process is shown in Figure 13.1. Thus, it is of no consequence whether proteins are normally found on the inner or outer aspects of the virion (or infected cells) or, indeed, whether they form part of circulating virions at all: an example of the latter is HBeAg. Any protein can be degraded by cellular proteinases and the derived peptides transported to the surface of the hepatocyte with the MHC molecule. There are constraints on this system, however. The peptide/MHC molecule binding is a specific one. Therefore, as there are a limited number of MHC molecules, it follows that only some of the infinite number of possible foreign peptides can be presented. It may be that not all the HBV proteins contain such peptides, and, thus, only certain of them can act as cytotoxic T-cell targets. Secondly, certain types of MHC molecules are found within and between particular population groups; thus, dissimilar peptides are presented by different people. These aspects will make the study of this field, in particular the study of cytotoxic T-cell escape mutants, a very difficult one.

HBsAg, HBcAg, and HBeAg have all been put forward as containing the major cytotoxic T-cell epitope. Some recent evidence indicates that the core antigen contains one of these targets. Experiments with vaccinia recombinants show that a region encompassing amino acids 18 to 27 acts as a target in in-vitro systems that present peptides associated with MHC class 1 HLA A2[11] antigens.

PRE-CORE/CORE AND PRE-S/S GENE BIOLOGY

Figure 13.2**A** shows that there are three translational start codons (ATG) within the surface gene. Translation beginning at any of these terminates at a single stop codon (TAG); therefore three proteins can be made, all having HBsAg at their carboxyl terminus.

Similarly, Figure 13.2**B** shows the translational products of the pre-core/

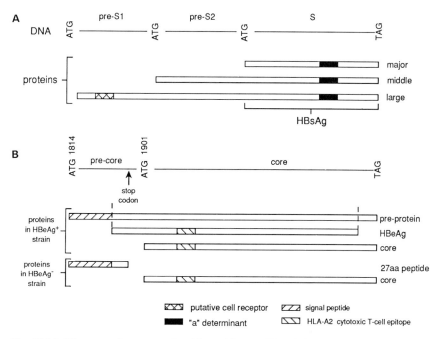

Fig. 13.2A Three proteins are translated from this gene. Translation can begin at one of three ATGs (translational start codon), all terminating at the single TAG. All three proteins contain HBsAg. The position of the 'a' determinant and the putative viral attachment protein (in pre-S1) are shown. **B** In an HBeAg-positive strain, translation beginning at the first ATG results in a long pre-protein that is cleaved within the endoplasmic reticulum, resulting in HBeAg: this is secreted onto the surface of the hepatocyte and into the serum. It is not part of the virion. The signal peptide (the first 19 amino acids) enables this secretion to take place. Translation at the second ATG results in HBcore, essential for nucleoprotein and therefore virion production. In HBeAg-negative strains, a stop codon at position 1896 at the end of the pre-core results in early termination of translation of HBeAg. However, HBcore production is unaffected; thus, virion production continues unabated. The HLA-A2 restricted cytotoxic T-cell epitope in the core is shown.

core region. It is important to note that two separate proteins can be generated. If translation begins at the first ATG, a long protein is produced that is cleaved at both ends within the endoplasmic reticulum. This is secreted into the serum as HBeAg. There is some evidence, both from transfection experiments in cultured cells[12] and from liver biopsies (using electron microscopy)[13] that HBeAg is found on the surface of cells: it could thus act as a target for the humoral response. If translation begins at the second ATG, then the core, or major nucleocapsid protein, is produced. As this does not contain a signal sequence (like HBeAg) at the beginning, it is not secreted. Thus, it is clear that a translationally functional pre-core region is vital for the synthesis of HBeAg, but not for viral particles.[14]

Selection and pathogenicity of pre-core variants

It is well established that nonsense mutations (resulting in stop codons) in the pre-core region occur commonly in anti-HBe positive patients.[15-17] Sequential studies have shown that the wild-type strain is present during the HBeAg positive phase, replaced after seroconversion to anti-HBe by the variant.[18] During the intervening period, a mixture is present. In the majority a stop codon is generated at position 1896, though a number of variants have been described that have a similar effect on translation, for example, loss of the pre-core ATG.[18, 19] Such examples are shown in Figure 13.3. This phenomenon thus explains the situation of a viral coded protein being switched off while virus continues to circulate. It would seem that this is a regular event in the interaction between HBV and its host, as it has been described from various parts of the world.

HBeAg may function as an immune modulator; this would explain why it is produced in large amounts yet is not associated with the virion. If this is correct, it follows that when HBeAg production ceases, cellular immune activity increases against HBcAg, which shares epitopes with HBeAg, resulting in ongoing hepatitis. However, this model presupposes, with no

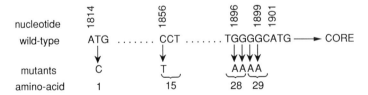

Fig. 13.3 Partial nucleotide and amino acid (aa) sequence of the pre-core region of HBV, showing representative mutants compared with the wild type. T to C at aa 1 (ref. 18) results in loss of the ATG; thus, no translation occurs. At aa 15 (ref. 23) is the proline-to-serine substitution described in the text. At the end of the pre-core, all four Gs have been documented to mutate to A. The first two result in translational stop codons (either TAG or TGA). The A at 1898 is associated with the change at aa 15 and that at 1899 with the A at 1896.

evidence, that a soluble protein (HBeAg) can protect a short peptide (derived from HBcAg) presented in association with MHC class 1 to the cytotoxic T cell. A protective role for HBeAg could, however, be envisaged if the immune attack is antibody mediated. As the balance tips with time in favour of the immune system, so hepatocytes with HBeAg on their surface will be destroyed. Those with pre-core deficient strains would survive: pre-core variants would thus be a form of humoral escape mutant. It seems unlikely that they are cellular escape mutants, because HBcAg is still produced, resulting in short peptides that may be identical to those derived from HBeAg.

Selection of variants occurs both in patients with progressive disease after seroconversion (seen particularly in Mediterranean countries and the Far East; these patients have high-level viraemia and often go on to cirrhosis) and in those who are in the process of clearing the virus. Their relationship to pathogenicity is therefore unclear. At least two studies[15,20] have documented that patients who clear HBV often have a mixture of wild-type and mutant strains, while those with progressive activity almost invariably have mutated strains alone. A further study has shown that selection of the mutant strain in anti-HBe positive patients resulted in peaks of enzyme activity and ongoing disease.[21] However, it seems difficult to distinguish between the effects of selection of the mutant and the presence of anti-HBe, as they are so often found together.

So, what dictates the further clinical course in those who select the mutant? The difference between those who recover and those who progress must reside in the latter group's inability to clear the other antigens of the virus. The Mediterranean subgroup of patients have high-level viraemia, yet have an active immune response, reflected in the raised transaminases. There may be a deficient cytotoxic T-cell response, or, alternatively, T-cell escape mutants (possibly in the core protein, for which some preliminary evidence is available – the author's unpublished observations) are sequentially selected, clearance of the previous strains being marked by peaks of activity. This process is outlined in Figure 13.4. Those who clear the virus seem able to mount an adequate initial response. There is no evidence that the strain infecting these groups of patients is fundamentally different.

A pre-core mutant that produces HBeAg

Two groups have described a variant with a proline to serine substitution at amino acid 15 of pre-core. Liang et al[22] found this strain in a patient with no serological markers of HBV, but with DNA detectable by polymerase chain reaction. On infecting a chimpanzee, the usual markers ensued, with persistence in the liver. A weak IgG, but not IgM, anti-HBc response occurred. A number of changes were seen around the genome, but the researchers paid particular attention to the serine at amino acid 15, discussing whether it might be related to the failure to produce IgM anti-HBc.

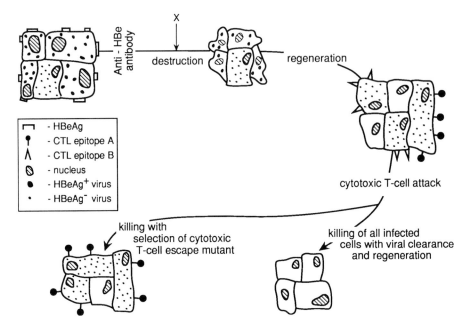

Fig. 13.4   Diagrammatic representation of the proposed immune response against a block of hepatocytes that are infected with HBV. Anti-HBe recognizes HBeAg-producing strains, killing cells infected with them, probably via killer cells. Those cells that are infected with HBeAg-negative mutant strains survive. After regeneration of the hepatocytes, all infected cells have mutant strains. A cytotoxic T-cell response is mounted against the infected cells, probably against core peptides: some people have a strong response, killing all infected hepatocytes and clearing the virus, while others do not, allowing subsequent virion replication cycles to produce mutants in T-cell epitopes. The response kills cells infected with the original strain, but allows those with the mutant to grow through. It is likely that this selection process continues against other epitopes until the virus is eventually cleared. Point X is the point at which a putatively strong immune response would occur during fulminant hepatitis.

However, the epitopes to which anti-HBc reacts are not believed to reside in the pre-core region, and in the Chinese isolates described below,[23] a normal anti-HBc response was seen. Carman et al[23] studied Chinese patients from Hong Kong. This strain was seen in half of the anti-HBe-positive patients with progressive disease, the others having the stop codon mutation. These two mutations were never found in the same patient, implying that they have similar biological significance.

A number of aspects make this 'Chinese' strain interesting. Firstly, the serine substitution was found during the HBeAg-positive phase of the illness, whereas the stop codon is seldom if ever seen at that stage. The second feature is the mutual exclusivity of the two mutations and the fact that, even after many years of anti-HBe positivity, the stop codon never emerged in those with the serine substitution. Thirdly, there is the finding that those patients who were infected with the serine-containing strain during the HBeAg-positive phase went on to severe disease after sero-conversion. The relationship of this strain to virulence, particularly in the light of the third point, and its transmissibility need further study. The question of whether this is a circulating strain or whether it is selected early in the HBeAg-positive phase (and, if so, what is the selection pressure?) also needs to be addressed. Figure 13.3 shows the position of this mutation in the pre-core region.

Pre-core variants and fulminant hepatitis

There is a strong epidemiological association with the pre-core stop codon variant and the fulminant course of HBV infection. It has been recognized for some time that infants infected by anti-HBe-positive mothers can have severe acute disease. Furthermore, anti-HBe-positive patients have been the index case in outbreaks of fulminant disease. A number of groups[24-27] have now shown that anti-HBe-positive patients with this form of the infection have circulating pre-core variants. The sequence of other genes in the infective contact is very similar to that in those with the fulminant disease, implying that the isolate has been transmitted. It would seem that if a person receives an infective dose of HBV that is unable to produce HBeAg, the disease produced in the immunologically naive person is very severe, probably because of the absence of the modulating effect of HBeAg. However, some results contrast with this finding. Carman et al[24] studied both HBeAg- and anti-HBe-positive patients with fulminant disease and found a perfect correlation with strain and HBe serology, showing that HBeAg-positive cases are not caused by the pre-core mutant. Interestingly, the variants found by Liang et al[27] occurred in HBeAg-positive patients: it is possible that this reactivity was due to degraded core particles, which are known to reveal HBeAg epitopes. An alternative hypothesis is, therefore, that an excessive immune response (probably genetically determined) against the normal strain occurs, resulting in a fulminant course, clearance of the virus, seroconversion to anti-HBe, and selection of the pre-core variant. This mechanism would occur at point X in Figure 13.4. However, until transmission experiments are performed in animal models, the correct mechanism will remain unclear.

In contrast, patients with acute resolving hepatitis are generally not infected with mutants.[18,26] Two studies,[28,29] however, have shown an association, and this conflict will need to be resolved.

Relationship to interferon therapy

Success with interferon can be predicted by a peak of transaminases after initiation of therapy. This implies an enhanced immune response, and it is known that those with some hepatitic activity before therapy will respond best. It may therefore be that those with immune pressure on HBV, and thus in the process of losing HBeAg and selecting a pre-core variant, will respond. If so, responders (those who lose HBeAg) would have variants as their major species after seroconversion.

Four groups have now studied this aspect, with conflicting results. Takeda et al[30] have found that the presence of variant as a mixture with wild type in pretreatment sera predicts long-term remission. Those who have wild type alone may respond to therapy, but relapse later. However, this study was performed on only one patient in each group. Xu et al,[31] using African sera, found no patient that selected variant strains after interferon therapy, but it is not known whether such strains occur naturally in this area.

We studied Italian patients.[32] In particular, we were interested in the Mediterranean subgroup of anti-HBe-positive chronic hepatitis patients, who are believed to respond poorly to interferon. No significant correlation was found between response, either short- or long-term, and sequence in this group (not all these patients are infected with variants). However, there was a trend towards poorer response in those *with* the mutant, in keeping with the findings in other Italian patients[33] (see below), but in contrast with the results in Japanese patients.[30] In the second part of this study, HBeAg-positive patients on interferon therapy were compared to a control HBeAg-positive group to correlate the emergence of mutant with seroconversion to anti-HBe. The natural seroconverters seemed to select mutant strains at an earlier stage to the treated group. The third phase of this study compared the pretreatment sequence of HBeAg-positive patients who responded to those who did not. Once again, no differences were noted between the two groups. Thus, we could not confirm the findings of Takeda et al[30] and must conclude that sequencing the pretreatment sequence does not aid in selection of candidates for therapy with interferon. Brunetto et al[33] also studied Italian patients, finding that, of HBeAg-positive subjects, those with mixed isolates were just as likely to respond as those with wild type alone. Of anti-HBe-positive patients, three of six responders (two others had mixtures) and 11 of 16 non-responders (the rest had mixtures) had variants as a single species.

Pre-S variants

A number of groups have begun to analyse the pre-S regions in chronic carriers. Brechot's group in France[34] have studied serial samples from an HBeAg-positive patient over 6 years. In the initial samples, wild-type sequences were found. However, with time, important changes appeared in both the pre-core/core and pre-S regions. In the pre-core region, the stop codon mutation was noted, this time in the context of a 36-base pair insertion at the end of the pre-core. A very similar insertion has been described by another group,[35] leading to interesting questions about its origin, as it bears no resemblance to other known sequences, HBV or otherwise. It may be that a specific recombination event has occurred with the human genome. Three types of pre-S genomes were present at the later stages. The first consisted of the wild type. In the second, deletions in the pre-S1 region led to a stop codon, leading to a truncated protein. However, the cell binding area is translated, as this is found before the stop codon. In addition, both the pre-S1 and pre-S2 regions had numerous point mutations and deletions, leading to significant divergence from the initial strain. The third type of genome consisted of a recombination between wild type and mutant. In the last sample studied, the second type of genome had become the majority.

Sanantonio et al[36] have noted multiples of three base pair deletions (thus, the region remains in frame) from the pre-S2 region in chronic carriers, both HBeAg and anti-HBe positive. In all cases, the pre-S2 start codon was mutated out, thereby inhibiting production of this protein. Figure 13.5 outlines some of these changes.

The study of this region is at an early stage; therefore conclusions are difficult. B- and T-cell antigenic sites have been identified in pre-S1, pre-S2, and HBs. Thus, it seems that this region may also be under selective pressure and that these changes represent escape mutations. As the putative cell binding region of pre-S1 is intact in all the above variants, these strains should be viable.

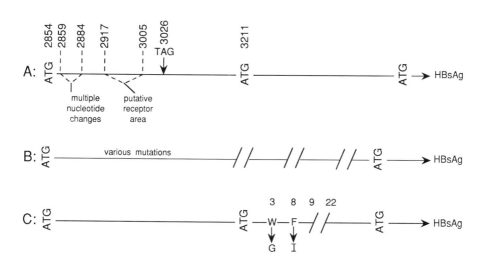

Fig. 13.5 Three examples of pre-S mutants. **A** (ref. 34) shows multiple changes in the pre-S1 with a novel translational stop codon (TAG). The putative viral attachment area is intact. **B** (ref. 36) has changes distributed widely throughout pre-S: the ATG of pre-S2 has been mutated out and further deletions have been noted in pre-S2. In **C** (ref. 43) pre-S2 has aa changes, as shown at positions 8 and 9 and a deletion from aa 9 to 22. This patient also had significant changes in the 'a' determinant, as detailed in Figure 13.6.

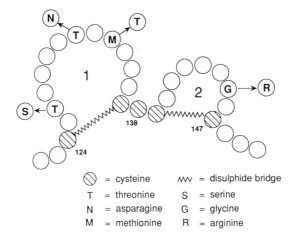

$\bigcirc$ = cysteine $\wedge\wedge$ = disulphide bridge

T = threonine   S = serine

N = asparagine   G = glycine

M = methionine   R = arginine

Fig. 13.6   Amino acids of the 'a' determinant. Two loops are formed from disulphide bridges between cysteine residues. Loop 1 has been changed (ref. 43), as shown in a patient with cocirculating HBsAg and anti-HBs. Loop 2 had a glycine-to-arginine change (ref. 40) in a vaccinated patient who went on to chronic carriage.

Surface variation

The cell receptor is thought to be on either HBsAg or pre-S1.[37] Thus, any pressure on neutralization epitopes in these regions leading to variant selection would have to occur in non-receptor peptides for the virion to remain viable. Major protective epitopes are located in HBsAg, and this molecule is therefore employed in HBV vaccine. The 'a' antigenic determinant, which is common to all HBV isolates and to which most of the polyclonal anti-HBs bind, is believed to consist of two loops, formed by disulphide bridges[38] (Fig. 13.6). This represents an ideal site for the emergence of escape mutants.

A glycine-to-arginine substitution has been seen at amino acid 145 of HBsAg in monoclonal antibody treated liver transplant recipients[39] as well as in at least two vaccinees, respectively, from Italy[40] and Singapore,[41] with good levels of anti-HBs, who developed chronic hepatitis. The Italian case[40] was an infant born to a chronic carrier mother, who was shown to have the normal sequence. Binding of monoclonal antibodies that have previously been mapped to this region was dramatically reduced (Fig. 13.6), implying that the change is antigenically significant.

There is no published evidence that this variant has been transmitted to other human beings (though it has infected chimpanzees), nor that it occurs commonly in vaccinees. However, breakthroughs occur in most large-scale vaccination trials – for example, that undertaken in Gambia[42] – and some of these become carriers. It is not known whether these patients have a mutated genome or whether other factors such as timing of the vaccine play a role. Whether this particular mutation is the only important one also remains to be elucidated. However, as a measure to limit its emergence in an increasingly vaccinated world, a yeast-derived mutated HBsAg has been synthesized and is undergoing preliminary evaluation in animals (J Petre, October 1991, personal communication).

Other mutations of this region have been described in chronic carriers. For example, Moriyama et al[43] reported a patient with anti-HBs who was an HBeAg-positive carrier. There were both amino acid substitutions and a large deletion in pre-S2. However, of relevance here the substitutions noted in the first loop of the 'a' determinant: positions 126, 131, and 133 were different from previously described sequences (Fig. 13.6). Monoclonal antibody binding studies were not performed, and thus changed antigenicity was not formally proven. As with the Italian vaccine-induced mutant, the changes were stable over years and formed the only, or major, proportion of sequences present. It may thus be that merely changing the vaccine at position 145 will not adequately suppress the emergence of escape mutants but that other strategies, such as inclusion of pre-S epitopes, may be necessary, especially if the cell receptor protein is included. Disquietingly, sequences have been found that are not detectable on some standard diagnostic assays.

In an attempt at defining other important epitopes of HBsAg, we have studied the evolution of HBsAg under polyclonal antibody pressure in five liver transplant recipients receiving immunoglobulin.[44] Patients were selected for this study if they infected their new liver despite therapy: three were shown to be HBV-DNA positive, either by polymerase chain reaction (PCR), a very sensitive technique, or by dot blot hybridization, during therapy. These three are therefore likely candidates for the presence of escape mutants. Mutations, as compared to the pretreatment sequence, were seen to be clustered in two areas. Interestingly, most of the mutations resulted in amino acid substitutions, a result not to be expected of random mutation events. Whether these mutations had any relevance to graft infection is not clear; it may, rather, have been that immunoglobulin levels were not adequate to neutralize any virus.

CONCLUSIONS

The field is a rapidly growing one and has already led to some interesting observations about important epitopes and pathogenesis of disease. We are likely to derive insights into the mechanisms of cytotoxic T-cell escape and the role of such changes on virulence. One wonders whether these diverse changes are seen sequentially in individuals or whether different people select variants from different regions of the genome, depending, perhaps, on their MHC type. On a practical level, a new vaccine is being developed and changes are being made to the diagnostic assays for detection of HBsAg so that these novel sequences are not overlooked. However, it must be remembered that not all mutations are important: some will not lead to an amino acid change; others may not have any effect on replication. It is possible for non-viable genomes to be encapsulated and to leave the hepatocyte: therefore, findings of single mutants in a population of normal strains must be analysed with care. With the rapid DNA amplification and sequencing techniques available, we can expect this to be an intriguing and fruitful area in the future.

ACKNOWLEDGEMENTS

My thanks go to Professor Howard Thomas, St Mary's Hospital, London, for allowing me to work in his department and for sharing his innovative ideas with me.

REFERENCES

1 Thomas DB, Burt DS, Barnett BC, Graham CM, Skehel JJ. B and T cell recognition of influenza haemagglutinin. In: Cold Spring Harbor Symposium on Quantitative Biology: Immunological Recognition 1989; 54: 487
2 Pircher H, Moskophidis D, Rohrer U, Bürki K, Hengartner H, Zinkernagel RM. Viral escape by selection of cytotoxic T cell-resistant virus variants in vivo. Nature 1990; 346: 629–633
3 Phillips RE, Rowland-Jones S, Nixon DF et al. Human immunodeficiency virus genetic variation that can escape cytotoxic T cell recognition. Nature 1991; 354: 453–459
4 Carman WF, Thomas HC. Genetic variation in hepatitis B virus. Gastroenterology 1992; 102: 711–719
5 Carman WF, Thomas HC. Defined genetic variants of HBV. Rev Med Virol 1991; 1: 29–39
6 Milich DR, McLachlan A, Chisari FV, Kent SBH, Thornton GB. Immune response to the pre-S1 region of the hepatitis B surface antigen [HBsAg]: a pre-S1 specific T cell response can bypass nonresponsiveness to the pre-S2 and S regions of HBsAg. J Immunol 1986; 137: 315–322
7 Itoh Y, Takai E, Ohnuma H et al. A synthetic peptide vaccine involving the product of the pre-S 2 region of hepatitis B virus: protective efficacy in chimpanzees. Proc Natl Acad Sci USA 1986; 83: 9174–9178
8 Murray K, Bruce SA, Wingfield P, van Eerd P, de Reus A, Schellekens H. Protective immunisation against hepatitis B with an internal antigen of the virus. J Med Virol 1987; 23: 101–107
9 Budkowska A, Dubreuil P, Maillard P, Poynard T, Pillot J. A biphasic pattern of anti-pre-S responses in acute hepatitis B virus infection. Hepatology 1990; 12: 1271–1277
10 Pignatelli M, Waters J, Lever A, Iwarson S, Gerety R, Thomas HC. Cytotoxic T-cell responses to the nucleocapsid proteins of HBV in chronic hepatitis. J Hepatol 1987; 4: 15–21
11 Penna A, Chisari FV, Bertoletti A et al. Cytotoxic T lymphocytes recognize an HLA-A2 restricted epitope within the hepatitis B virus nucleocapsid antigen. J Hepatol 1991; 13: S59
12 Schlicht H-J, von Brunn A, Theilmann L. Antibodies in anti-HBe-positive patient sera bind to an HBe protein expressed on the cell surface of human hepatoma cells: implications for virus clearance. Hepatology 1991; 13: 57–61
13 Yamada G, Takaguchi K, Matsueda K et al. Immunoelectron microscopic observation of intrahepatic HBeAg in patients with chronic hepatitis B. Hepatology 1990; 12: 133–140
14 Schlicht HJ, Salfeld J, Schaller H. The duck hepatitis B virus pre-C region encodes a signal sequence which is essential for synthesis and secretion of processed core proteins but not for virus formation. J Virol 1987; 61: 3701–3709
15 Carman WF, Jacyna MR, Hadziyannis S et al. Mutation preventing formation of e antigen in patients with chronic HBV infection. Lancet 1989; 2: 588–591

16 Brunetto MR, Stemmler M, Schodel F et al. Identification of HBV variants which cannot produce precore-derived HBeAg and may be responsible for severe hepatitis. Ital J Gastroenterol 1989; 21: 151–154

17 Tong S, Li J, Vitvitski L, Trépo C. Active hepatitis B virus replication in the presence of anti-HBe is associated with viral variants containing an inactive pre-C region. Virology 1990; 176: 596–603

18 Okamoto H, Yotsumoto S, Akahane Y et al. Hepatitis B viruses with pre-core region defects prevail in persistently infected hosts along with seroconversion to the antibody against e antigen. J Virol 1990; 64: 1298–1303

19 Fiordalisi G, Cariani E, Mantero G et al. High genomic variability in the pre-C region of hepatitis B virus in anti-HBe, HBV-DNA positive chronic hepatitis. J Med Virol 1990; 31: 297–300

20 Naoumov NV, Schneider R, Grötzinger T et al. Precore mutants hepatitis B virus infection and liver disease. Gastroenterology 1992; February

21 Brunetto MR, Giarin MM, Oliver F et al. Wild-type and e antigen-minus hepatitis B viruses and course of chronic hepatitis. Proc Natl Acad Sci USA 1991; 88: 4186–4190

22 Liang TJ, Blum HE, Wands JR. Characterization and biological properties of a hepatitis B virus isolated from a patient without hepatitis B virus serologic markers. Hepatology 1990; 12: 204–212

23 Carman WF, Ferrao M, Lok ASF, Ma OCK, Lai CL, Thomas HC. Pre-core sequence variation in Chinese isolates of hepatitis B virus. J Infect Dis 1992; 165: 127–133

24 Carman WF, Fagan EA, Hadziyannis S et al. Association of a pre-core variant of HBV with fulminant hepatitis. Hepatology 1991; 14: 219–222

25 Kosaka Y, Takase K, Kojima M et al. Fulminant hepatitis B: induction by hepatitis B virus mutants defective in the precore region and incapable of encoding e antigen. Gastroenterology 1991; 324: 1087–1094

26 Omata M, Ehata T, Yokosuka O, Hosoda K, Ohto M. Mutations in the precore region of hepatitis B virus DNA in patients with fulminant and severe hepatitis. N Engl J Med 1991; 324: 1699–1704

27 Liang TJ, Hasegawa K, Rimon N, Wands JR, Ben-Porath E. A hepatitis B virus mutant associated with an epidemic of fulminant hepatitis. N Engl J Med 1991; 324: 1705–1709

28 Carman WF, Hadziyannis S, Karayiannis P et al. Association of the precore variant of HBV with acute and fulminant hepatitis B infection. In: Hollinger FB, Lemon S, Margolis K, eds. Viral hepatitis and liver disease. Baltimore, Md: Williams and Wilkins, 1991: pp 216–219

29 Hasegawa K, Huang J, Wands JR, Obata H, Liang TJ. Association of hepatitis B viral precore mutations with fulminant hepatitis B in Japan. Virology 1991; 185: 460–463

30 Takeda K, Akahane Y, Suzuki H et al. Defects in the precore region of the HBV genome in patients with chronic hepatitis B after sustained seroconversion from HBeAg to anti-HBe induced spontaneously or with interferon therapy. Hepatology 1990; 12: 1284–1289

31 Xu J, Brown D, Harrison T, Lin Y, Dusheiko G. Are hepatitis B virus pre-core defective mutants a determinant of response to interferon? J Hepatol 1991; 13: S81

32 Carman WF, Fattovich G, McIntyre G, Alberti A, Thomas HC. Pre-core HBV mutants: response to interferon therapy. J Hepatol 1991; 13: S16

33 Brunetto MR, Saracco G, Oliveri F et al. HBV heterogeneity and response to interferon. J Hepatol 1991; 13: S15

34 Tran A, Kremsdorf D, Capel F et al. Emergence of and takeover by hepatitis B virus (HBV) with rearrangements in the pre-S/S and pre-C/C genes during chronic HBV infection. J Virol 1991; 65: 3566–3574

35 Bhat RA, Ulrich PP, Vyas GN. Molecular characterisation of a new variant of hepatitis B virus in a persistently infected homosexual man. Hepatology 1990; 11: 271–276

36 Sanantonio T, Jung MC, Schneider R, Pastore G, Pape GR, Will H. Identification of HBV pre-S mutants and their intrafamilial spreading. J Hepatol 1991; 13: S69

37 Petit M, Dubanchet S, Capel F, Voet P, Dauguet C, Hauser P. HepG2 cell binding activities of different hepatitis B virus isolates: inhibitory effect of anti-HBs and anti-preS1 (21–47). Virology 1991; 180: 483–491

38 Brown SE, Howard CR, Zuckerman AJ, Steward MW. Affinity of antibody responses in man to hepatitis B vaccine determined with synthetic peptides. Lancet 1984; 2: 184–187

39 McMahon G, McCarthy LA, Dottavio D, Ostberg L. Surface antigen and polymerase gene variation in hepatitis B virus isolates from a monoclonal antibody treated liver

transplant patient. In: Hollinger FB, Lemon S, Margolis K, eds. Viral hepatitis and liver disease. Baltimore, Md: Williams and Wilkins, 1991: pp 219–221

40 Carman WF, Zanetti AR, Karayiannis P et al. Vaccine-induced escape mutant of hepatitis B virus. Lancet 1990; 336: 325–329

41 Zanetti AR, Tanzi E, Harrison TJ, Manzillo G, Zuckerman AJ. Hepatitis B virus escape mutants. Meeting on Genetic Heterogeneity of Hepatitis Viruses, Sestriere, Italy 1991; B17.

42 Whittle HC, Inskip H, Hall AJ, Mendy M, Downes R, Hoare S. Vaccination against hepatitis B and protection against chronic viral carriage in The Gambia. Lancet 1991; 337: 747–750

43 Moriyama K, Nakajima E, Hohjoh H, Asayama R, Okochi K. Immunoselected hepatitis B virus mutant. Lancet 1991; 337: 125

44 Carman WF, McIntyre G, Muller R, Thomas HC. Evolution of HBV surface antigen sequence under polyclonal antibody pressure. J Hepatol 1991; 13: S17

14

Reviews and leaders

M. C. Allison

References to recent reviews and leading articles in gastroenterology on the following subjects are given on pages 241–250. The references are listed numerically.

INDEX TO REFERENCES

ABSCESSES, LIVER   31
ABSCESSES, PANCREATIC   15, 65
ABSORPTION
  calcium   167
  cholesterol   78
  ion transport   13
  short bowel   185
  vitamin B_{12} 166
ACHLORHYDRIA   98, 126
ACQUIRED IMMUNE DEFICIENCY
     SYNDROME
  anorectal manifestations   259
  colorectal surgery   206, 259
  gastrointestinal manifestations   84
  hepatobiliary manifestations   45
  pancreatic manifestations   37
ADENOMA–CARCINOMA
     SEQUENCE   210, 254
AGEING   21, 212
  biliary disease   119
  colonic motor activity   203, 251
  diarrhoea   113
  diverticular disease   57, 253
  faecal impaction   113, 203, 251
  gastritis   98
  gastrointestinal haemorrhage   189
  gastro-oesophageal reflux   50
  immunity   51
  inflammatory bowel disease   99
  liver disease   244
  malabsorption   113
  oesophageal disease   50
  pancreatic disease   119
  peptic ulcer   88
  volvulus   186
ALACTASIA   1
ALCOHOL
  hepatoma   164

pathogenesis of acute pancreatitis   215
pathogenesis of chronic pancreatitis   202, 215
pathogenesis of liver disease   240
small intestinal mucosa   174
ALCOHOLIC LIVER DISEASE
  hepatoma   164
  nutritional management   144
ALPHA-FETOPROTEIN   230
AMBULATORY pH MONITORING   68, 266
5-AMINO SALICYLIC ACID   107, 173, 178, 191, 248
ANAL SPHINCTER   221, 251
ANGELCHIK PROSTHESIS   109
ANGINA VS. OESOPHAGEAL PAIN   238, 266
ANGIODYSPLASIA   189
ANO-RECTUM
  Crohn's disease   143
  Hirschsprung's disease   72, 260
  immunocompromised patients   259
  physiology   221, 251
ANTACIDS
  gastro-oesophageal reflux   220
  stress ulcer, prophylaxis   205
ANTIBIOTICS
  bowel preparation   219
  Helicobacter pylori   90
  for infective diarrhoea   10
ANTIGENS
  intestinal handling   145
  tumour-associated   223
ANTI-INFLAMMATORY DRUGS
  duodenal ulcer   88, 218
  gastric emptying   56
  gastric mucosal damage   98, 102, 183, 218, 228

ANTI-INFLAMMATORY DRUGS
    (contd)
    gastric ulcer   88, 218
    gastrointestinal haemorrhage   189
    intestinal mucosal damage   183
    oesophageal diseases   50
    misoprostol prophylaxis   102
ANUS
    carcinoma   see Cancer–anus
    Crohn's disease   143
    innervation   221
    physiology   221, 251
ASBESTOS AND COLORECTAL
    CANCER   256
ASCITES
    pancreatic   15
    peritoneovenous shunt   162
ASPIRIN AND THE STOMACH   218,
    228
ASTHMA, AND GASTRO-
    OESOPHAGEAL REFLUX   9, 92,
    131, 238
AUTOIMMUNE MECHANISMS
    in inflammatory bowel disease   216
    in liver disease   85, 156
AUTONOMIC NERVOUS SYSTEM
    control of motility and secretion   203
    motility disorders   150, 203
AZATHIOPRINE IN
    INFLAMMATORY BOWEL
    DISEASE   173

BACTERIA
    colorectal cancer   196
    diarrhoea   10
    DNA probes   53
    effect of antimicrobials   10
    enteric colonization   128
    gastroenteritis   101
    gut flora   198
    infectious enteritis   81
    therapeutic use   82
BACTERIAL VACCINES   137
BARRETT'S OESOPHAGUS   109, 179
BENZODIAZEPINE RECEPTORS   42
BETA-ADRENERGIC BLOCKADE,
    PORTAL HYPERTENSION   135,
    170
BILE PHYSIOLOGY   121, 165
BILE REFLUX
    and postgastrectomy cancer   168
    gastro-oesophageal reflux   93
    into pancreatic duct   157
BILIARY CIRRHOSIS, PRIMARY
    drug treatment   30, 122
    liver transplantation   6
    pathogenesis   85, 156
BILIARY TRACT
    ageing   21

AIDS   45
    diseases   157
    motility   97
    physiology   165
BISMUTH COMPOUNDS   94, 146
    dyspepsia   8
    Helicobacter pylori   90
BLOOD COAGULATION–
    INFLAMMATORY BOWEL
    DISEASE   249
BLOOD SUPPLY   see Circulation
BOWEL PREPARATION, SURGERY
    219
BRAIN, CONTROL OF GUT
    FUNCTION   229
BRANCHED-CHAIN AMINO ACIDS
    144, 160
BROWN BOWEL SYNDROME   116
BUDD-CHIARI SYNDROME   38, 129
BULIMIA NERVOSA   75

CAECAL VOLVULUS   186
CA 19-9 TUMOUR-ASSOCIATED
    ANTIGEN   223
CALCIUM CHANNEL BLOCKERS
    188, 267
CANCER, ANUS   95
CANCER, BILE DUCT   31, 157
CANCER, COLORECTUM
    aetiology   256
    asbestos   256
    bacteria   196
    chemotherapy   62, 76
    Crohn's disease   178
    diet   108, 196
    dysplasia   103
    inflammatory bowel disease   103, 178
    lasers   76, 148
    palliation   76, 148
    polypectomy   254
    radiotherapy   62, 76, 194
    screening   255
    surgery   11, 62, 76
    tumour markers   265
CANCER, GALL BLADDER   258
CANCER, LIVER   see Hepatoma
CANCER, OESOPHAGUS
    Barrett's oesophagus   179
    combined modality therapy   163
    lasers   184
    palliation   28
    photodynamic therapy   184
    primary small cell   33
    radiotherapy   4, 163
    surgery   4, 28, 163
CANCER, PANCREAS   49
    aetiology   104
    biology   180
    chemotherapy   155

CANCER, PANCREAS (contd)
  computerized tomography 27
  cystadenocarcinoma 27
  palliation 106, 120
  surgery 49, 96, 155
  tumour markers 223
CANCER, SMALL BOWEL 210
CANCER, STOMACH
  chemotherapy 18
  gastrectomy 110, 141
  postgastrectomy 168
CARCINOEMBRYONIC ANTIGEN
  265
CARCINOGENESIS
  bowel cancer 210, 256
  hepatoma 164
  pancreatic cancer 180
CARCINOIDS, GASTRIC 126, 182
CHEMOTHERAPY
  colorectal cancer 62, 76
  gastrointestinal lymphoma 91
  hepatoma 47
  pancreatic cancer 49, 155
  stomach cancer 18
CHEST PAIN 238, 266
CHILDHOOD
  Crohn's disease 136
  cystic fibrosis 12
  gastroenteritis 35, 105
  gastro-oesophageal reflux 227
  hepatitis vaccines 73
  lactose intolerance 1
  oral rehydration 24, 200
  vaccines for diarrhoea 137
CHOLANGITIS, PRIMARY
      SCLEROSING 157
CHOLECYSTECTOMY 58, 87, 181,
  258
CHOLECYSTOKININ 97
CHOLERA VACCINE 137
CHOLESTEROL
  intestinal regulation 78
CIGARETTE SMOKING see Smoking
CIMETIDINE 77, 205
CIRCULATION
  disturbance in liver failure 213
  gut 190
  portal hypertension 188
CIRRHOSIS see Liver disease
CISAPRIDE 151, 152
CLOSTRIDIUM DIFFICILE
  antibiotic-associated colitis 82
  diarrhoea, elderly 113
COELIAC DISEASE
  diagnosis 5
  molecular basis 124
  pathophysiology 145
COLECTOMY FOR CONSTIPATION
  60

COLITIS
  antibiotic-associated 82, 113
  biopsy diagnosis 259
  collagenous 222
  diversion 192
  immunocompromised patients 259
  ischaemic 190
  microscopic 127
  ulcerative see Ulcerative colitis
COLON
  angiodysplasia 189
  dysfunction in elderly 251, 253
  endometriosis 269
  fermentation 196
  motility 203
  motility disorder 139, 177, 203, 264
  mucosal metabolism 133, 196
  obstruction 186
  pneumatosis cystoides 193
  sexually transmitted disease 259
  stercoral perforation 211
  volvulus 186
COLONOSCOPY
  malignant polyp removal 254
  surveillance in ulcerative colitis 103, 178
COLORECTAL CANCER see Cancer,
  colorectum
COLORECTAL POLYPOSIS
  colonoscopic treatment 254
  familial 172
  markers 172
  risk of colorectal cancer 210
COLORECTAL SURGERY
  acquired immune deficiency syndrome
  206
  bowel preparation 219
  cancer 11, 62, 76
  constipation 60
  Crohn's disease 262
  ileo-anal pouch function 138
  transanal resection 11
  volvulus 186
COMPUTERIZED AXIAL
      TOMOGRAPHY
  acute pancreatitis 17, 224
  liver diseases 31
  pancreatic masses 27
CONSTIPATION
  elderly 251
  Hirschsprung's disease 72, 260
  irritable bowel 235
  surgical treatment 60
CORTICOSTEROIDS IN
      INFLAMMATORY BOWEL
      DISEASE 173
CROHN'S DISEASE 178
  aetiology 169, 178
  anal lesions 143
  cerebrovascular complications 123

CROHN'S DISEASE (contd)
　corticosteroids　173
　cyclosporin　173
　differential diagnosis　46
　enteral nutrition　136
　immunology in　178
　immunosuppressive drugs　173
　in elderly　99
　intestinal permeability　169
　metronidazole　173
　nutritional disturbance　136
　oral contraceptive　250
　parenteral feeding　136
　pathogenesis　178, 216, 249, 250
　procoagulant activity　249
　quality of life　83
　recrudescence following resection　262
　relapse　36
　smoking　250
　sulphasalazine and analogues　173
CYCLOSPORIN, CROHN'S DISEASE
　　173
CYSTADENOMA/
　　CYSTADENOCARCINOMA　27
CYSTIC FIBROSIS　12
CYTOPROTECTION OF GASTRIC
　　MUCOSA　102

DEFENCE MECHANISMS,
　　GASTRODUODENAL　130,
　　228
DEGLUTITION, PHYSIOLOGY　112
DEGLUTITION DISORDERS　112,
　　238
DELTA VIRUS　69
DIABETES–EFFECT ON GUT　117,
　　195
DIAGNOSIS
　acute pancreatitis　17
　coeliac disease　5
　cystic fibrosis　12
　diarrhoea in AIDS　84
　early gastric cancer　110
　endometriosis　46, 269
　foreign body ingestion　161
　gall bladder disease　268
　gastro-oesophageal reflux　68, 227,
　　266
　Hirschsprung's disease　72, 260
　irritable bowel　209, 235
　intestinal infection　53
　intestinal ischaemia　190
　liver tumours　31
　microscopic colitis　127
　pancreatic abscess　17
　pancreatic cancer　27
　protozoan diarrhoea　101
　sexually transmitted disease　259
　Zollinger-Ellison syndrome　246

DIARRHOEA
　acquired immune deficiency syndrome
　　84
　antibiotic-associated　82, 113
　antimicrobials for infectious diarrhoea
　　10
　bismuth for　94
　collagenous colitis　222
　diabetic　195
　elderly　113
　infectious enteritis　81
　irritable bowel　235
　oral rehydration　24, 200
　parasitic　81
　postvagotomy　64
　viral gastroenteritis　35, 105
DIET
　fibre　108
　irritable bowel　79
　lactose intolerance　1
　pancreatic cancer　104
　short bowel　185
DIVERSION COLITIS　192
DIVERTICULOSIS　57
　colonic　57, 253
　duodenal　16
　Meckel's　241
DNA PROBES, DIAGNOSIS OF
　　INTESTINAL INFECTION　53
DOMPERIDONE　152
DRUGS
　aminosalicylic acid derivatives　107, 173,
　　191
　antisecretory drugs　199, 208
　beta-adrenergic blockers　135, 170
　bismuth compounds　94, 146
　cisapride　151
　gastric emptying　56
　Helicobacter pylori　90
　irritable bowel　26, 79
　inflammatory bowel disease　173
　octreotide　100
　oesophageal damage　74
　olsalazine　248
　omeprazole　32, 114, 149
　peptic ulcer　77
　portal hypertension　135, 159, 170, 188
　prokinetic agents　151, 152
　prostaglandins　102, 208
　sucralfate　153
DUODENAL ULCER
　aetiology　43, 217, 218
　bismuth compounds　94
　drugs for　34, 77
　elderly　88, 189
　haemorrhage　39, 176, 189
　Helicobacter pylori　25, 154, 175, 242
　histamine H_2-blockade　34, 77
　long-term management　34

DUODENAL ULCER (contd)
  non-steroidal anti-inflammatory drugs
      218
  omeprazole   114, 149, 199
  pathophysiology   130, 217
  relapse   34
  sucralfate   153
  treatment of NSAID-induced ulcers
      218
  trials of drug treatments   34
  vagotomy   19
DUODENUM
  diverticulosis   16
  epidermal growth factor 130
  physiology   130
DYSPEPSIA, ROLE OF BISMUTH   8
DYSPHAGIA IN ELDERLY   50
DYSPLASIA, INFLAMMATORY
      BOWEL DISEASE   103

EATING DISORDERS   75
ELDERLY   see Ageing
ELECTROMYOGRAPHY,
      PELVIC   221
EMPTYING   see Gastric emptying
ENDOMETRIOSIS   46, 269
ENDOPROSTHESIS
  carcinoma of pancreas   49, 106
  chronic pancreatitis   41
ENDOSCOPY   161
  early diagnosis gastric cancer   110
  electrocoagulation   176
  ERCP   see ERCP
  gastrointestinal haemorrhage   39, 176
  heater probe   39, 176
  injection sclerotherapy non-variceal
      bleeds   176
  intervention in chronic pancreatitis   22,
      41
  lasers   39, 176
  percutaneous gastrostomy   158
ENDOTOXINS   198
ENTERAL FEEDING
  alcoholic liver disease   144
  Crohn's disease   136
  percutaneous endoscopic gastrostomy
      158
  short bowel   185
ENTERITIS
  bacterial   81
  tuberculous   81
  vaccines   137
ENTEROCOLITIS, C. DIFFICILE   82,
      113
ENTEROCHROMAFFIN CELLS   32,
      126, 182
ENZYMOLOGY OF PANCREAS   17
EPIDEMIOLOGY
  acute pancreatitis   215

chronic pancreatitis   21, 215
colorectal cancer   255, 256
Crohn's disease   250
diverticular disease   57
gallstones   71
hepatoma   214
pancreatic cancer   104
peptic ulcer   242
EPIDERMAL GROWTH FACTOR   93,
      130
ERCP
  acute gallstone pancreatitis   48, 120
  chronic pancreatitis   41, 120
  elderly   119
  palliation obstructive jaundice   106, 120

FAECAL INCONTINENCE
  after ileoanal anastomosis   138
  in elderly   251
  pathophysiology   221
FAMOTIDINE   77
FATTY ACIDS   78, 133, 196
FIBRE   108
  diverticular disease   253
  fermentation, flora, and flatus   196
FIBROLAMELLAR HEPATOMA   197
FISTULA, OCTREOTIDE THERAPY
      100
FLUMAZENIL   42
FLUOROURACIL
  colorectal cancer   62, 76
  pancreatic cancer   155
FULMINANT HEPATIC FAILURE
      44, 52, 263
FUNCTIONAL BOWEL DISORDERS
      see Irritable bowel
FUNDOPLICATION   109, 231

GALANIN   187
GALL BLADDER   97, 121, 268
GALLSTONES
  asymptomatic   87
  complications   157
  diagnostic imaging   268
  epidemiology   71
  extracorporeal lithotripsy   29
  ileus   61
  management   58
  pathophysiology   97, 121, 239
  pancreatitis   181
  pigment stones   239
  problems in elderly   119
  surgery   58, 87, 181, 258
GASTRECTOMY
  cancer risk   168
  gastric cancer   110, 141
  gastric lymphoma   91
GASTRIC ACID
  antisecretory agents   77, 182, 208

GASTRIC ACID (contd)
  control of secretion 208, 252
  omeprazole 32, 114, 149, 199
  pathogenesis of duodenal ulcer 43
  stress ulcer 40
  Zollinger-Ellison syndrome 80
GASTRIC EMPTYING
  central control 229
  diabetic neuropathy 117, 195
  drug effects 56, 152
  in disease states 55
GASTRIC MUCOSA
  ageing 21, 98
  aspirin 183, 218, 228
  cytoprotection 102
  defence mechanisms 130, 228
  drug effects 183, 218, 228
  enterochromaffin cells 120
  non-steroidal anti-inflammatory drugs
      183, 218
  parietal cell physiology 199, 208
  prostaglandins 228
  secretion of mucus 228
  stress ulcer 40, 205
  watermelon stomach 171
GASTRIC ULCER
  aetiology 43, 217, 218
  bismuth compounds 94
  colloidal bismuth 94
  drug-induced 218
  drugs for 77
  elderly 88, 189
  haemorrhage 39, 176, 189
  omeprazole 32, 114, 149, 199
  pathophysiology 228
  prostaglandins 228
  sucralfate 153
  treatment of NSAID-induced
      ulcers 218
GASTRIC VARICES 2
GASTRIN
  effect of antisecretory drugs 32, 126,
      182, 208
  physiology 252
  relation to gastric carcinoids 32
  Zollinger-Ellison syndrome 246
GASTRITIS
  aetiology 98
  in elderly 98
  Helicobacter pylori 154, 182
GASTROENTERITIS
  bacterial 101
  protozoan 101
  viral 35, 105
GASTROINTESTINAL
  HAEMORRHAGE see
      Haemorrhage, gastrointestinal
GASTRO-OESOPHAGEAL REFLUX
  aetiology 6

antacids 220
children and infants 227
clinical features 238
complications 131
detection 266
drug damage 74
histamine H_2-antagonists 77, 220
in elderly 50
oesophageal pH monitoring 68
omeprazole 114, 149, 220
pathophysiology 93, 112
prokinetic drugs 151, 152
respiratory disorders 9, 92, 131, 238
surgery 109, 230
GASTROPARESIS 117, 151, 195
GASTROSTOMY, PERCUTANEOUS
    ENDOSCOPIC 158
GLIADIN ANTIBODIES 5
GLUCAGONOMA 118
GLUTEN-SENSITIVE
    ENTEROPATHY see Coeliac
    disease
GROWTH FACTORS 130
GROWTH FAILURE,
    INFLAMMATORY BOWEL
    DISEASE 136
GUT HORMONES
  control of gut function 234
  irritable bowel 26
  islet cell tumours 118
  pancreatic cancer 180
  somatostatin 100

HAEMORRHAGE,
    GASTROINTESTINAL
  colonic diverticulosis 57
  drug treatment 226
  electrocoagulation 176
  endoscopy 161, 176
  heater probe 39, 176
  in elderly 189
  injection sclerotherapy for non-variceal
      bleeding 176
  laser treatment 39, 176
  oesophageal ulcer 131, 238
  peptic ulcer 39, 88, 176
  prevention 135
  stress ulcers 40
  use of vasopressin 226
  variceal 2, 257
  watermelon stomach 171
HEATER PROBES 39, 176
HELICOBACTER PYLORI
  bismuth compounds 94, 146
  drug treatment 90, 182
  duodenal ulcer 25, 154, 175, 242
  gastritis 98
HEPATIC ENCEPHALOPATHY
  benzodiazepine receptors 42

HEPATIC ENCEPHALOPATHY (contd)
  fulminant hepatic failure   44, 263
  in alcoholic liver disease   144
HEPATIC VEIN THROMBOSIS   38,
    129
HEPATITIS
  and hepatoma risk   214
  chronic viral   69, 233
  viral, classification   7
  viral, interferon treatment   66, 70, 115,
    233
  viral, vaccines   73
HEPATOMA   214
  fibrolamellar   197
  hormonal treatment   47
  imaging   31
  in elderly   244
  interstitial treatment   147
  pathogenesis   164
  tumour markers   230
HIRSCHSPRUNG'S DISEASE   72, 260
HISTAMINE AND THE STOMACH
    252
HISTAMINE H$_2$-ANTAGONISTS   77,
    208
  duodenal ulcer   34
  mucosal protection   102
  oesophagitis   220
  stress ulcer prophylaxis   205
HISTOPATHOLOGY   see Intestinal
    mucosa
HORMONES, GUT   see Gut hormones
HYPERLIPIDAEMIA AND
    PANCREATITIS   237

ILEAL POUCH, ANAL
    ANASTOMOSIS   138, 142
ILEUM   see Small intestine
ILEUS, POSTOPERATIVE   140
IMMUNITY AND NUTRITION   51
IMMUNOLOGY
  antigen handling by small intestine   145
  coeliac disease   124
  chronic viral hepatitis   69, 233
  inflammatory bowel disease   178, 216
  liver disease   156
  mucosal immunity   247
  primary biliary cirrhosis   85
IMMUNOSUPPRESSIVES
  inflammatory bowel disease   173
INFLAMMATORY BOWEL DISEASE
    178
  5-amino salicylic acid   107, 173, 191, 248
  cancer   178
  cerebrovascular complications   123
  corticosteroids   173
  immunology   178, 216
  immunosuppressive drugs   173
  in elderly   99

metronidazole   173
olsalazine   248
oral contraceptive   250
pathogenesis   178, 216, 249, 250
procoagulant activity   249
quality of life   83
relapse   36
smoking   250
sulphasalazine   107, 173, 191
INSULINOMA   118
INTERFERON
  viral hepatitis   7, 66, 70, 115, 233
INTESTINAL MUCOSAL
    ABSORPTION   see Absorption
INTESTINAL MUCOSA
  ageing   21
  antigen handling   145
  bacterial overgrowth   128
  brown bowel syndrome   116
  calcium absorption   167
  cholesterol metabolism   78
  drug effects   183
  effect of alcohol   174
  endotoxins   198
  fermentation   196
  immunology   247
  lactose intolerance   1
  metabolism   133
  permeability   169
  transport of ions   13
  vitamin B$_{12}$ metabolism   166
INTESTINAL OBSTRUCTION
  gallstone ileus   61
  Hirschsprung's disease   72
  postoperative ileus   140
  volvulus   186
INTESTINE, IMMUNOLOGY   see
    Immunology
INTRAEPITHELIAL
    LYMPHOCYTES   247
ION TRANSPORT   13, 167
IRRITABLE BOWEL   264
  diagnosis   209, 235
  gut hormones   26
  motility studies   139, 150, 177
  psychological stress   261
  therapy   26, 79
ISCHAEMIA, INTESTINAL   113,
    190
ISLET CELL TUMOURS   118
  computerized tomography   27
  gastrinomas   246
  metastatic   20

JAUNDICE
  malignant obstructive   106
JEJUNUM   see Small intestine

LACTOSE INTOLERANCE   1

LASER
  cancer palliation   148
  for liver tumours   147
  gastrointestinal haemorrhage   39, 176
LAXATIVES   251
LITHOTRIPSY, EXTRACORPOREAL
    29, 58
LIVER DISEASES
  acquired immune deficiency syndrome
    45
  alcoholic   240
  autoimmune mechanisms   156
  in elderly   244
  in pregnancy   207
  nutritional management   144, 160
  risk factors for surgery   86
  ursodeoxycholic acid   30, 122
  vasodilatation in   213
LIVER FAILURE
  acute   44, 263
  vasodilatation in   213
LIVER FUNCTION IN PORTAL
    HYPERTENSION   188
LIVER IMAGING   31
LIVER POLYCYSTIC DISEASE   245
LIVER REGENERATION   204
LIVER TRANSPLANTATION   111
  Budd-Chiari syndrome   129
  fulminant hepatic failure   44, 52, 263
  graft rejection   14
  metastatic neuroendocrine tumours   20
  primary biliary cirrhosis   6
  Wilson's disease   225
LIVER TUMOURS
  imaging   31
  treatment   147
LYMPHOCYTES,
    INTRAEPITHELIAL   247
LYMPHOMA, PRIMARY GUT   3, 91

MAGNETIC RESONANCE IMAGING
    31
MALABSORPTION   113
  bacterial overgrowth   128
  brown bowel syndrome   116
  Crohn's disease   136
MONOMETRY
  anorectal   221
  oesophageal   266
MECKEL'S DIVERTICULUM   241
MESENTERIC ISCHAEMIA   190
METOCLOPRAMIDE   152
METRONIDAZOLE
  Helicobacter pylori   90
  inflammatory bowel disease   173
MICROSCOPIC COLITIS   127
MISOPROSTOL   102
MOTILITY
  anal sphincter   221

central control   229
colon   203
gut hormones   234
ileo-colonic junction   177
neuropeptides   187
oesophagus   112
orocaecal transit   89
sphincter of Oddi   97, 236
MOTILITY DISORDERS
  biliary   97, 236
  cisapride therapy   151
  colonic   203
  diabetes   117, 195
  gastric emptying   117
  incontinence of faeces   221, 251
  irritable bowel   139, 150, 177, 264
  oesophageal   112, 243, 266
  oesophageal spasm   243
  postoperative ileus   140
  sphincter of Oddi   97, 236
MOTILITY TESTING, ANORECTAL
    221
MUCOSA, SMALL BOWEL   see
    Intestinal mucosa

NEUROBIOLOGY OF INTESTINAL
    MUCOSA   187
NEUROENDOCRINE TUMOURS   20
NEUROPEPTIDES   187, 229
NITRATES IN PORTAL
    HYPERTENSION   159
NITROSAMINES   168
NON-A, NON-B HEPATITIS   see
    Hepatitis
NON-STEROIDALS   see Anti-
    inflammatory drugs
NORWALK AGENT   35
NUTCRACKER OESOPHAGUS   243
NUTRITION
  alcoholic liver disease   144
  Crohn's disease   136
  immunity   51
  short bowel   185

OBSTRUCTION   see Intestinal
    obstruction
OCTREOTIDE   100
OESOPHAGEAL PAIN   238, 266
OESOPHAGEAL VARICES
  beta blockers   135, 170
  haemorrhage   189
  nitrates   159
  operative management   2
  sclerotherapy   201, 232, 257
OESOPHAGITIS
  acquired immune deficiency
    syndrome   84
  drug-induced   74
  drug treatment   77, 131, 220

OESOPHAGITIS (contd)
  haemorrhage 189
  omeprazole   114, 149, 220
  pathophysiology 93
  radiation-induced 59
  reflux 131, 266
OESOPHAGUS
  ageing 50
  ambulatory pH monitoring 68
  Barrett's 109, 179
  drug damage 74
  motility 112
  motility disorders 112, 243, 266
  motility testing, clinical applications 266
  oesophagectomy 4, 28, 163
  radiation damage 59
  reflux surgery 109, 230
  spasm 243, 266
  surgery 4, 28, 163
OESOPHAGUS, CANCER   see Cancer,
    oesophagus
OLSALAZINE 248
OMEPRAZOLE   114, 149
  effect on gastric acid and plasma gastrin
    32, 126, 182, 208
  oesophagitis 220
  therapeutic role 208
  Zollinger-Ellison syndrome 80
OPPORTUNISTIC INFECTIONS
    259
OROCAECAL TRANSIT   89

PAEDIATRICS   see Childhood
PALLIATION
  hepatoma 147
  laser 148
  oesophageal cancer 4, 28
  pancreatic cancer 49, 106, 155
PANCREAS
  acquired immune deficiency syndrome
    37
  ageing 21, 113
  cystic neoplasms 27
  physiology 134
PANCREAS, CANCER   see Cancer,
    pancreas
PANCREAS, EXOCRINE FUNCTION
  ageing 113
  physiology 134
PANCREAS, SURGERY
  acute pancreatitis 15, 65, 181
  cancer 49, 96, 155
  chronic pancreatitis 22, 96, 125
  pancreatic duct endoprosthesis 41
PANCREATIC
    MASSES–COMPUTERIZED
    TOMOGRAPHY 27
PANCREATITIS, ACUTE
  abscess formation 65

acquired immune deficiency syndrome
    37
  alcohol 215
  complications 15, 132, 181
  diagnosis 17
  ERCP 48, 120
  hyperlipidaemia 237
  pathogenesis 157, 215, 237
  prediction of severity 224
  pseudocysts 15, 181
  splenic vein thrombosis 132
  surgery 15, 65, 181
PANCREATITIS, CHRONIC
  alcoholic pathogenesis 215
  complications 15
  endoscopic treatment 41, 120
  epidemiology 23
  in elderly 23, 119
  pain 125
  pancreatic duct endoprosthesis 41, 120
  pathogenesis 202, 215
  surgery 22, 125
PARASITES 101, 259
PARENTERAL NUTRITION
  Crohn's disease 136
  short bowel 185
PARIETAL CELL PHYSIOLOGY   199
PEPTIC ULCER
  aetiology 43, 217, 218
  cimetidine 77
  colloidal bismuth 94
  drugs for 77
  elderly 88, 189
  haemorrhage 39, 176, 189
  Helicobacter pylori 25, 154, 177, 242
  non-steroidal anti-inflammatory drugs
    218
  omeprazole 114, 149, 199
  pathophysiology 130, 217
  ranitidine 77
  stress-induced 205
  sucralfate 153
  surgery 19
  treatment of NSAID-induced ulcers
    218
PERCUTANEOUS ENDOSCOPIC
    GASTROSTOMY   see
    Gastrostomy
PERFORATION
  colon, stercoral 211
  peptic ulcer 88
PERIANAL CROHN'S DISEASE   143
PERITONEOVENOUS SHUNT   162
PHOTODYNAMIC THERAPY   184
PIGMENT GALLSTONES   239
PNEUMATOSIS CYSTOIDES
    INTESTINALIS   193
POLYCYSTIC DISEASE   245
POLYPOSIS SYNDROMES   172, 210

POLYPS, COLORECTAL   see Colorectal
   polyposis
PORTACAVAL SHUNTS   2, 129
PORTAL HYPERTENSION   188
   drug treatment   135, 159, 170
PORTAL VEIN THROMBOSIS   38
POSTOPERATIVE COMPLICATIONS
   antireflux surgery   109, 231
   cancer after peptic ulcer surgery   168
   gastrectomy   141
   ileal pouches after protocolectomy   138,
      142
   ileus   140
   liver transplantation   14
   oesophageal surgery for cancer   163
   palliation of obstructive jaundice   106
   pancreatectomy   96
   patients with liver disease   86
   peritoneovenous shunt   162
   septicaemia   198
   vagotomy and pyloroplasty   64
POTASSIUM OESOPHAGEAL
   DAMAGE   74
POUCHITIS AFTER COLECTOMY
   AND ANASTOMOSIS   142
PREDNISOLONE   see Corticosteroids
PREGNANCY
   colonic motility   203
   liver diseases   207
PRIMARY BILIARY CIRRHOSIS   see
   Biliary cirrhosis
PROBIOTICS–THERAPEUTIC USE
   82
PROKINETIC AGENTS   151, 152
PROPRANOLOL, PORTAL
   HYPERTENSION   135, 170
PROSTAGLANDINS
   antisecretory effect   208
   gall baldder   121
   gastric mucosa, cytoprotection   102, 130,
      183
   intestinal mucosa   183
   stress ulcer prophylaxis   205
PROTEIN–CALORIE
   MALNUTRITION   51
PSEUDOCYSTS, PANCREATIC   15,
   132
PSEUDOMEMBRANOUS
   ENTEROCOLITIS   82
PSYCHIATRY
   eating disorders   75
   irritable bowel   261

QUINOLONES
   acute diarrhoea   10
   Helicobacter pylori   90

RADIATION DAMAGE,
   OESOPHAGUS   59

RADIOLOGY, OESOPHAGEAL
   DISEASE   266
RADIOTHERAPY
   anal carcinoma   95
   colorectal cancer   62, 76, 194
   oesophageal cancer   4, 163
   pancreatic cancer   155
RANITIDINE   77
RECURRENCE OF CROHN'S
   DISEASE   262
REFLUX, GASTRO-OESOPHAGEAL
   see Gastro-oesophageal reflux
REGENERATION OF LIVER   204
REHYDRATION, ORAL   24, 200
ROTAVIRUS   105, 137

SCLERODERMA AND GASTRO-
   OESOPHAGEAL REFLUX   67
SCLEROTHERAPY
   non-variceal haemorrhage   176
   treatment of variceal bleeding   201, 232,
      257
SCREENING
   gastrointestinal malignancy   255
   inflammatory bowel disease and
      dysplasia   103, 178
SEXUALLY TRANSMITTED
   DISEASES   259
SHORT BOWEL   185
SMALL BOWEL
   bacterial overgrowth   128
   effect of alcohol   174
   ischaemia   190
   lymphoma   3
   motility disorders   139
   obstruction   61
SMALL CELL OESOPHAGEAL
   CANCER   33
SMOKING AND CROHN'S DISEASE
   250
SMOOTH MUSCLE
   brown bowel syndrome   116
   motility disorders   139, 203
   oesophageal sphincters   112, 243
   physiology   203, 267
SOMATOSTATIN
   effects on exocrine pancreas   134
   long-acting analogue   see Octreotide
   producing tumours   118
   therapeutic uses   100
SPASM, OESOPHAGEAL   243
SPHINCTEROTOMY, ENDOSCOPIC
   48
SPHINCTERS
   anal   221, 251
   Oddi, dyskinesia   97, 236
   oesophageal   112
SPLENIC VEIN THROMBOSIS
   131

STAGING
  gastric cancer   110
STENTS   see Endoprosthesis
STERCORAL PERFORATION   211
STOMACH, CANCER   see Cancer,
     stomach
STOMAL VARICES   63
STRESS
  irritable bowel   261
  peptic ulcer   40, 205
  ulcer prophylaxis   205
SUCRALFATE   153
SULPHASALAZINE   107, 191
SWALLOWING   see Deglutition

T LYMPHOCYTES   247
TRANSANAL RESECTION   11
TRANSPLANTATION   see under
     individual organs
TUBERCULOSIS, ENTERIC   81
TUMOUR MARKERS
  colorectal cancer   265
  hepatoma   230
  pancreatic cancer   223

ULCERATIVE COLITIS   178
  aetiology   178
  5-amino salicylic acid   173, 191, 248
  cerebrovascular complications   123
  colonic mucosal metabolism   133
  corticosteroids   173
  early diagnosis colorectal cancer   103,
     178
  ileo-anal pouch function   138, 142
  immunology   178, 216
  immunosuppressive drugs   173
  in elderly   99
  olsalazine   248
  pathogenesis   216
  quality of life   83
  relapse   36

sulphasalazine   107, 173, 191
ULTRASOUND
  acute pancreatitis   17
  biliary   267
  intraoperative   54
  liver diseases   31
URSODEOXYCHOLIC ACID FOR
     LIVER DISEASE   30, 122

VACCINES
  enteric infections   137
  viral hepatitis   73
VAGAL INNERVATION   150, 203
VAGOTOMY   19
  adverse effects   64
VARICES
  gastric   2
  oesophageal   see Oesophageal varices
  stomal   63
VASODILATATION IN LIVER
     FAILURE   213
VASODILATORS
  portal hypertension   159
VASOPRESSIN, VARICEAL
     HAEMORRHAGE   226
VIRAL GASTROENTERITIS   35, 105
VIRAL HEPATITIS   see Hepatitis
VIRAL VACCINES   137
VITAMIN B_{12} BINDING PROTEINS
     166
VOLVULUS, COLONIC   186

WATERMELON STOMACH   171
WILSON'S DISEASE   225

ZOLLINGER-ELLISON SYNDROME
     246
  antisecretory drugs   77
  gastro-oesophageal reflux   67
  omeprazole   80, 149
  pathology   118

REFERENCES

 1 Editorial. Lactose intolerance. Lancet 1991; 338: 663–664
 2 Editorial. Emergency portacaval shunts. Lancet 1991; 337: 952
 3 Editorial. Primary gut lymphomas. Lancet 1991; 337: 1384–1385
 4 Editorial. Radiotherapy or surgery for squamous cell oesophageal carcinoma? Lancet 1991; 337: 1318–1319
 5 Editorial. Diagnosis of coeliac disease. Lancet 1991; 337: 590
 6 Editorial. Is PBC cured by liver transplantation? Lancet 1991; 337: 272–273
 7 Editorial. The A to F of viral hepatitis. Lancet 1990; 336: 1158–1160
 8 Editorial. Bismuth and dyspepsia. Lancet 1990; 336: 472–473 (10 refs)
 9 Editorial. Reflux and respiratory symptoms. Lancet 1990; 336: 282–283 (21 refs)
10 Editorial. Quinolones in acute non-travellers' diarrhoea. Lancet 1990; 336: 282 (21 refs)
11 Editorial. Endoscopic transanal resection. Lancet 1990; 336: 411–412
12 Editorial. Cystic fibrosis: prospects for screening and therapy. Lancet 1990; 335: 79–80

13 Editorial. Methods of investigating intestinal transport. JPEN 1991; 15: 93S–98S

14 Adams DH, Neuberger JM. Patterns of graft rejection following liver transplantation. J Hepatol 1990; 10: 113–119 (28 refs)

15 Adler J, Barkin JS. Management of pseudocysts, inflammatory masses, and pancreatic ascites. Gastroenterol Clin North Am 1990; 19: 863–871 (62 refs)

16 Afridi SA, Fichtenbaum CJ, Taubin H. Review of duodenal diverticula. Am J Gastroenterol 1991; 86: 935–938 (38 refs)

17 Agarwal N, Pitchumoni CS, Sivaprasad AV. Evaluating tests for acute pancreatitis. Am J Gastroenterol 1990; 85: 356–366 (77 refs)

18 Ajani JA, Ota DM, Jackson DE. Current strategies in the management of locoregional and metastatic gastric carcinoma. Cancer 1991; 67 (suppl 1): 260–265 (35 refs)

19 Alexander-Williams J. A requiem for vagotomy (editorial). BMJ 1991; 302: 547–548

20 Alsina AE, Bartus S, Hull D, Rosson R, Schweizer RT. Liver transplant for metastatic neuroendocrine tumor. J Clin Gastroenterol 1990; 12: 533–537 (19 refs)

21 Altman DF. Changes in gastrointestinal, pancreatic, biliary, and hepatic function with ageing. Gastroenterol Clin North Am 1990; 19: 227–234 (35 refs)

22 Ammann RW. A critical appraisal of interventional therapy in chronic pancreatitis. Endoscopy 1991; 23: 191–193 (18 refs)

23 Ammann RW. Chronic pancreatitis in the elderly. Gastroenterol Clin North Am 1990; 19: 905–914 (52 refs)

24 Avery ME, Snyder JD. Oral therapy for acute diarrhoea. The underused simple solution. N Engl J Med 1990; 323: 891–894 (43 refs)

25 Axon AR. Duodenal ulcer: the villain unmasked? (editorial). BMJ 1991; 302: 919–921

26 Bailey LD Jr, Stewart WR Jr, McCallum RW. New directions in the irritable bowel syndrome. Gastroenterol Clin North Am 1991; 20: 335–349 (72 refs)

27 Balthazar EJ, Chako AC. Computed tomography of pancreatic masses. Am J Gastroenterol 1990; 85: 343–349 (31 refs)

28 Bancewicz J. Cancer of the oesophagus. BMJ 1990; 300: 3–4 (20 refs)

29 Barkun AN, Ponchon T. Extracorporeal biliary lithotripsy. Review of experimental studies and a clinical update. Ann Intern Med 1990; 112: 126–137 (72 refs)

30 Bateson MC. New directions in primary biliary cirrhosis (editorial). BMJ 1990; 301: 1290–1291

31 Bennett WF, Bova JG. Review of hepatic imaging and a problem-oriented approach to liver masses. Hepatology 1990; 12: 761–765 (61 refs)

32 Berlin RG. Omeprazole. Gastrin and gastric endocrine cell data from clinical studies. Dig Dis Sci 1991; 36: 129–136 (73 refs)

33 Beyer KL, Marshall JB, Diaz-Arias AA, Loy TS. Primary small-cell carcinoma of the esophagus. Report of 11 cases and review of the literature. J Clin Gastroenterol 1991; 13: 135–141 (58 refs)

34 Bianchi-Porro G, Parente F. Long term treatment of duodenal ulcer. A review of management options. Drugs 1991; 41: 38–51 (91 refs)

35 Blacklow NR, Greenberg HB. Viral gastroenteritis. N Engl J Med 1991; 325: 252–264 (196 refs)

36 Blumberg RS. Relapse of chronic inflammatory bowel disease. 'A riddle wrapped in a mystery inside an enigma'. Gastroenterology 1990; 98: 792–796 (44 refs)

37 Bonacini M. Pancreatic involvement in human immunodeficiency virus infection. J Clin Gastroenterol 1991; 13: 58–64 (74 refs)

38 Boughton BJ. Hepatic and portal vein-thrombosis (editorial). BMJ 1991; 302: 192–193

39 Bown S. Bleeding peptic ulcers (editorial). BMJ 1991; 302: 1417–1418

40 Bresalier RS. The clinical significance and pathophysiology of stress-related gastric mucosal hemorrhage. J Clin Gastroenterol 1991; 13 (suppl 2): S35–S43 (100 refs)

41 Burdick JS, Hogan WJ. Chronic pancreatitis: selection of patients for endoscopic therapy. Endoscopy 1991; 23: 155–159 (55 refs)

42 Butterworth RF, Pomier-Layrargues G. Benzodiazepine receptors and hepatic encephalopathy. Hepatology 1990; 11: 499–501 (25 refs)

43 Bynum TE. Non-acid mechanisms of gastric and duodenal ulcer formation. J Clin Gastroenterol 1991; 13 (suppl 2): S56–S64 (114 refs)

44 Capocaccia L, Angelico M. Fulminant hepatic failure. Clinical features, etiology, epidemiology, and current management. Dig Dis Sci 1991; 36: 775–779 (28 refs)

45 Cappell MS. Hepatobiliary manifestations of the acquired immune deficiency syndrome. Am J Gastroenterol 1991; 86: 1–15 (299 refs)

46 Cappell MS, Friedman D, Mikhail N. Endometriosis of the terminal ileum simulating the clinical, roentgenographic, and surgical findings in Crohn's disease. Am J Gastroenterol 1991; 86: 1057–1062 (55 refs)

47 Carr BI, Van Thiel DH. Hormonal manipulation of human hepatocellular carcinoma. A clinical investigative and therapeutic opportunity. J Hepatol 1990; 11: 287–289 (30 refs)

48 Carr-Locke DL. Acute gallstone pancreatitis and endoscopic therapy. Endoscopy 1990; 22: 180–183 (47 refs)

49 Carter DC. Cancer of the pancreas. Gut 1990; 31: 494–496 (42 refs)

50 Castell DO. Esophageal disorders in the elderly. Gastroenterol Clin North Am 1990; 19: 235–254 (57 refs)

51 Chandra RK. 1990 McCollum Award Lecture. Nutrition and immunity: lessons from the past and new insights into the future. Am J Clin Nutr 1991; 53: 1087–1101 (119 refs)

52 Chapman RW, Forman D, Peto R, Smallwood R. Liver transplantation for acute hepatic failure? Lancet 1990; 335: 32–35 (33 refs)

53 Char S, Farthing MJ. DNA probes for diagnosis of intestinal infection. Gut 1991; 32: 1–3 (35 refs)

54 Charnley RM, Hardcastle JD. Intraoperative abdominal ultrasound. Gut 1990; 31: 368–369 (26 refs)

55 Chaudhuri TK, Fink S. Gastric emptying in human disease states. Am J Gastroenterol 1991; 86: 533–538 (61 refs)

56 Chaudhuri TK, Fink S. Update: pharmaceuticals and gastric emptying. Am J Gastroenterol 1990; 85: 223–230 (79 refs)

57 Cheskin LJ, Bohlman M, Schuster MM. Diverticular disease in the elderly. Gastroenterol Clin North Am 1990; 19: 391–403 (15 refs)

58 Cheslyn-Curtis S, Russell RC. New trends in gallstone management. Br J Surg 1991; 78: 143–149 (79 refs)

59 Chowhan NM. Injurious effects of radiation on the esophagus. Am J Gastroenterol 1990; 85: 115–120 (29 refs)

60 Christiansen J. Surgical treatment of severe constipation. Scand J Gastroenterol 1991; 26: 225–230 (47 refs)

61 Clavien PA, Richon J, Burgan S, Rohner A. Gallstone ileus. Br J Surg 1990; 77: 737–742 (42 refs)

62 Cohen AM, Minsky BD. Aggressive surgical management of locally advanced primary and recurrent rectal cancer. Current status and future directions. Dis Colon Rectum 1990; 33: 432–438 (50 refs)

63 Conte JV, Arcomano TA, Naficy MA, Holt RW. Treatment of bleeding stomal varices. Report of a case and review of the literature. Dis Colon Rectum 1990; 33: 308–314 (35 refs)

64 Cuschieri A. Postvagotomy diarrhoea: is there a place for surgical management? Gut 1990; 31: 245–246 (23 refs)

65 D'Egidio A, Schein M. Surgical strategies in the treatment of pancreatic necrosis and infection. Br J Surg 1991; 78: 133–137 (54 refs)

66 Davis GL. Recombinant alpha-interferon treatment of non-A and non-B (type C) hepatitis: review of studies and recommendations for treatment. J Hepatol 1990; 11 (suppl 1): S72–S77 (23 refs)

67 Day JP, Richter JE. Medical and surgical conditions predisposing to gastroesophageal reflux disease. Gastroenterol Clin North Am 1990; 19: 587–607 (91 refs)

68 de Caestecker JS, Heading RC. Esophageal pH monitoring. Gastroenterol Clin North Am 1990; 19: 645–669 (131 refs)

69 Desmet VJ. Immunopathology of chronic viral hepatitis. Hepatogastroenterology 1991; 38: 14–21 (136 refs)

70 Di Bisceglie AM, Hoofnagle JH. Antiviral therapy of chronic viral hepatitis. ACG Committee on FDA-Related Matters. Am J Gastroenterol 1990; 85: 650–654 (40 refs)

71 Diehl AK. Epidemiology and natural history of gallstone disease. Gastroenterol Clin North Am 1991; 20: 1–19 (117 refs)

72 Doig CM. Hirschsprung's disease – a review. Int J Colorectal Dis 1991; 6: 52–62 (169 refs)

73 Eddleston A. Modern vaccines. Hepatitis. Lancet 1990; 335: 1142–1145 (28 refs)
74 Eng J, Sabanathan S. Drug-induced esophagitis. Am J Gastroenterol 1991; 86: 1127–1133 (100 refs)
75 Fairburn CG, Peveler RC. Bulimia nervosa and a stepped care approach to management. Gut 1990; 31: 1220–1222 (51 refs)
76 Fazio VW. Curative local therapy of rectal cancer. Int J Colorectal Dis 1991; 6: 66–73 (65 refs)
77 Feldman M, Burton ME. Histamine₂-receptor antagonists. Standard therapy for acid-peptic diseases. New Eng J Med 1990; 323: 1672–1680 and 1749–1755 (90 refs)
78 Field FJ, Kam NT, Mathur, SN. Regulation of cholesterol metabolism in the intestine. Gastroenterology 1990; 99: 539–551 (89 refs)
79 Friedman G. Treatment of the irritable bowel syndrome. Gastroenterol Clin North Am 1991; 20: 313–333 (55 refs)
80 Frucht H, Maton PN, Jensen RT. Use of omeprazole in patients with Zollinger-Ellison syndrome. Dig Dis Sci 1991; 36: 394–404 (79 refs)
81 Fry RD. Infectious enteritis. A collective review. Dis Colon Rectum 1990; 33: 520–527 (73 refs)
82 Fuller R. Probiotics in human medicine. Gut 1991; 32: 439–442 (42 refs)
83 Garrett JW, Drossman DA. Health status in inflammatory bowel disease. Biological and behavioral considerations. Gastroenterology 1990; 99: 90–96 (59 refs)
84 Gazzard BG. Practical advice for the gastroenterologist dealing with symptomatic HIV disease. Gut 1990; 31: 733–735 (39 refs)
85 Gershwin ME, Mackay IR. Primary biliary cirrhosis: paradigm or paradox for autoimmunity? Gastroenterology 1991; 100: 822–833 (90 refs)
86 Gholson CF, Provenza JM, Bacon BR. Hepatologic considerations in patients with parenchymal liver disease undergoing surgery. Am J Gastroenterol 1990; 85: 487–496 (68 refs)
87 Gibney EJ. Asymptomatic gallstones. Br J Surg 1990; 77: 368–372 (85 refs)
88 Gilinsky NH. Peptic ulcer disease in the elderly. Gastroenterol Clin North Am 1990; 19: 255–271 (100 refs)
89 Gilmore IT. Orocaecal transit time in health and disease. Gut 1990; 31: 250–251 (31 refs)
90 Glupczynski Y, Burette A. Drug therapy for *Helicobacter pylori* infection: problems and pitfalls. Am J Gastroenterol 1990; 85: 1545–1551 (55 refs)
91 Gobbi PG, Dionigi P, Barbieri F et al. The role of surgery in the multimodal treatment of primary gastric non-Hodgkin's lymphomas. A report of 76 cases and review of the literature. Cancer 1990; 65: 2528–2536 (54 refs)
92 Goldman JM, Bennett JR. Gastro-oesophageal reflux and asthma; a common association, but of what clinical importance? Gut 1990; 31: 1–3 (17 refs)
93 Goldstein JL, Schlesinger PK, Mozwecz HL, Layden TJ. Esophageal mucosal resistance. A factor in esophagitis. Gastroenterol Clin North Am 1990; 19: 565–586 (136 refs)
94 Gorbach SL. Bismuth therapy in gastrointestinal diseases. Gastroenterology 1990; 99: 863–875 (138 refs)
95 Gordon PH. Current status – perianal and anal canal neoplasms. Dis Colon Rectum 1990; 33: 799–808 (84 refs)
96 Grace PA, Pitt HA, Longmire WP. Pylorus-preserving pancreatoduodenectomy: an overview. Br J Surg 1990; 77: 968–974 (76 refs)
97 Grace PA, Poston GJ, Williamson RC. Biliary motility. Gut 1990; 31: 571–582 (196 refs)
98 Green LK, Graham DY. Gastritis in the elderly. Gastroenterol Clin North Am 1990; 19: 273–292 (137 refs)
99 Grimm IS, Friedman LS. Inflammatory bowel disease in the elderly. Gastroenterol Clin North Am 1990; 19: 361–389 (148 refs)
100 Grosman I, Simon D. Potential gastrointestinal uses of somatostain and its synthetic analogue octreotide. Am J Gastroenterol 1990; 85: 1061–1072 (149 refs)
101 Guerrant RL, Bobak DA. Bacterial and protozoal gastroenteritis. N Engl J Med 1991; 325: 327–340 (228 refs)
102 Guslandi M. Gastric cytoprotection. What does it really mean for the prescriber? Drugs 1991; 41: 507–513 (78 refs)

103 Gyde S. Screening for colorectal cancer in ulcerative colitis: dubious benefits and high costs. Gut 1990; 31: 1089–1092 (21 refs)
104 Haddock G, Carter DC. Aetiology of pancreatic cancer. Br J Surg 1990; 77: 1159–1166 (138 refs)
105 Haffejee IE. The pathophysiology, clinical features and management of rotavirus diarrhoea. Q J Med 1991; 79: 289–299 (139 refs)
106 Hatfield AR. Palliation of malignant obstructive jaundice – surgery or stent? Gut 1990; 31: 1339–1340 (11 refs)
107 Hayllar J, Bjarnason I. Sulphasalazine in ulcerative colitis: in memoriam? Gut 1991; 32: 462–463 (28 refs)
108 Heaton KW. Dietary fibre. BMJ 1990; 300: 1479–1480 (47 refs)
109 Hill LD, Aye RW, Ramel S. Antireflux surgery. A surgeon's look. Gastroenterol Clin North Am 1990; 19: 745–775 (39 refs)
110 Hioki K, Nakane Y, Yamamoto M. Surgical strategy for early gastric cancer. Br J Surg 1990; 77: 1330–1334 (100 refs)
111 Hockerstedt K. Liver transplantation today. Scand J Gastroenterol 1990; 25: 1–10 (63 refs)
112 Holloway RH, Dent J. Pathophysiology of gastroesophageal reflux. Lower esophageal sphincter dysfunction in gastroesophageal reflux disease. Gastroenterol Clin North Am 1990; 19: 517–535 (93 refs)
113 Holt PR. Diarrhea and malabsorption in the elderly. Gastroenterol Clin North Am 1990; 19: 345–359 (71 refs)
114 Holt S, Howden CW. Omeprazole. Overview and opinion. Dig Dis Sci 1991; 36: 385–393 (93 refs)
115 Hoofnagle JH. Alpha-interferon therapy of chronic hepatitis B. Current status and recommendations. J Hepatol 1990; 11 (suppl 1): S100–S107 (33 refs)
116 Horn T, Svendsen LB, Nielsen R. Brown-bowel syndrome. Review of the literature and presentation of cases. Scand J Gastroenterol 1990; 25: 66–72 (43 refs)
117 Horowitz M, Edelbroek M, Fraser R, Maddox A, Wishart J. Disordered gastric motor function in diabetes mellitus. Recent insights into prevalence, pathophysiology, clinical relevance, and treatment. Scand J Gastroenterol 1991; 26: 673–684 (76 refs)
118 Howard TJ, Stabile BE, Zinner MJ, Chang S, Bhagavan BS, Passaro E Jr. Anatomic distribution of pancreatic endocrine tumors. Am J Surg 1990; 159: 258–264 (96 refs)
119 Ingber S, Jacobson IM. Biliary and pancreatic disease in the elderly. Gastroenterol Clin North Am 1990; 19: 433–457 (92 refs)
120 Irani SK. Endoscopic management of pancreatic disorders. Gastroenterol Clin North Am 1990; 19: 975–997 (111 refs)
121 Jacyna MR. Interactions between gall-bladder bile and mucosa; relevance to gall-stone formation. Gut 1990; 31: 568–570 (48 refs)
122 James OF. Ursodeoxycholic acid treatment for chronic cholestatic liver disease. J Hepatol 1990; 11: 5–8 (46 refs)
123 Johns DR. Cerebrovascular complications of inflammatory bowel disease. Am J Gastroenterol 1991; 86: 367–370 (45 refs)
124 Kagnoff MF. Understanding the molecular basis of coeliac disease. Gut 1990; 31: 497–499 (32 refs)
125 Karanjia ND, Reber HA. The cause and management of the pain of chronic pancreatitis. Gastroenterol Clin North Am 1990; 19: 895–904 (39 refs)
126 Karnes WE Jr, Walsh JH. The gastrin hypothesis. Implications for antisecretory drug selection. J Clin Gastroenterol 1990; 12 (suppl 2): S7–S12 (70 refs)
127 Kingham JG. Microscopic colitis. Gut 1991; 32: 234–235 (14 refs)
128 Kirsch M. Bacterial overgrowth. Am J Gastroenterol 1990; 85: 231–237 (74 refs)
129 Klein AS, Cameron JL. Diagnosis and management of the Budd Chiari syndrome. Am J Surg 1990; 160: 128–133 (59 refs)
130 Konturek SJ. Role of growth factors in gastroduodenal protection and healing of peptic ulcers. Gastroenterol Clin North Am 1990; 19: 41–65 (130 refs)
131 Kozarek RA. Complications of reflux esophagitis and their medical management. Gastroenterol Clin North Am 1990; 19: 713–731 (126 refs)
132 Lankisch PG. The spleen in inflammatory pancreatic disease. Gastroenterology 1990; 98: 509–516 (72 refs)

133 Latella G, Caprilli R. Metabolism of large bowel mucosa in health and disease. Int J Colorectal Dis 1991; 6: 127–132 (72 refs)
134 Layer P, van der Ohe M, Muller MK, Beglinger C. Effects of somatostatin on the exocrine pancreas. Scand J Gastroenterol 1991; 26: 129–136 (90 refs)
135 Lebrec D. Current status and future goals of the pharmacologic reduction of portal hypertension. Am J Surg 1990; 160: 19–25
136 Lennard-Jones JE. Nutrition in Crohn's disease. Ann R Coll Surg Engl 1990; 72: 152–154 (24 refs)
137 Levine MM. Modern vaccines. Enteric infections. Lancet 1990; 335: 958–961 (17 refs)
138 Levitt MD, Lewis AA. Determinants of ileoanal pouch function. Gut 1991; 32: 126–127 (40 refs)
139 Lind CD. Motility disorders in the irritable bowel syndrome. Gastroenterol Clin North Am 1991; 20: 279–295 (75 refs)
140 Livingston EH, Passaro EP Jr. Postoperative ileus. Dig Dis Sci 1990; 35: 121–132 (142 refs)
141 Macintyre IM, Akoh JA. Improving survival in gastric cancer: review of operative mortality in English language publications from 1970. Br J Surg 1991; 78: 771–776 (108 refs)
142 Madden MV, Farthing MJ, Nicholls RJ. Inflammation in ileal reservoirs: 'pouchitis'. Gut 1990; 31: 247–249 (37 refs)
143 Marks CG. Anal lesions in Crohn's disease. Ann R Coll Surg Engl 1990; 72: 158–159 (6 refs)
144 Marsano L, McClain CJ. Nutrition and alcoholic liver disease. JPEN 1991; 15: 337–344 (80 refs)
145 Marsh MN. Grains of truth: evolutionary changes in small intestinal mucosa in response to environmental antigen challenge. Gut 1990; 31: 111–114 (21 refs)
146 Marshall BJ. The use of bismuth in gastroenterology. The ACG Committee on FDA-Related Matters. American College of Gastroenterology. Am J Gastroenterol 1991; 86: 16–25 (76 refs)
147 Masters A, Steger AC, Bown SG. Role of interstitial therapy in the treatment of liver cancer. Br J Surg 1991; 78: 518–523 (52 refs)
148 Mathus-Vliegen EM, Tytgat GN. Analysis of failures and complications of neodymium: YAG laser photocoagulation in gastrointestinal tract tumors. A retrospective survey of 18 years' experience. Endoscopy 1990; 22: 17–23 (49 refs)
149 Maton PN. Omeprazole. N Engl J Med 1991; 324: 965–975 (181 refs)
150 Mayer EA, Raybould HE. Role of visceral afferent mechanisms in functional bowel disorders. Gastroenterology 1990; 99: 1688–1704 (121 refs)
151 McCallum RW. Cisapride: a new class of prokinetic agent. The ACG Committee on FDA-related matters. American College of Gastroenterology. Am J Gastroenterol 1991; 86: 135–149 (80 refs)
152 McCallum RW. Gastric emptying in gastroesophageal reflux and the therapeutic role of prokinetic agents. Gastroenterol Clin North Am 1990; 19: 551–564 (57 refs)
153 McCarthy DM. Sucralfate. N Engl J Med 1991; 325: 1017–1025 (159 refs)
154 McKinlay AW, Upadhyay R, Gemmell CG, Russell RI. *Helicobacter pylori*: bridging the credibility gap. Gut 1990; 31: 940–945 (91 refs)
155 Merrick HW, Dobelbower RR Jr. Aggressive therapy for cancer of the pancreas. Does it help? Gastroenterol Clin North Am 1990; 19: 935–962 (114 refs)
156 Meyer zum Buschenfelde KH, Lohse AW, Manns M, Poralla T. Autoimmunity and liver disease. Hepatology 1990; 12: 354–363 (152 refs)
157 Misra SP, Dwivedi M. Pancreaticobiliary ductal union. Gut 1990; 31: 1144–1149 (76 refs)
158 Moran BJ, Taylor MB, Johnson CD. Percutaneous endoscopic gastrostomy. Br J Surg 1990; 77: 858–862 (32 refs)
159 Moreau R, Lebrec D. Nitrovasodilators and portal hypertension. J Hepatol 1990; 10: 263–267 (45 refs)
160 Morgan MY. Branched chain amino acids in the management of chronic liver disease. Facts and fantasies. J Hepatol 1990; 11: 133–141 (32 refs)
161 Morrissey JF, Reichelderfer M. Gastrointestinal endoscopy (1). N Engl J Med 1991; 325: 1142–1149 (122 refs)

162 Moskovitz M. The peritoneovenous shunt: expectations and reality. Am J Gastroenterol 1990; 85: 917–929 (105 refs)

163 Muller JM, Erasmi H, Stelzner M, Zieren U, Pichlmaier H. Surgical therapy of oesophageal carcinoma. Br J Surg 1990; 77: 845–857 (174 refs)

164 Naccarato R, Farinati F. Hepatocellular carcinoma, alcohol and cirrhosis: facts and hypotheses. Dig Dis Sci 1991; 36: 1137–1142 (81 refs)

165 Nathanson MH, Boyer JL. Mechanisms and regulation of bile secretion. Hepatology 1991; 14: 551–566 (170 refs)

166 Neale G. B12 binding proteins. Gut 1990; 31: 59–63 (26 refs)

167 Norman AW. Intestinal calcium absorption: a vitamin D-hormone-mediated adaptive response. Am J Clin Nutr 1990; 51: 290–300 (44 refs)

168 Northfield TC, Hall CN. Carcinoma of the gastric stump: risks and pathogenesis. Gut 1990; 31: 1217–1219 (42 refs)

169 Olaison G, Sjodahl R, Tagesson C. Abnormal intestinal permeability in Crohn's disease. A possible pathogenic factor. Scand J Gastroenterol 1990; 25: 321–328 (81 refs)

170 Olsson R. Beta-receptor blocking treatment in portal hypertension. Scand J Gastroenterol 1990; 25: 641–646 (56 refs)

171 Park RH, Russell RI. Watermelon stomach. Br J Surg 1991; 78: 395–396 (24 refs)

172 Parks TG. Extracolonic manifestations associated with familial adenomatous polyposis. Ann R Coll Surg Engl 1990; 72: 181–184 (22 refs)

173 Peppercorn MA. Advances in drug therapy for inflammatory bowel disease. Ann Intern Med 1990; 112: 50–60 (152 refs)

174 Persson J. Alcohol and the small intestine. Scand J Gastroenterol 1991; 26: 3–15 (133 refs)

175 Peterson WL. *Helicobacter pylori* and peptic ulcer disease. N Engl J Med 1991; 324: 1043–1048 (97 refs)

176 Peterson WL. Bleeding peptic ulcer. Epidemiology and nonsurgical management. Gastroenterol Clin North Am 1990; 19: 155–170 (92 refs)

177 Phillips SF, Camilleri M. The ileocecal area and the irritable bowel syndrome. Gastroenterol Clin North Am 1991; 20: 297–311 (52 refs)

178 Podolsky DK. Inflammatory bowel disease. N Engl J Med 1991; 325: 928–937 and 1008–1016 (250 refs)

179 Polepalle SC, McCallum RW. Barrett's esophagus. Current assessment and future perspectives. Gastroenterol Clin North Am 1990; 19: 733–744 (47 refs)

180 Poston GJ, Gillespie J, Guillou PJ. Biology of pancreatic cancer. Gut 1991; 32: 800–812 (268 refs)

181 Poston GJ, Williamson RC. Surgical management of acute pancreatitis. Br J Surg 1990; 77: 5–12 (146 refs)

182 Pounder R, Smith J. Drug-induced changes of plasma gastrin concentration. Gastroenterol Clin North Am 1990; 19: 141–153 (119 refs)

183 Price AH, Fletcher M. Mechanisms of NSAID-induced gastroenteropathy. Drugs 1990; 40 (suppl 5): 1–11 (59 refs)

184 Puolakkainen P, Ramo J, Schroder T. Photodynamic therapy in gastroenterology. Scand J Gastroenterol 1990; 25: 417–421 (31 refs)

185 Purdum PP, Kirby DF. Short-bowel syndrome: a review of the role of nutrition support. JPEN 1991; 93–101 (99 refs)

186 Rabinovici R, Simansky DA, Kaplan O, Mavor E, Manny J. Cecal volvulus. Dis Colon Rectum 1990; 33: 765–769 (36 refs)

187 Rattan S. Role of galanin in the gut. Gastroenterology 1991; 100: 1762–1768 (69 refs)

188 Reichen J. Liver function and pharmacological considerations in pathogenesis and treatment of portal hypertension. Hepatology 1990; 11: 1066–1078 (209 refs)

189 Reinus JF, Brandt LJ. Upper and lower gastrointestinal bleeding in the elderly. Gastroenterol Clin North Am 1990; 19: 293–318 (100 refs)

190 Reinus JF, Brandt LJ, Boley SJ. Ischemic diseases of the bowel. Gastroenterol Clin North Am 1990; 19: 319–343 (39 refs)

191 Riley SA, Turnberg LA. Sulphasalazine and the aminosalicylates in the treatment of inflammatory bowel disease. Q J Med 1990; 75: 551–562 (57 refs)

192 Roediger WE. The starved colon – diminished mucosal nutrition, diminished absorption, and colitis. Dis Colon Rectum 1990; 33: 858–862 (57 refs)

193 Rogy MA, Mirza DF, Kovats E, Rauhs R. Pneumatosis cystoides intestinalis (PCI). Int J Colorectal Dis 1990; 5: 120–124 (55 refs)

194 Rosenthal SA, Trock BJ, Coia LR. Randomized trials of adjuvant radiation therapy for rectal carcinoma: a review. Dis Colon Rectum 1990; 33: 335–343 (48 refs)

195 Rothstein RD. Gastrointestinal motility disorders in diabetes mellitus. Am J Gastroenterol 1990; 85: 782–785 (39 refs)

196 Royall D, Wolever TM, Jeejeebhoy KN. Clinical significance of colonic fermentation. Am J Gastroenterol 1990; 85: 1307–1312 (69 refs)

197 Ruffin, MT IV. Fibrolamellar hepatoma. Am J Gastroenterol 1990; 85: 577–581 (44 refs)

198 Saadia R, Schein M, MacFarlane C, Boffard KD. Gut barrier function and the surgeon. Br J Surg 1990; 77: 487–492 (91 refs)

199 Sachs G, Munson K, Hall K, Hersey SJ. Gastric H^+, K^+-ATPase as a therapeutic target in peptic ulcer disease. Dig Dis Sci 1990; 35: 1537–1544 (33 refs)

200 Sack DA. Use of oral rehydration therapy in acute watery diarrhoea. A practical guide. Drugs 1991; 41: 566–573 (45 refs)

201 Sarin SK, Kumar A. Sclerosants for variceal sclerotherapy: a critical appraisal. Am J Gastroenterol 1990; 85: 641–649 (91 refs)

202 Sarles H, Bernard JP, Gullo L. Pathogenesis of chronic pancreatitis. Gut 1990; 31: 629–632 (72 refs)

203 Sarna SK. Physiology and pathophysiology of colonic motor activity. Dig Dis Sci 1991; 36: 827–862 and 998–1018 (537 refs)

204 Schaffner F. Structural and functional aspects of regeneration of human liver. Dig Dis Sci 1991; 36: 1282–1286 (43 refs)

205 Schiessel R, Feil W, Wenzl E. Mechanisms of stress ulceration and implications for treatment. Gastroenterol Clin North Am 1990; 19: 101–120 (65 refs)

206 Scholefield JH, Northover JM, Carr ND. Male homosexuality, HIV infection and colorectal surgery. Br J Surg 1990; 77: 493–496 (74 refs)

207 Schorr-Lesnick B, Lebovics E, Dworkin B, Rosenthal WS. Liver diseases unique to pregnancy. Am J Gastroenterol 1991; 86: 659–670 (136 refs)

208 Schubert ML, Shamburek RD. Control of acid secretion. Gastroenterol Clin North Am 1990; 19: 1–25 (147 refs)

209 Schuster MM. Diagnostic evaluation of the irritable bowel syndrome. Gastroenterol Clin North Am 1991; 20: 269–278 (35 refs)

210 Sellner F. Investigations on the significance of the adenoma-carcinoma sequence in the small bowel. Cancer 1990; 66: 702–715 (272 refs)

211 Serpell JW, Nicholls RJ. Stercoral perforation of the colon. Br J Surg 1990; 77: 1325–1329 (66 refs)

212 Shamburek RD, Farrar JT. Disorders of the digestive system in the elderly. N Engl J Med 1990; 322: 438–443 (87 refs)

213 Sherlock S. Vasodilatation associated with hepatocellular disease: relation to functional organ failure. Gut 1990; 31: 365–367 (43 refs)

214 Simonetti RG, Camma C, Fiorello F, Politi F, D'Amico G, Pagliaro L. Hepatocellular carcinoma. A worldwide problem and the major risk factors. Dig Dis Sci 1991; 36: 962–972 (126 refs)

215 Singh M, Simsek H. Ethanol and the pancreas. Current status. Gastroenterology 1990; 98: 1051–1062 (131 refs)

216 Snook J. Are the inflammatory bowel diseases autoimmune disorders? Gut 1990; 31: 961–963 (41 refs)

217 Soll AH. Pathogenesis of peptic ulcer and implications for therapy. N Engl J Med 1990; 322: 909–916 (66 refs)

218 Soll AH, Weinstein WM, Kurata J, McCarthy D. Nonsteroidal anti-inflammatory drugs and peptic ulcer disease. Ann Intern Med 1991; 114: 307–319 (80 refs)

219 Solla JA, Rothenberger DA. Preoperative bowel preparation. A survey of colon and rectal surgeons. Dis Colon Rectum 1990; 33: 154–159 (41 refs)

220 Sontag SJ. The medical management of reflux esophagitis. Role of antacids and acid inhibition. Gastroenterol Clin North Am 1990; 19: 683–712 (104 refs)

221 Speakman CT, Kamm MA. The internal and sphincter – new insights into faecal incontinence. Gut 1991; 32: 345–346 (26 refs)

222 Stampfl DA, Friedman LS. Collagenous colitis: pathophysiologic considerations. Dig Dis Sci 1991; 36: 705–711 (42 refs)

223 Steinberg W. The clinical utility of the CA 19-9 tumor-associated antigen. Am J Gastroenterol 1990; 85: 350–355 (43 refs)

224 Steinberg WM. Predictors of severity of acute pancreatitis. Gastroenterol Clin North Am 1990; 19: 849–861 (60 refs)

225 Sternlieb I. Perspectives on Wilson's disease. Hepatology 1990; 12: 1234–1239 (70 refs)

226 Stump DL, Hardin TC. The use of vasopressin in the treatment of upper gastrointestinal haemorrhage. Drugs 1990; 39: 38–53 (112 refs)

227 Sutphen JL. Pediatric gastroesophageal reflux disease. Gastroenterol Clin North Am 1990; 19: 617–629 (86 refs)

228 Szabo S. Mechanisms of gastric mucosal injury and protection. J Clin Gastroenterol 1991; 13 (suppl 2): S21–S34 (73 refs)

229 Tache Y, Garrick T, Raybould H. Central nervous system action of peptides to influence gastrointestinal motor function. Gastroenterology 1990; 98: 517–528 (132 refs)

230 Taketa K. Alpha-fetoprotein: re-evaluation in hepatology. Hepatology 1990; 12: 1420–1432 (174 refs)

231 Taylor TV, Holt S. Antireflux surgery. BMJ 1990; 300: 1603–1604 (19 refs)

232 Terblanche J. Has sclerotherapy altered the management of patients with variceal bleeding? Am J Surg 1990; 160: 37–42 (45 refs)

233 Thomas HC. The hepatitis B virus and the host response. J Hepatol 1990; 11 (suppl 1): S83–S89 (42 refs)

234 Thompson JC. Humoral control of gut function. Am J Surg 1991; 161: 6–18 (69 refs)

235 Thompson WG. Symptomatic presentations of the irritable bowel syndrome. Gastroenterol Clin North Am 1991; 20: 235–247 (71 refs)

236 Toouli J. Clinical relevance of sphincter of Oddi dysfunction. Br J Surg 1990; 77: 723–724 (8 refs)

237 Toskes PP. Hyperlipidemic pancreatitis. Gastroenterol Clin North Am 1990; 19: 783–791 (32 refs)

238 Traube M. The spectrum of the symptoms and presentations of gastroesophageal reflux disease. Gastroenterol Clin North Am 1990; 19: 609–616 (52 refs)

239 Trotman BW. Pigment gallstone disease. Gastroenterol Clin North Am 1991; 20: 111–126 (108 refs)

240 Tsukamoto H, Gaal K, French SW. Insights into the pathogenesis of alcoholic liver necrosis and fibrosis: status report. Hepatology 1990; 12: 599–608 (88 refs)

241 Turgeon DK, Barnett JL. Meckel's diverticulum. Am J Gastroenterol 1990; 85: 777–781 (41 refs)

242 Tytgat GN, Rauws EA. *Campylobacter pylori* and its role in peptic ulcer disease. Gastroenterol Clin North Am 1990; 19: 183–196 (68 refs)

243 Valori RM. Nutcracker, neurosis, or sampling bias? Gut 1990; 31: 736–737 (34 refs)

244 Van Dam J, Zeldis JB. Hepatic diseases in the elderly. Gastroenterol Clin North Am 1990; 19: 459–472 (126 refs)

245 Vauthey JN, Maddern GJ, Blumgart LH. Adult polycystic disease of the liver. Br J Surg 1991; 78: 524–527 (88 refs)

246 Vinayek R, Frucht H, Chiang HC, Maton PN, Gardner JD, Jensen RT. Zollinger-Ellison syndrome. Recent advances in the management of the gastrinoma. Gastroenterol Clin North Am 1990; 19: 197–217 (84 refs)

247 Viney J, MacDonald TT, Spencer J. Gamma/delta T cells in the gut epithelium. Gut 1990; 31: 841–844 (34 refs)

248 Wadworth AN, Fitton A. Olsalazine. A review of its pharmacodynamic and pharmacokinetic properties, and therapeutic potential in inflammatory bowel disease. Drugs 1991; 41: 647–664 (96 refs)

249 Wakefield A, Cohen Z, Levy G. Procoagulant activity in gastroenterology. Gut 1990; 31: 239–241 (35 refs)

250 Wakefield AJ, Sawyerr AM, Hudson M, Dhillon AP, Pounder RE. Smoking, the oral contraceptive pill, and Crohn's disease. Dig Dis Sci 1991; 36: 1147–1150 (51 refs)

251 Wald A. Constipation and fecal incontinence in the elderly. Gastroenterol Clin North Am 1990; 19: 405–418 (52 refs)

252 Waldum HL, Sandvik AK, Brenna E, Petersen H. Gastrin-histamine sequence in the

regulation of gastric acid secretion. Gut 1991; 32: 698–701 (61 refs)

253 Watters DA, Smith AN. Strength of the colon wall in diverticular disease. Br J Surg 1990; 77: 257–259 (34 refs)

254 Waye JD, Haggitt RC. Controversies, dilemmas, and dialogues. When is colonoscopic resection of an adenomatous polyp containing a 'malignancy' sufficient? Am J Gastroenterol 1990; 85: 1564–1568 (33 refs)

255 Weil J, Langman MJ. Screening for gastrointestinal cancer: an epidemiological review. Gut 1991; 32: 220–224 (42 refs)

256 Weiss W. Asbestos and colorectal cancer. Gastroenterology 1990; 99: 876–884 (54 refs)

257 Westaby D, Williams R. Status of sclerotherapy for variceal bleeding in 1990. Am J Surg 1990; 160: 32–36 (47 refs)

258 Wetter LA, Way LW. Surgical therapy for gallstone disease. Gastroenterol Clin North Am 1991; 20: 157–169 (77 refs)

259 Wexner SD. Sexually transmitted diseases of the colon, rectum, and anus. The challenge of the nineties. Dis Colon Rectum 1990; 33: 1048–1062 (161 refs)

260 Wheatley MJ, Wesley JR, Coran AG, Polley TZ Jr. Hirschsprung's disease in adolescents and adults. Dis Colon Rectum 1990; 33: 622–629 (45 refs)

261 Whitehead WE, Crowell MD. Psychologic considerations in the irritable bowel syndrome. Gastroenterol Clin North Am 1991; 20: 249–267 (59 refs)

262 Williams JG, Wong WD, Rothenberger DA, Goldberg SM. Recurrence of Crohn's disease after resection. Br J Surg 1991; 78: 10–19 (128 refs)

263 Williams R, Gimson AE. Intensive liver care and management of acute hepatic failure. Dig Dis Sci 1991; 36: 820–826 (28 refs)

264 Wingate DL. The irritable bowel syndrome. Gastroenterol Clin North Am 1991; 20: 351–362 (54 refs)

265 Woolfson K. Tumor markers in cancer of the colon and rectum. Dis Colon Rectum 1991; 34: 506–511 (47 refs)

266 Wu WC. Ancillary tests in the diagnosis of gastroesophageal reflux disease. Gastroenterol Clin North Am 1990; 19: 671–682 (41 refs)

267 Yu J, Bose R. Calcium channels in smooth muscle. Gastroenterology 1991; 100: 1448–1460 (91 refs)

268 Zeman RK, Garra BS. Gallbladder imaging. The state of the art. Gastroenterol Clin North Am 1991; 20: 127–156 (49 refs)

269 Zwas FR, Lyon DT. Endometriosis. An important condition in clinical gastroenterology. Dig Dis Sci 1991; 36: 353–364 (120 refs)

Index

Abdominal aortic aneurysms, peptic ulcer
   bleeding, 138
Abdominal bloating, functional, 49, 57–58.
Achlorhydria, 32
Acid secretion, and *Helicobacter pylori*
   infection, 42
Acid/pepsin damage, protective
   mechanisms, 36
Adenomatous Polyposis Coli (APC) gene,
   154, 155
   kindred 353, colorectal cancer, 155
Adolescence, and gluten intolerance, 121
Adrenaline, bleeding peptic ulcer, 141, 143,
   145–146
AIDS, gastrointestinal bleeding, 139
Alcohol injection, bleeding peptic ulcer,
   141–142, 145–146
Alcoholic liver disease
   anti-HCV prevalence, 206
   see also Cirrhosis
Alexithymia, 55
Alpha interferon
   fluorouracil combination, 161, 162
   hepatitis C, 209, 210–212
Amantidine, 106
5-Aminosalicylic acid (5-ASA), 5–6
   Crohn's disease, 7–8
   enemas, 7
   mechanism of action, 6
   side-effects, 8
Aminotransferase (ALT)
   acute hepatitis C infection, 199
   chronic hepatitis C infection, 200, 201
Andenomatous polyposis, familial (FAP),
   151, 152, 153
   associated tumours, 152
   presymptomatic screening, 154–155
Aneuploidy, ulcerative colitis,
   premalignancy, 18
Antigliadin antibodies, coeliac disease, 124
Antioxidants, pancreatitis, 91, 95
α-1-antitrypsin, faecal clearance, Crohn's
   disease, 5
Anxiety
   irritable bowel syndrome, 65

non-ulcer dyspepsia, 66
and rectal sensitivity, 56
Aplastic anaemia, NANBH, 206
Apolipoprotein B, RNA editing, 79
Ascorbic acid, gastric secretion, *Helicobacter
   pylori* effects, 41
Autoimmune hepatitis, anti-HCV positivity,
   205
Azathioprine, 9–10

Balloon dilatation, endoscopic, Crohn's
   disease, 15–16
Beclomethasone, enemas, 9
Beger's operation, 94, 96–97
Behaviour therapy, irritable bowel syndrome
   (IBS), 68–69
Beta blockers
   complications, 188
   haemodynamic changes, 177–180
   variceal bleeding prevention, clinical
     trials, 182–184
   versus no treatment, variceal rebleed
     prevention, 184–186
   versus sclerotherapy, variceal rebleed
     prevention, 186–188
Betamethasone, 9
Bile acids
   enzymes, cloning, 80–81
   hepatocyte uptake, 81
   metabolism, molecular biology, 80–81
   synthesis, circadian rhythm, 80
Biliary drainage, endoscopic, chronic
   pancreatitis, 93
Bladder, irritability, 57
Bleeding peptic ulcer, thermal/injection
   methods, experimental studies,
   145–146.
Blood donors, hepatitis C prevalence,
   202
Blood transfusion, post-transfusion hepatitis
   C, 203, 207
Borborygmi, 49
Bristol stool-form scale, 51
Bromocriptine, 106

c-Ki-*ras* genes, 18
Cell migration, and HGF-SF, 77
Chest pain, oesophageal origin, 56
Children, immunodeficiency, hepatic lectin
 in opsonic defect, 77–79
Chloride transport, cystic fibrosis, 125
Cholangitis
 pancreatic head obstructions, 93
 sclerosing, inflammatory bowel disease,
 18–19
Cholecystokinin (CCK), cDNA, 76
Cholesterol 7α-hydroxylase, molecular
 biology, 80–81
Chromosome alterations, colorectal cancer,
 156–157
Cimetidine, 129
Cirrhosis
 azygous blood flow, propranolol effects,
 179
 chronic hepatitis C, 208
 and duodenal ulcer, 106
 propranolol, WHVP/HVPG effects,
 177–180
 vasopressin effects, 175–176
Coeliac disease, 119–125
 antibody measurement, 124
 antigliadin antibodies, 124
 cystic fibrosis association, 127, 129
 definition, 120
 diagnostic criteria, 119–120
 diagnostic problems, 120–121
 ESPGAN diagnostic criteria, 120
 gluten challenge, 120–121
 HLA associations, 123
 immunological aspects, 123–124
 intraepithelial lymphocytes, 123
 investigations, 122–124
 jejunal biopsy, 121–122
 latency, 121
 trigger factors, 121
 and ulcerative colitis, 2
 upper intestinal permeability, 123
Cognitive behavioural therapy, irritable
 bowel syndrome, 69
Colipase
 cDNA, 75–76
 pancreatic, 75–76
Colon cancer, adjuvant therapy, 162–
 163
Colonoscopy, colorectal cancer screening,
 153–154
Colorectal cancer
 adjuvant therapy, 162–164
 chromosome alterations, 156–157
 common, hereditary factors, 152–153
 dietary factors, 157, 159
 epidemiology, 157, 159
 genetic alterations, 155–157
 genetic model, 157, 158
 genetics, 151–157

liver metastases, regional chemotherapy,
 161
 management, 159–164
 metastases, treatment, 159–162
 mortality, 151
 non-polyposis, hereditary, 152
 predispositions, inherited, 152–153
 proto-oncogene activation, 155
 screening
 high risk patients, 153–154
 ulcerative colitis, 16–18
 tumour-suppressor gene inactivation,
 155–157
Constipation, functional, 49
Core-biopsy, ultrasound-guided, 87
Corticosteroids, new, inflammatory bowel
 disease, 9
Cow's-milk-protein intolerance, cystic
 fibrosis association, 127
Crohn's disease, 38
 balloon dilatation, 15–16
 colitis, surgery, 14
 cystic fibrosis association, 127–128
 elemental and enteral diets, 10–11
 faecal α-1-antitrypsin clearance, 5
 fistulas, surgery, 15
 IgA secretion reduction, 3
 ileal pouch-related, 13
 magnetic resonance imaging, 5
 maintenance treatment, 8
 malignancy risks, 18
 Mycobacterium paratuberculosis, 2
 perianal, 15
 postoperative recurrence, 14
 skip lesions, 15
 strictureplasty, 14–15
 surgery, 13–16
 total parenteral nutrition (TPN), 11–12
 vascular injury/focal arteritis, 4
Cryoglobulinaemia, anti-HCV prevalence,
 206
CT scans, contrast-enhanced, pancreatic
 cancer, 87
Cyclosporin (CyA), 10
Cystic fibrosis (CF), 98, 125–130
 associated diseases, 127–130
 GI complications, 126–127
 omeprazole, 129
 transmembrane regulator (CFTR), 98,
 125
Cytokines
 Helicobacter pylori infection, 31
 inflammatory bowel disease, 3

DCC mutations, colorectal cancer, 156–157
Delta-F508
 cystic fibrosis, 125–126
 geographical distribution, 125–126
Deoxycholic acid, rectal sensitivity, 53

Depression
  irritable bowel syndrome, 65
  non-ulcer dyspepsia, 66
Diarrhoea, functional, 49
Diuretics, WHPV/HVPG effects, 182
Drug abuse, and HCV transmission,
    203–204, 205
Duodenal ulcer
  aetiology, 105–107
  antral gastritis association, 36
  dietary aspects, 105
  dopaminergic brain-gut axis, 106
  gastric metaplasia association, 36
  gastro-duodenal motility, 108–109
  Helicobacter pylori, 34–38, 43, 105–107
  hypnotherapy, 68
  NSAIDs, 112–113
  omeprazole, 109–112
  recurrence rate, 38
  surgery, 113–114
Duodenitis
  Helicobacter pylori, 36–37
  metaplasia association, 36–37
Dyspepsia, functional, 56
Dyspepsia, non-ulcer (NUD), 63
  Helicobacter pylori, 38–39, 43
  psychological factors, 66–67
Dysplasia, ulcerative colitis, 16–18
  DNA analysis, 17–18

Electrocoagulation, bipolar, bleeding peptic
    ulcer, 142, 143, 146
Elemental diet, Crohn's disease, 10–11
ELISA, hepatitis C virus, 198, 201
Encephalopathy, hepatic, and beta blockers,
    188
Endoscopy
  inflammatory bowel disease, 4
  postprocedure *Helicobacter pylori*
    infection, 30
Enteral diet, Crohn's disease, 10–11
Enterogastric reflux, postoperative,
    scintigraphy, 113
Enterovesical fistulas, Crohn's disease, 15
Ethanolamine, bleeding peptic ulcer, 141,
    146
Exclusion diets, irritable bowel syndrome,
    59

Faecal occult blood, screening, colorectal
    cancer, 153–154
Famotidine, 108, 140
FAP *see* Adenomatous polyposis, familial
    (FAP)
Fats, dietary, pancreatic cancer, 85
Finney side-to-side strictureplasty, 14
Fish oils, dietary therapy, inflammatory
    bowel disease, 12

Flaviviruses, 196
Fluorodeoxyuridine, in liver metastases,
    161, 162
5-Fluorouracil, 87
  biomodulation, 160–161
  combination therapy, 160–161
  metastatic colorectal cancer, 160–161
Folinic acid, 160
Frusemide, WHPV/HVPG effects, 182
Functional bowel diseases, definitions, 49
Functional gastrointestinal disorders
  aetiology, 64–67
  psychological factors, 63–71
  psychological treatments, 67–69

G protein-linked receptors, 74–75
Gardner's syndrome, 85
  and familial adenomatous polyposis,
    152
Gastrectomy, partial, duodenal ulcer,
    113–114
Gastric cancer
  aetiological factors, 39–41
  Helicobacter pylori, 39–42
Gastric ulcer
  bleeding vessel undersewing, 147–148
  Helicobacter pylori, 38, 43
  NSAIDs, 112
Gastritis
  atrophic, 34
  autoimmune, 33, 35
  chronic, 32–35
  eosinophilic, 33–34
  Helicobacter pylori-associated, 27, 29–30,
    31–32, 33
  hypochlorhydric, 27, 29–30
    pathogenesis, 31–32, 33
  lymphocytic, 33–34
  reactive (reflux-type), 33–34
Gastro-duodenal motility, duodenal ulcer,
    108–109
Gastrointestinal bleeding
  prophylaxis, 112–113
  see also Peptic ulcer bleeding; Variceal
    bleeding
Gastrointestinal neoplasia, morbidity/
    mortality, 151
Gastropathy
  congestive, 184
  portal hypertension, 184
Giardiasis, cystic fibrosis association, 127
Glucagonoma syndrome, 85
Gluten intolerance, transient, 121
Glycine/taurine ratios, duodenal bile acids,
    cystic fibrosis, 130
Glypressin
  in acute variceal bleeding, 174–175
  nitroglycerin combination, 174–175
Granisetron, 58

H$^+$K$^+$-ATPase, gastric, 75
H$_2$-receptor antagonists, 140
  duodenal ulcer recurrence, 38
  tolerance, 108
H$_2$-receptor gene, 74–75
Haemophiliacs, hepatitis C, 204
HBeAg
  as immune modulator, 220–221
  synthesis, 220
    pre-core mutant, 221–223
HBsAg
  epitopes, 226–227
  glycine-to-arginine substitution, 226–227
  in HBV vaccine, 226
Heart surgery, peptic ulcer bleeding, 138
Heater probe, bleeding peptic ulcer, 141,
  143
Heinecke-Mikulicz strictureplasty, 14
Helicobacter pylori, 27–43
  carbohydrate-associated receptor
    adherence, 27
  chronic gastritis, 34–35
  detection, 28
  duodenal ulcer, 34–38, 105–107
  duodenitis, 36–37
  epidemiology, 28–29, 30
  gastric B-cell lymphoma, 42
  gastric cancer, 39–42
  gastric ulcer, 38
  non-ulcer dyspepsia, 38–39
  omeprazole effects, 111–112
  pathogenicity mechanisms, 31–42
  postendoscopy syndrome, 30
  species, 27
  toxic ammonia effects, 34
  transmission, 29–31
  treatment, 42–43
Hepatitis
  chronic active (CAH), 208
  chronic persistent (CPH), 208
Hepatitis B, concurrent hepatitis C, 205–206
Hepatitis B virus (HBV)
  'Chinese' strain, 222–223
  escape mutants, 217
  immune response against, 217–219
  pre-core variants
    fulminant infection, 223
    selection and pathogenicity, 220–221,
    222
  pre-core/core and pre-S/S gene biology,
    219–227
  pre-S variants, chronic carriers, 224–225
  surface variation, 226–227
  vaccine, and carriers, 227
  variants, 217–230
  and interferon therapy, 223–224
Hepatitis C virus (HCV), 195–216
  acute infection
    clinical features, 206–207
    management, 209

serological diagnosis, 199–200
  alpha interferon, 209, 210–212
  antibodies, 197–198
  chronic infection
    clinical features, 207–208
    management, 209–210
    serological diagnosis, 200–201
  community-acquired transmission,
    203–204
  diagnosis, 197–201
  genomic diversity, 197
  genomic RNA, 196
  high-risk populations, 204
  intrafamilial transmission, 201–202
  maternal-infant transmission, 202
  nosocomial/occupational exposure, 204
  population studies, 202
  post-transfusion infection, 203, 207
  proteins, 196–197
  recombinant immunoblot assays, 198, 201
  RNA testing, 198–201
  subclinical infection, 207
  transmission, 201–202
  virology, 195–197
Hepatitis E virus (HEV), 195
Hepatocellular carcinoma (HCC)
  anti-HCV prevalence, 206
  chronic hepatitis C, 208
  genetic changes, 165
Hepatocyte growth factor (HGF), 76–77
  scatter factor (HGF–SF), 76–77
Hepatocytes, cytotoxic T cell interaction,
  218
Herpes simplex virus, duodenal ulcer, 106
HIV infection, HCV infection coexistence,
  201, 206
HLA, coeliac disease, 123
5-Hydroxytryptamine (5-HT)
  antagonists, 58
  irritable bowel syndrome, 57
Hypergastrinaemia, in *Helicobacter pylori*
  infection, 39
Hyperoxygen radicals, *Helicobacter pylori*
  infection, 31
Hyperpepsinogenaemia
  duodenal ulcer, 105, 106
  Helicobacter pylori, 106
Hypnotherapy, irritable bowel syndrome,
  59, 67–68

IgA deficiency, coeliac disease, 124
IgG anti-HBcAg response, 221
Ileal pouch-anal anastomosis, ulcerative
  colitis, 13
Immunosuppressive agents, inflammatory
  bowel disease, 9–10
Inflammatory bowel disease
  abnormal metabolic pathways, 4
  clinical assessments, 4–5

Inflammatory bowel disease (*contd*)
 dietary fish oils, 12
 epidemiology, 1–2
 genetics, 2
 hypnotherapy, 68
 immune mechanisms, 2–4
 immunosuppressive agents, 9–10
 infectious agents, 2
 models, 4
 new corticosteroid preparations, 9
 pathogenesis, 1–4
 salicylates, 5–9
 sclerosing cholangitis, 18–19
 smoking, 1
 see also Crohn's disease; Ulcerative colitis
Interferon, hepatitis B virus variants,
  223–224
Interferon-alpha
 fluorouracil combination, 161, 162
 hepatitis C, 209, 210–212
Interleukins, 106
Intestinal carcinomas, cystic fibrosis
  association, 128
Intestine, sensory system, 56–58
Intragastric acidity
 control, 107–114
 nocturnal, 107
Intravariceal pressure, reduction,
  propranolol, 179
Irritable bowel syndrome (IBS), 49–62
 behaviour therapy, 68–69
 consulters/non-consulters, differences,
  53–54
 defaecatory symptoms, 50–51
 definitions, 49
 diagnosis, 50
 and intestinal sensory system, 56–58
 Manning criteria, 50
 mechanism of symptoms, 55–56
 non-gastrointestinal symptoms, 55
 prevalence, 51–52
 psychological factors, 54–55, 57
  aetiological aspects, 64–67
  influence on referral, 65–66
 psychological therapy, 59, 67–69
 sensitized receptors, 57, 58
 somatic/visceral pain thresholds, 52–53
 treatment, 58–59
Irritable stomach syndrome, 56
Isosorbide 5-mononitrate
 propranolol combination, HVPG effects,
  181
 renal function effects, 180
Isotype scanning, inflammatory bowel
  disease, 4–5

Jaundice, pancreatic head obstruction,
  93
Jejunal biopsy, coeliac disease, 121–122

Kausch-Whipple procedure, 87, 94
Kidney function, and beta blockers, 188

Lactoferrin, 4
Lectin, hepatic, opsonic defect in
  immunodeficiency, 77–79
Leukotrienes, duodenal ulcer, 106
Life events, non-ulcer dyspepsia, 66
Lipase, pancreatic, 75
Lithostathine, 89–90
Lithotripsy, extracorporeal shock-wave
  (ESWL), pancreatic stones, 91, 93
Liver
 chronic disease, anti-HCV prevalence, 205
 molecular biology, 76–77
Liver function, and beta blockers, 188
Liver metastases, regional chemotherapy,
  161
 systemic therapy combination, 161–162
Liver transplantation, postoperative
  hepatitis C, 204
Lymphoma, B-cell, *Helicobacter pylori*, 42
Lynch syndromes, 85, 152, 153, 154

Magnetic resonance imaging, Crohn's
  disease, 5
Malabsorption
 in cystic fibrosis, 128–130
 pancreatic enzyme supplements, 129
Manning criteria, irritable bowel syndrome,
  50
Mannose-binding protein
 deficiency, opsonization defect, 77–79
 gene, 78–79
MEN-1, 85
Menetrier's disease, 33–34
6-Mercaptopurine, 9
Methotrexate, 10, 160
Misoprostol, 112, 129, 137
Molecular biology, in gastroenterology,
  73–83
Molsidomine, in portal hypertension,
  181–182
Mycobacterium paratuberculosis, Crohn's
  disease, 2

Nadolol
 HVPG reduction, 180
 variceal bleeding prevention, clinical
  trials, 182–184
Nasogastric aspirate, peptic ulcer bleeding,
  137
Neurotic bowel, 56
Nicotine, ulcerative colitis, 10
Nitroglycerin
 glypressin combination, 174–175
 vasopressin combination, 175–176

Nitrovasodilators
portal pressure effects, 180–181
propranolol combination, HVPG effects, 181
Non-A, non-B (NANB) hepatitis, 195–212
associated diseases, 205–206
fulminant, 204
post-transfusion, 203, 207
see also Hepatitis C virus (HCV)
NSAIDs
duodenal ulcer, 112–113
gastric ulcer, 112
peptic ulcer bleeding, 135, 137
Nutrition, cystic fibrosis, 128

Obsessional trait, irritable bowel syndrome, 65
Octreotide, 90–91
in acute variceal bleeding, 171–174
Oesophagus, spasm, 63
Olsalazine, 5
side-effects, 8
3-omega fatty acids, 12
Omeprazole, 129, 140
adverse effects, 111
cystic fibrosis, 129
in duodenal ulceration, 109–112
genotoxicity, 111
ranitidine comparisons, 109–111
Ondansetron, 58
Open-heart surgery, peptic ulcer bleeding, 138
Opsonization defect, mannose-binding protein, 77–79

p53 mutations, colorectal cancer, 156–157
Pain thresholds, somatic/visceral, irritable bowel syndrome, 52–53
Pancreas
divisum, 95, 97
fistulas, octreotide, 90–91
molecular biology, 75–76
pseudocysts
endoscopic cystogastrostomy/ endocystoduodenostomy, 93
octreotide, 91
stones, 89
ES/ESWL therapy, 91, 93
Pancreatectomy, pylorus/duodenum preserving, 94, 96–97
Pancreatic cancer
associated autosomal dominant disorders, 85
autocrine control, 86
curative resection/adjuvant therapy, 87, 89
diagnosis and staging, 86–87
epidemiology/aetiology, 85
genetic aspects, 85

growth factors/oncogenes, 85–86
hormonal/paracrine control, 86
palliation, endoscopic surgery versus surgical bypass, 87, 88
Pancreatic enzymes
gene regulation, 75–76
supplementation, cystic fibrosis, 129
Pancreatic stone protein (PSP), 89–90
Pancreatic thread protein, 90
Pancreaticoduodenectomy, pylorus-preserving, 87–88
Pancreatitis, acute, 90, 94–95, 98
gallstones, 95
necrotizing, 94–95
pancreas divisum, 95, 97
Pancreatitis, chronic, 89–94
classification/aetiology, 89–90
endoscopic management, 91–93
free radical activity, 90
medical treatment, 90–93
neuritis association, 93–94
new operations, 93–94
Pancreatopathy
hypertensive, 89
obstructive, 89
Pepsinogen F, 73–74
Pepsinogens, genes, 73–74
Peptic ulcer bleeding, 135–150
associated conditions, 138–139
clinical investigations, 137–138
drug treatment, 140–141
trial numbers, 141
endoscopic stigmata, 137–138
endoscopic treatment, 135
consensus statement, 144–145
meta-analyses, 145
randomized controlled trials, 141–142
randomized uncontrolled trials, 142–144
trial numbers, 144
epidemiology, 136
hospitalization costs, 148
mortality, 136
pathophysiology, 139
recurrent, pH and drug therapy, 140–141
surgery, 147–148
Swain theories, 139
see also Duodenal ulcer; Gastric ulcer
Peptic ulcers, perforation, 139
Pernicious anaemia
autoantibodies, 75
gastric atrophy/cancer, 39
Pestiviruses, 196
pH, duodenal, cystic fibrosis, 129
N-(phosphonacetyl)-L-aspartate (PALA), 160, 162
Plasminogen activation factor, 95
Platelet-activating factors, duodenal ulcer, 106
Polidocanol, 143

Polymerase chain reaction (PCR), *Helicobacter pylori* detection, 28
Polymorphonuclear leucocytes, inflammatory bowel disease, 3–6
Polyunsaturated fats, pancreatic cancer, 85
Portal hypertension
  gastropathy, propranolol, 184
  molsidomine, 181–182
  nitrovasodilators, 181–182
  pharmacotherapy, 171–191
  pressure lowering drugs, 177
  see also Variceal bleeding
Postendoscopy syndrome, *Helicobacter pylori*, 30
Pouchitis, 13
Prednisolone, enemas, 9
Proctalgia fugax, 63
Propranolol
  azygous blood flow effects, cirrhosis, 179
  hepatic encephalopathy induction, 188
  intravariceal pressure reduction, 179
  nitrovasodilator combination, 181
  non-responders and portal pressure, 178–179, 181
  portal hypertension gastropathy, 184
  variceal bleeding prevention, clinical trials, 182–184
  WHVP/HVPG effects in cirrhotics, 177–180
Prostaglandin E$_2$, 106
Protein, X, 90
Proton pump, 75
Pseudomonas infection, cystic fibrosis, 126
Pulse rate, and HVPG, 178
Pyloroplasty, bleeding peptic ulcer, 147

Ranitidine, 108, 129, 137
  bismuth citrate, 113
  omeprazole comparisons, 109–111
Rectal cancer
  adjuvant therapy, 163–164
  postoperative radiotherapy/chemotherapy combination, 164
Rectovaginal fistulas, Crohn's disease, 15
Retinal pigment epithelium, congenital hypertrophy, FAP, 152
Reviews and leaders
  index, 231–241
  references, 241–251
Ribavirin, hepatitis C, 212
RNA editing, 79
Russell's operation, 94

Salicylates, new preparations
  inflammatory bowel disease, 5–9
  pharmacokinetics, 5–6

Scatter factor (SF), 76–77
Sclerosing cholangitis
  HLA association, 19
  inflammatory bowel disease, 18–19
Sclerotherapy
  injection, complications, 146
  versus beta blockers, variceal rebleed prevention, 186–188
Secretin, cDNA, 76
Smoking
  gastric cancer, 114
  inflammatory bowel disease, 1
  intragastric acidity effects, 107–108
  pancreatic cancer, 85
Somatization, irritable bowel syndrome, 54–55
Somatoform autonomic dysfunction, 63–64
Somatostatin
  in acute variceal bleeding, 171–174
  other agent comparisons, 172–174
  transfusion requirement effects, 172
Sphincterotomy, endoscopic
  acute pancreatitis, 95, 98
  chronic pancreatitis, 91–92
Spironolactone, WHPV/HVPG effects, 182
Steatorrhoea, pancreatic, 128
Stomach
  molecular biology, 73–75
  proteases and receptors, 73–75
Stress
  denial, irritable bowel syndrome, 54–55
  duodenal ulcer, 105
  non-ulcer dyspepsia, 66
Strictureplasty, Crohn's disease, 14–15
Sucralfate, 38, 108
Sulphasalazine, 5, 14

Thalassaemia major, hepatitis C, 204
Total parenteral nutrition (TPN), Crohn's disease, 11–12
Tranexamic acid, 140
Trypsin inhibitors, 95
Tumour necrosis factor (TNF), antagonists, 95

Ulcerative colitis
  malignancy, 16–18
  nicotine, 10
  surgery, 12–13
Ultrasonography, endoluminal (endoscopic), pancreatic cancer, 86
Urea, carbon-labelled, breath tests, 28
Urea:creatinine ratio, peptic ulcer bleeding, 137
Urease, *Helicobacter pylori*, 27
Ursodeoxycholic acid, 130

Vagotomy
  bleeding peptic ulcer, 147
  duodenal recurrence, 113
  laparoscopic, 114
  omeprazole comparisons, 109, 110
Variceal bleeding
  acute, drug therapy, 171–176
  prevention, 176–188
    beta blocker clinical trials, 182–184
  recurrence, prediction index, 180
  recurrence prevention, 176–188
    beta blockers/no treatment, 184–186
    beta blockers/sclerotherapy, 186–188
Vasodilators
  arterial baroreceptor activation, 180

  and pulmonary wedge pressure, 180
  see also Nitrovasodilators
Vasopressin, bleeding varices, 175–176
Vomiting, psychogenic, 63

Wedge hepatic venous pressure (WHVP),
    somatostatin/octreotide effects,
    171–172

d-Xylose absorption test, coeliac disease, 123

Zollinger-Ellison syndrome, 36, 38, 107

Books are to be returned on or before
the last date below.

LIBREX —